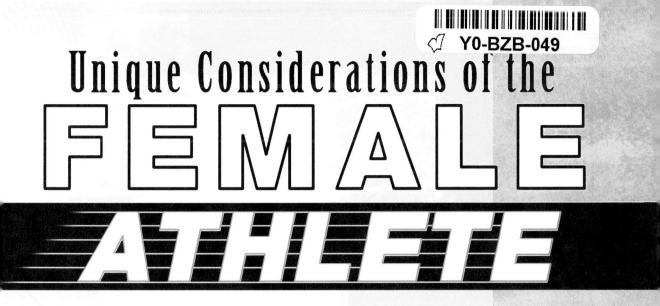

Unique Considerations of the
FEMALE
ATHLETE

MICHAEL BRUNET

Unique Considerations of the
FEMALE
ATHLETE

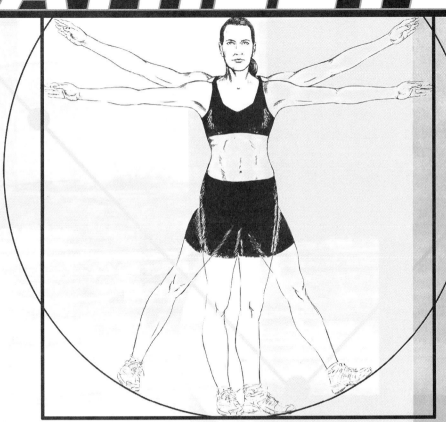

MICHAEL BRUNET

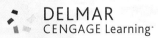

DELMAR
CENGAGE Learning

Australia • Brazil • Japan • Korea • Mexico • Singapore • Spain • United Kingdom • United States

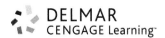
DELMAR
CENGAGE Learning

Unique Considerations of the Female Athlete
Michael Brunet

Vice President, Career and Professional Editorial: Dave Garza

Director of Learning Solutions: Matthew Kane

Acquisitions Editor: Mathew Seeley

Managing Editor: Marah Bellegarde

Senior Product Manager: Darcy M. Scelsi

Editorial Assistant: Samantha Zullo

Vice President, Career and Professional Marketing: Jennifer McAvey

Marketing Manager: Kristin McNary

Marketing Coordinator: Erica Ropitsky

Production Director: Carolyn Miller

Content Project Manager: Ken McGrath

Art Director: Jack Pendleton

Library of Congress Control Number: 2008938427

ISBN-13: 978-1-401-89781-9

ISBN-10: 1-4018-9781-9

Delmar
Street address
City, State ZIP
USA

Cengage Learning is a leading provider of customized learning solutions with office locations around the globe, including Singapore, the United Kingdom, Australia, Mexico, Brazil, and Japan. Locate your local office at:
international.cengage.com/region

Cengage Learning products are represented in Canada by Nelson Education, Ltd.

For your lifelong learning solutions, visit **delmar.cengage.com**

Visit our corporate website at **www.cengage.com**

Printed in Canada.
1 2 3 4 5 6 7 11 10 09 08

Dedication

I dedicate this book to my wife, Desiree and my daughter, Mallory.
I am forever indebted to you for your selflessness.

Contents

Preface

In the last few decades, the number of female athletes has grown exponentially which could arguably be tied with the passing of Title IX of the Educational Amendments Act in 1972. Title IX assures that girls and women have equal opportunity to participate in interscholastic and intercollegiate sports. Although there has been a rise in female athlete participation, medical preparedness to handle the unique conditions of the female athlete has not increased. We, as health care professionals, are in a constant stage of "catch up" as we have focused the many previous years of heath care on male athletes.

It is commonly known that men and women differ, but from a sports medicine knowledge base we are only scratching the surface of these differences. Women's bodies act differently with competitive physiological stress. These differences span from anatomical, physiological, and psychological. It is well documented that female athletes struggle with body image issues more than men and that the younger generation displays more evidence of body dissatisfaction than ever before. The female athlete experiences other gender specific consequences to exercise. For example, too much exercise can lead to menstrual cycle disturbances, poor bone health, and even child bearing complications. In reference to the lack of published female specific issues, the American College of Sports Medicine coined the term the female athlete triad (triad) in the early 90's. The triad consists of disordered eating, amenorrhea, and osteoporosis and can hinder any aged female athlete. Today now multiple national and international organizations have position stands on the triad.

The intent of this book is to shed some light on issues and pathologies specific to the female athlete. An Online Companion to the book provides additional information including discussion questions and PowerPoint presentations for each of the chapters The Online Companion may be accessed from: delmarlearning.com/companions, click on the Allied Health discipline tab. The title of the book should appear in the list. Click on that to access the content.

Contributors

Anh-Dung "Yum" Nguyen, PhD, ATC
Post Doctoral Research Assistant
Applied Neuromechanical Research
Laboratory
University of North Carolina at
Greensboro
Greensboro, North Carolina

Barb Hoggenboom, EdD, PT SCS, ATC
Associate Professor, Physical Therapy
Grand Valley State University
Allendale, Michigan

David Giardina, ATC, PTA
Metro Physical Therapy
Chalmette, Louisiana

David Kahler, MD
Associate Professor of Orthopaedic Surgery
Orthopaedic Trauma
University of Virginia,
Charlottesville, Virginia

Dawn Weatherwax-Fall, RD, CSSD, LD,
ATC, CSCS
Owner
Sports Nutrition 2 Go
Liberty Township, Ohio www.sn2g.com

James Cole, MD
Louisiana Oncology Associates
Hematology / Oncology
Lafayette, Louisiana

John MacKnight, MD
Associate Professor of Clinical Internal
Medicine and Clinical Orthopaedic Surgery

Co-Medical Director for Sports Medicine
Primary Care Team Physician
University of Virginia
Charlottesville, VA

John Storment, MD
Fertility and Women's Health Center of
Louisiana
New Orleans, Louisiana

Jolene Bennett, MA, PT, OCS, ATC
Grand Valley State University,
Allendale, MI

Margaret Grace Kuhn, MD
Resident
Washington University
St Louis, Missouri

Mike Brunet, PhD, ATC, CPT, STS
Assistant Professor, Program Director
Athletic Training
Louisiana College
Pineville, Louisiana
Owner, Precision Health and
Consulting
www.myprecisionservices.com

Ron Thomspon, PhD
Academy for Eating Disorders
Bloomington, Indiana

Ron Thompson, PhD, FAED
Psychologist
Bloomington Center for Counseling and
Human Development
Bloomington, Indiana

Roberta Trattner Sherman, PhD, FAED
Psychologist
Bloomington Center for Counseling and
Human Development
Bloomington, Indiana

Sandra J Shultz, PhD, ATC
Fellow of American College of Sports
Medicine
Fellow of National Athletic Trainer's
Association
Associate Professor and Director of
Graduate Studies
University of North Carolina at
Greensboro,
Department of Exercise and Sport
Science Greensboro, North Carolina

Sherri Bartz, PhD, ATC, CSCS
Assistant Professor Grand Valley State
University
Allendale, Missouri

Sherry Werner, BS, MS, PhD
Tulane Institute of Sports Medicine
Tulane, Louisiana

Turner A "Tab" Blackburn Jr, MEd, PT, ATC
VP, Clemson Sports Medicine and
Rehabilitation
Director, Sports Plus Physical Therapy
of Manchester Georgia
Adjunct Assistant Professor, University
of St. Augustine

Reviewers

David Berry, BS, MAT, MA, PhD
Salem State College
Salem, Massachusetts

Kirk Brown, PhD, LAT, ATC
The University of North Carolina at
Wilmington
Wilmington, North Carolina

Roger Clark, PhD, ATC
Colorado State University Pueblo
Pueblo, Colorado

Lori Dewald, EdD, ATC, CHES
University of Minnesota Duluth
Duluth, Minnesota

Michael Goforth, MS, ATC
Virginia Tech
Blacksburg, Virginia

Kathleen Laquale, PhD, LATC, LDN
Bridgewater State College
Bridgewater, Massachusetts

Deidre Leaver-Dunn, PhD, ATC
The University of Alabama
Tuscaloosa, Alabama

Kent Scriber, EdD, ATC, PT
Ithaca College
Ithaca, New York

Introduction to the Female Athlete

CHAPTER 1

Women and Sport Participation

Mike Brunet, PhD, ATC, CPT, STS

Introduction

Women do not have a long history of participating in organized sports, but since the and the 20th century their participation in sports has grown exponentially. However, research of gender-specific issues related to women and sports has not been well researched and documented until last 30 years. As researchers devote more time to studying the specific gender nuances in women's athletics the knowledge base continues to grow and women now participate in sports more safely and with better results.

History of Women in Sport

Women have not always been accepted in sport participation. Before 1800 it was believed that women were too fragile to participate in sports. For example, bike riding was considered too strenuous. However in the late 1800s, bicycling became an important political symbol for women and bike races were documented as early as 1885. Elizabeth Cady Stanton wrote that "many a woman is riding to the suffrage on a bicycle." The bicycle enabled women from all social strata to travel-alone or with male companions.[4] By the turn of the century, nearly 30,000 American women owned and rode bicycles (Figure 1-1). This is important because it symbolized many things like freedom, transportation, and physical activity.

From the early 1900s to the mid 1930s, women's participation in athletics rose, as the number of sports available to them increased. Cycling became an acceptable activity for women as it was now associated with transportation in addition to being a piece of exercise equipment. It is commonly known that cycling does take physical exertion, but for a woman to perform such a task might have lead to pathological situations. Since riding was associated with transport, this practice was acceptable. What differentiates this era from the previous is the construction of indoor facilities and the working class, not just the upper class, organized some of these sporting activities. In the mid 1800s YWCA was formed and gymnasiums were constructed. Community support was a major step forward in the history of women's sports. Women began to play more strenuous sports such as racquetball, volleyball, field hockey, and swimming. Participation in these sports would have been unheard of years before due to their rigorous nature. It was during this time that women's professional sport participation began to emerge. In 1922, Glena Collett won six amateur golf titles, Gertrude Ederle beat the English Channel swimming record by two hours in 1926 (Figure 1-2), and Helen Wills monopolized women's tennis through the 1930s.

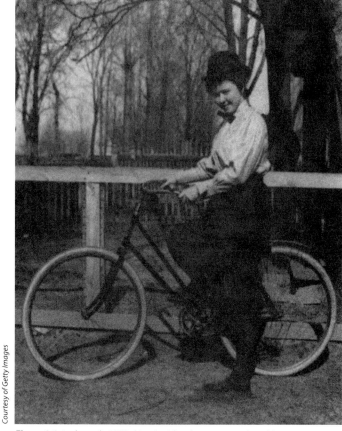

Courtesy of Getty Images

Figure 1-1 In the early 1800s bicycle riding became popular with women. It allowed women more independence and mobility in society.

The early 1900s also saw the birth of basketball, which did for groups of women what the bicycle accomplished for the individual woman.[4] By the 1920s, women's colleges like Mount Holyoke and Wellesley offered organized sports for women. The addition of these sports were justified by the colleges who argued that exercise would enhance a women's physical attributes as a laborer in the work force.[4]

After 1980s, a decline in the emphasis of women's participation occurred. Individuals in higher education thought it was "unfeminine" for women to participate in vigorous activities. This lead to the downplaying of female sport participation. For instance, the Women's Division of the National Amateur Athletic Federation maintained that competition would "harm the nervous system, encourage rowdiness, and lead to injury and exploitation."[4] It was further stated that a women's role as a mother was more important than sport and that men and women should not compete together.[4] Interestingly

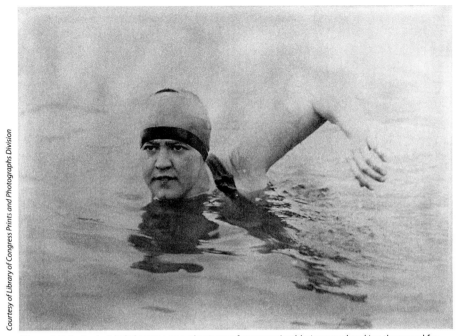

Courtesy of Library of Congress Prints and Photographs Division

Figure 1-2 Gertrude Ederle became an early pioneer for women's athletics upon breaking the record for swimming the English channel.

enough, some men began to redefine the female athlete and view them as sexy and romantic.[4] Of the few sports women still participated in at this time, gymnastics was the most popular sport due to its mild form of calisthenics.

When World War II broke out in 1941 women were asked to perform tasks that predominantly had been done by men in the past. Women's participation in sport flourished once again during this period, not only due to less subjection of pressures being emitted from higher education, but now they had to replace men in society due to war. The number of organized tournaments for women rose as a result of working class women's involvement in vigorous sports. It was during 1940s that spot apparel was adapted for particular sports.

In the early 1950s, there was an overall decline in female participation in sport, but since the end of the 1950s to the present, there has been a precipitous increase. Now female athletes are enrolling in colleges and universities at an ever increasing rate. There are laws (Title IX enactment from the Educational Assistance Act of 1972)[1] that mandate that college and university campuses establish equal numbers of men's and women's sports. There are also now government and town organizations that are responsible for organizing, administrating, and overseeing particular sporting events.

During 1960, it was apparent that women were letting go of the association of fitness and such began promoting themselves as participants in competitive sports. In 1944, the Division for Girls and Women's Sports joined the U.S. Olympic Development Committee in an effort to train female Olympians and the Commission on Intercollegiate Athletics for Women was founded. This commission was brought about to govern college games and tournaments.

In 1970s, women's sport involvement in international sports was growing as well. In the 1992 Olympics, more than 3000 women participated. At the 1996 Olympic games, more than 3800 females participated (a 27% increase).[6]

So where was the turning point in women's role in athletics? One author[4] writes that it was the "battle of the sexes," or the tennis matches between Bobby Riggs and Billie Jean King in 1973 in which King won all three sets. From then on, it was evident that women and sport were a formidable force.

Analyzing the Statistics

With all of these innovations and milestones of the last 150 years, one might think that just as many female athletes participate in sport as there are male athletes. The NCAA Gender-Equity report shows differently. This report provides the *average* number of sport participants at different size academic institutions. From 1991-2003, the NCAA reports that more females participated in collegiate sports than ever before, but still the numbers are not as great as male sport participants. For instance, the NCAA Division 1 level reports that male athletes made up 69% of the participants on average, where as female athletes only made up 31%. During the 2002-2003 school year, 56% were male athletes and 44% were female athletes. At the NCAA Division II level, 68% of the sport participants were male and 32% were female athletes during the 1991-92 competitive season, but the 2002-03 season revealed a 60% male participation and 40% female participation. The NCAA Division III level showed similar results. During the 1991-1992 season, 65% of the sport participants were male and 35% were female versus 58% male and 42% female during the 2002-03 season. Though men's and women's sport participation is not a 1:1 ratio, it is easy to see an increase in female sport participation.

Women's Health in Athletics

It is important to note that even though there has been a precipitous rise in women's participation in sports over the last few decades, their participation has not been paralleled by sport preparedness. This disconnect can set the stage for injuries.[2] Due to a brief and relatively recent history of the development of women's sports in North America, it is easy to see why some complex injuries suffered by female athletes' have not been tracked properly. This puts the medical community at a disadvantage because it has not had the same time to research gender specific conditions as it has to research many of the male specific pathologies. Some of these gender specific conditions, or pathologies, include biomechanical differences, breast health, infertility issues, orthopedic conditions, and the alarmingly high incidence of anterior cruciate ligament ruptures. Each of these topics will be discussed in detail throughout this book.

Summary

As women's participation in sports continues to increase the need for additional research into women's health in sport participation needs to increase. An increased knowledge of gender specific conditions and pathologies will help the women athletes of the future to participate in athletics more safely and more effectively.

Additional Readings

1. Brumberg, Joan Jacobs. *The Body Project: An Intimate History of American Girls.* New York: Random House; 1997.

2. Hargreaves, Jennifer. *Sporting Females: Critical Issues in the History and Sociology of Women's Sports.* London, New York: Routledge; 1994.

3. Smith, Lissa. *Nike Is a Goddess: The History of Women in Sports.* New York: Atlantic Monthly Press; 1998.

References

1. Education Amendments of 1972, PL 92-318, Title IX. *Prohibitions of Sex Discrimination,* July 1, 1972.

2. Griffin, Letha Y. The female athlete. In: Delee JC, and Drez D (Eds.). *Orthopedic Sports Medicine: Principles and Practice.* Philadelphia, Pennsylvania: W. B. Saunders Publisher; 1994: 356-373.

3. NCAA Gender-Equity Survey Results, 1991-2003. Available at: NCAA.org.

4. Nelson MB. Introduction: Who We might become. In: Smith L (Ed.). *Nike Is a Goddess: The History of Women in Sports.* Atlantic Monthly Press, New York; 1998.

5. Smith L (Ed.). *Nike Is a Goddess: The History of Women in Sports.* Atlantic Monthly Press, New York; 1998.

6. Warren HC. *Dictionary of Psychology.* Boston: Houghton Mifflin Co; 1934.

CHAPTER 2

Gender Differences in Anatomy

Sandra J. Shultz PhD, ATC, CSCS

Anh-Dung Nguyen PhD., ATC

Introduction

Prior to the onset of puberty, there are few anatomical differences between males and females. Prepubescent males and females younger than the age of 12 tend to have almost no differences in postural characteristics, muscle strength and flexibility, joint laxity, or body composition. However, with the onset of puberty, substantial anatomical differences begin to emerge in regard to stature, joint mobility, and body composition. Sex hormones, which also differ dramatically post-puberty, appear to be an important mediator of these anatomical differences. This chapter examines important sex differences in bone, joint, muscle, posture and other features as they emerge post puberty (Table 2-1). Because

TABLE 2-1 · **An Overview of Sex Differences in Anatomy**

ANATOMICAL VARIABLE	COMPARED TO MALES
Stature	Females are shorter in stature, and have relatively narrower shoulders, wider pelvis, and smaller chest diameter.
Sex Hormones	Females secrete more estrogen and males secrete more testosterone. These hormonal differences ultimately impact a variety of anatomical structures.
Bone and Ligament	Females have smaller bones, both in diameter and cortical thickness. Ligaments are also smaller consistent with smaller skeletal dimensions. Differences persist even once correcting for height and weight.
Joint	Females have greater general joint laxity and knee laxity. Greater laxity in females has also been documented at the ankle and shoulder.
Muscle	Females have: • Smaller muscle fiber and total muscle cross sectional area, and smaller pennation angles • Greater myotendon extensibility and compliance • Longer delays in muscle force generation • Equal muscle strength when equal amounts of muscle are compared
Body Composition	Females have less lean body mass and greater fat mass per unit of weight, resulting in approximately 6%-10% greater percentage of relative body.
Lower Extremity Posture	Females stand with greater anterior pelvic tilt, femoral internal rotation, knee hyperextension (genu recurvatum) and knee valgus.
Upper Extremity Posture	Females tend to stand with more rounded shoulders and greater carrying angle of the elbow.

many of these gender-specific anatomical differences have been implicated as possible risk factors for injury, the clinical implications of these sex differences will also be discussed.

Bone and Joint Anatomy

With the onset of puberty, females grow rapidly in the first 2–4 years then plateau, while males grow for a longer period of time. As such, females are shorter and generally have smaller statures and bone mass than males. Other differences following the onset of puberty include narrower shoulders, a wider pelvis, and a smaller chest diameter in females compared to males.[118]

Bone Structure

Age, pubertal stage, and body mass (both height and weight) are the most important determinants of bone mineral content and density.[9, 74] Bone mass increases rapidly through childhood and adolescents. As each sex matures, females accumulate bone at a more rapid rate until menarche (first menstrual cycle), then males begin to surpass females until about the age of 17–19.[25] Ultimately, males have larger bones (even once corrected for body height and weight), in both diameter and cortical thickness.[25] Peak bone mass occurs around 25–30 years of age, although, peak bone mass is achieved at some sites much earlier.[74] Peak bone mass is maintained fairly well until the age of 50, when it gradually declines with advancing age. Bone loss occurs faster in females than males, and in sedentary more than physically active individuals. Regardless of sex, height, and age, weight is an important predictor of bone mass, with both greater lean body mass and fat mass contributing to greater bone mass.[9]

As with most tissues, sex hormones play a critical role in bone growth, closure, and overall health throughout the lifespan, with estrogen appearing to have a greater effect than testosterone.[25] Bone density is adversely affected in females who have delayed menarche and amenorrhea, which has implications on bone health later in life. Estrogen deficiency post menopause is thought to be a primary factor in the development of osteoporosis in older women.

Ligament Structure

Ligaments connect bone to bone and are critical to the stability of the joint. Because they connect bone to bone, it stands to reason that a smaller bone structure would be related to smaller ligaments. Gender differences in ligament size have been largely studied at the knee due to the higher incidence of anterior cruciate ligament (ACL) injuries in females. These studies[7, 92, 105] consistently report a smaller ligament (both ACL and posterior cruciate ligament (PCL)) in females compared to males, and suggest these differences are largely related to sex differences in skeletal dimensions and weight. However, in one study, the sex differences persisted once correcting for total body weight, but not when correcting to lean body mass.[7] Given the greater relative higher proportion of fat mass to fat free mass in females compared to males, this finding would suggest that the female ACL is smaller in proportion to total body weight compared to males. Whether this relationship holds for other ligaments is unknown. Furthermore, it is not yet known if this sex difference poses a greater risk of ligament injury in the female.[45]

Joint Laxity

Joint laxity has been studied extensively in males and females, both at specific joints, as well as with more general measures of joint laxity. These sex differences appear to be mediated at least in part by sex hormones, and are often cited as a potential risk factor for musculoskeletal injury.

Joint Specific Laxity

Sex differences in joint laxity have been examined at multiple joints, including the shoulder, knee, and ankle. Because of the gender disparity in an ACL injury in females, anterior knee laxity has received the most attention regarding potential sex differences, with multiple investigations reporting findings of greater anterior knee laxity in females compared to males.[16, 43, 72, 91, 92, 101] Fewer investigations have examined sex differences at other joints, but appear to support increased joint laxity in females compared to males at the ankle[16, 117] and shoulder.[18]

Sex differences in joint laxity appear to be mediated in part by sex differences in endocrinology. Females have greater estrogen levels than males, and estrogen has been shown to have a profound effect on collagen tissue, specifically in regard to increased metabolic turnover,[36, 38, 49, 53, 56] increased elastin content, and decreased fiber diameter and density.[1, 34, 48] This has led to investigations examining changes in knee laxity across the menstrual cycle with changing sex hormone concentrations. While some have shown significant increases in knee laxity across the menstrual cycle,[31, 51, 101, 100] others have not.[16, 66, 115] These discrepancies are likely due to methodological differences in how data were sampled and how cycle phase was defined.[100] In one study examining sex differences in knee laxity across multiple days of the female's menstrual cycle, sex differences in knee laxity were found to be greatest during the early luteal phase of the female's menstrual cycle and least during the days of menses.[101]

General Joint Laxity

General joint laxity (GJL) is most often measured using the Beighton score,[12, 13, 21] which provides an overall sense of joint hypermobility based on bilateral examination of fifth finger extension beyond 90°, opposition of the thumb to the forearm, elbow hyperextension beyond 10°, knee hyperextension beyond 10°, and forward flexion of the trunk so that the palms of the hands rest on the floor. For each examination, a score of 0 or 1 is given depending on whether the criterion is met (score range 0–9). An overall score ≥4 is commonly used to classify individuals with hypermobility, however, others have used a higher, more conservative cutoff score.

Using these methods, females have greater GJL laxity compared to males and the difference is consistent across ages.[13, 63] Although GJL is greatest in infancy and declines as age increases, with the greatest decline during childhood, the decline in females tends to be slower than males.[17, 42] It has been reported that the greatest sex difference in GJL occurs around the age of 15, which may be explained by hormonal influences during puberty.[63] Although the influence of hormones on GJL has not been examined, the hormone relaxin has been hypothesized to influence this sex difference.[17] However, much work is needed to determine the effects of sex hormones on GJL.

Clinical Implications

Individuals with increased joint laxity are considered to be prone to orthopedic disorders, such as dislocations, subluxations, ligamentous injury, and early onset of osteoarthritis. The stability of a joint is greatly influenced by the tightness of the joint capsule and the ligaments surrounding the joint. When joint laxity is present, the muscles acting as dynamic stabilizers must compensate for reduced capsule-ligamentous stability.

Increased joint laxity has been associated with both acute and chronic injury.[13, 88, 114] This relationship is of particular concern in the athletic population where large forces are applied to the joints during sport activity. Lax and hyper-lax athletes have been observed to have an increase in musculoskeletal injury and joint sprains,[2, 82] particularly knee and ankle joint sprains.[30, 43] Knee laxity has also been implicated as a risk factor for knee osteoarthritis through its effects on the distribution of loads and stresses placed on the joint.[98]

Muscle

Gender differences in muscle have been observed both in the intrinsic characteristics of the muscle, as well as in the proportion of muscle to overall body weight. While females are often considered to be weaker than males, this is primarily due to sex differences in body composition, as there is no evidence of sex differences in muscle strength once equal amounts of muscle are compared.[118]

Body Composition

It is well recognized that adult males and females differ in body composition, reflected in the relative percentage of fat mass to fat free (muscle, bone) mass. These sex differences begin to appear post puberty (ages 12–14), as boys and girls do not differ substantially in height, weight, girth, bone width, or skinfold thickness before this time.[118] Following puberty however, female and male endocrinology begins to differ considerably, with females secreting more estrogen and males secreting more testosterone. These hormonal differences ultimately determine differences in body composition.[41] Testosterone is an anabolic steroid that increases bone formation and protein synthesis, which leads to greater bone and muscle mass development in males compared to females. Estrogen, on the other hand, appears to be a primary mediator of fat deposition and distribution.[8, 33] Higher estrogen levels have also been shown to decrease lean body mass by increasing the amount of serum hormone binding globulin (SHBG), a hormone that effectively binds circulating testosterone, making less testosterone bioactively available for protein synthesis.[41] Hence, sex differences in body composition begin to emerge post puberty, and are characterized by females having less fat free mass and greater fat mass, resulting in approximately 6%–10% greater percentage of relative body fat.[118] These sex differences suggest that a female, compared to a male of similar total body weight, has less muscle mass to move and control their total body weight against gravity during sport activities.

Muscle Structure

Gender differences in human muscle characteristics have been examined in a variety of muscles, including the vastus lateralis, gastrocnemius, and triceps brachii. Sex differences in muscle architecture and structure include females having smaller muscle fiber and total muscle cross sectional area,[5, 65, 71, 103, 108] smaller pennation angles,[65, 71] and decreased glycolytic enzymes.[103] These sex differences have been observed in both sedentary and physically active populations, and appear to hold across different sports.[5, 65] Although some studies have reported a greater proportion of Type I (slow twitch) to Type II (fast twitch) muscle fibers in females compared to males,[5, 103, 108] others have not.[108] Collectively, these sex differences in muscle characteristics may explain observed sex differences in myotendon extensibility and compliance,[65, 71] the time needed to develop tension within the muscle,[14, 22, 119] and metabolic responses to exercise.

As with body composition, gender differences in muscle characteristics are also thought to be hormone mediated.[103] As previously noted, testosterone is responsible for bone and muscle mass development, which would explain the greater cross sectional area in males compared to females. This in turn would explain the greater pennation angle of muscle fibers in males, as this angle has been shown to be highly correlated with cross sectional area.[65, 71] Sex hormones (estrogen and relaxin) are also thought to influence the elasticity of connective tissue in females,[15, 79, 99] which may lead to increased elasticity of the series elastic component, and explain longer delays in muscle force generation in females compared to males.[14, 119] The contention of a hormonal influence on series elasticity is further supported by Zhou et al,[122] who found gender differences in mechanical behavior of the leg extensors did not appear until after adolescence.

Lower Extremity Posture

When considering lower extremity posture, it appears that postural differences between males and females occur mainly in the proximal structures of the kinetic chain in the pelvis, hips, and knees. Based on the available literature and clinical observations, females tend to stand with a lower extremity posture of greater anterior pelvic tilt, femoral internal rotation, knee hyperextension (genu recurvatum), and knee valgus (Figure 2-1). Sex differences have not been observed in tibial torsion[86, 107] or foot pronation as measured by navicular drop[11, 52, 81, 113] and rearfoot angle.[10, 104]

Lower extremity posture is an important aspect to consider when evaluating sex differences in lower extremity function and injury, as malalignments may cause abnormal stress patterns or compensatory motions along the lower extremity kinetic chain. The malalignments may be related to muscle strength imbalances or influenced by the integrity of ligaments, joint capsule, or musculotendinous structures.

Pelvic Tilt

The neutral position of the pelvis is when the anterior superior iliac spines (ASIS) lie in the same transverse plane and are aligned in the same frontal

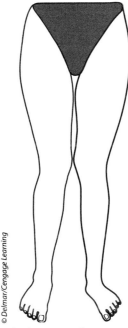

© Delmar/Cengage Learning

Figure 2-1 Females tend to stand with a lower extremity posture of greater anterior pelvic tilt, femoral internal rotation, knee hyperextension (genu recurvatum) and knee valgus.

plane as the pubic symphysis, and the same transverse plane as the posterior superior iliac spines (PSIS).[68] A deviation from this neutral position, termed pelvic tilt, is defined by the orientation of the ASIS and PSIS in the transverse plane (Figure 2-2). Pelvic tilt angles where the PSIS are above the horizontal in reference to the ASIS are considered an anterior pelvic tilt. This occurs as the ASIS moves anteriorly and inferiorly and the PSIS moves superiorly. Pelvic tilt angles where the PSIS are below the horizontal relative to the ASIS are considered a posterior pelvic tilt. This occurs as the ASIS moves posterior and superiorly and the PSIS moves inferiorly.[70, 83, 94]

Sex and Age Differences: Pelvic Tilt

Comparison of the mean values reported for the adult population appears to be similar across studies (range 9°–12°), regardless of the method or instrument used in the measurement.[4, 29, 39, 40, 73, 102] These normative values reflect a mean anterior tilt of the pelvis in normal adult subjects. While studies reporting normative values on males and females have not examined sex differences, one retrospective study of ACL injury risk factors supports this contention, finding females had greater anterior pelvic tilt than males regardless of injury status.[52] No studies were found that examined standing pelvic tilt angles across age groups, so it is unclear if pelvic tilt changes with maturation. Future research is needed on larger populations to confirm sex and age related differences in pelvic angles.

Clinical Implications: Pelvic Tilt

The imbalance of muscles acting on the pelvis can affect the posture of the body above and below the pelvis.[68] The relationship of pelvic tilt to the lumbar spine[29, 39, 68, 73] and sacral angle[35, 40] indicate that increased anterior pelvic tilt is often associated with increased lordosis (Figure 2-3). Factors thought to contribute to excessive anterior pelvic tilt and lumbo-pelvic instability include

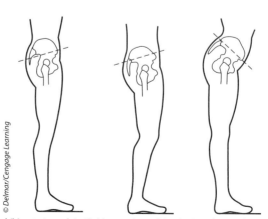

© Delmar/Cengage Learning

Figure 2-2 (a) Normal (b) anterior pelvic tilt (c) posterior pelvic tilt. Females tend to stand with more anterior pelvic tilt compared to males.

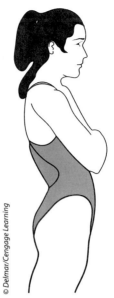

© Delmar/Cengage Learning

Figure 2-3 Increased lumbar lordosis is often associated with increased anterior pelvic tilt.

muscular tightness and shortening of the erector spinae and hip flexors, and elongation, inhibition, and weakening of the abdominals and gluteals.[23, 57, 67] Clinical perspectives suggest that excessive anterior pelvic tilt leads to alignment changes in the lower kinetic chain, including increased femoral internal rotation, genu valgus, genu recurvatum, and foot pronation.[23, 57, 62, 76] (See Figure 2-1.)

Femoral Torsion (Anteversion)

Torsion of the femur is defined as the angle formed between the axis of the femoral neck and a transverse line through the femoral condyles, also known as the transcondylar axis or plane.[27, 83] Forward projection of the femoral neck from the transcondylar plane is known as anteversion. Excessive anteversion in adulthood usually results from a lack of anteversion regression from infancy to adulthood.[78] Another factor considered to contribute to excessive anteversion is increased stress on the medial femoral growth plate through childhood. The source of this increased stress can come from regular sitting in the "reverse tailor's" position. Children often sit in this position while engaged in television viewing. This stress is further increased with frequent in-toe belly sleeping.[78]

Sex and Age Differences: Anteversion

Anteversion is greatest as an infant and gradually decreases with age.[27, 110] Normal anteversion at birth is approximately 35°–40° and decreases to approximately 12°–15° in adulthood.[78] While the American Orthopaedic Association[6] defines normal anteversion angle as 15°–20°, normal values reported in healthy subjects appear to be somewhat lower, with means ranging from

7° to 18°.[19, 64, 86, 87, 89, 95, 97, 102] While some studies reported a difference between sexes, with higher values in females compared to males,[19, 87] others have not.[64]

Clinical Implications: Anteversion

The most common problem associated with increased anteversion is an intoeing gait.[47, 107] This type of gait pattern can cause several gait abnormalities leading to compensations in other parts of the lower extremity, including medial rotation of the patella,[47] internal rotation of the tibia, and overpronation of the subtalar joint during walking.[107] As the child's gait improves with age, a compensatory external torsion of the tibia has been found to occur.[37] This compensatory tibial torsion has been shown to affect other lower extremity alignments. There is a correlation between femoral anteversion and quadriceps angle where the compensation of external tibial torsion leads to a higher quadriceps angle.[61]

Quadriceps Angle

The quadriceps angle or Q-angle is a clinical measurement that is used to represent the quadriceps muscle force on the patella in the frontal plane.[96] It represents the angle formed by the vectors for the combined pull of the quadriceps femoris and the patellar tendon (Figure 2-4).[59]

Sex and Age Differences: Q-angle

The American Orthopaedic Association[6] considers a Q-angle of 10° to be normal and angles 15°–20° to be abnormal. However, the mean values reported in the literature range from 8°–15° in males, and 12°–19° in females.[3, 46, 55, 58, 75, 120] Hence, Hvid[60] has suggested that angles greater than 15° for men and greater than 20° for women are clinically abnormal. While Q-angles have been reported in healthy

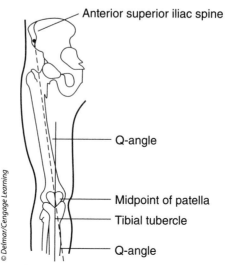

Anterior superior iliac spine

Q-angle

Midpoint of patella

Tibial tubercle

Q-angle

© Delmar/Cengage Learning

Figure 2-4 Measurement of quadriceps angle.

subjects ranging in age from 13–60 years old, there were no reported differences between age groups.

There is strong evidence to support greater Q-angles in females compared to males.[3, 46, 55, 58, 60, 120] The prevailing thought that larger Q-angles in females are a result of females having a wider pelvis has not been demonstrated.[46, 55] On the contrary, Horton and Hall[55] reported larger mean hip widths in males compared to females and did not find a relationship between increased hip width and Q-angle. While they suggested that males have longer femurs, would have lead to decreasing the hip width to femur length ratio compared to females, this data was inconclusive. Hence, the reasons for this difference are still unknown.

Clinical Implications: Q-angle

As previously mentioned, increased femoral anteversion is compensated by external rotation of the tibia.[61] Increased knee valgus, in standing, has also been suggested to influence Q-angle.[120] Both of these lower extremity malalignments would result in an increased Q-angle, with the tibial tuberosity positioned more lateral in the frontal plane. Conversely, a compensated internal rotation of the tibia due to over pronation of the foot[28, 109, 112] will position the tibial tuberosity more medial in the frontal plane, resulting in a decreased Q-angle measurement. Clinically, increased Q-angle has been associated with abnormal tracking of the patella resulting in various patallofemoral joint dysfunctions such as patellofemoral pain syndrome, chondromalacia, patella dislocations, and subluxations.

Tibiofemoral Angle

Tibiofemoral angle is formed by the intersection of a line that represents the long axis of the femur and a line that represents the long axis of the tibia in the frontal plane. The axes of each segment are defined by an anatomical axis and a mechanical axis respective to each segment. Moreland et al.[80] has described these axes in detail. The anatomical and mechanical axes of the tibia are the same and are represented by a line between the knee joint center and the ankle joint center. The mechanical axis of the femur represents a line from the center of the head of the femur to the knee joint center. The anatomical axis of the entire femur represents a line from the shaft of the femur through the knee joint center. Hence the anatomical axis of the femur has a greater valgus angulation of approximately 5°–7° relative to the mechanical axis.[84] When the femur and tibia are aligned in a straight line in the frontal plane, this is assumed to be the neutral position. Any deviation from this neutral position is commonly referred in terms of varus or valgus alignment of the knee (Figure 2-5).

Sex Differences: Tibiofemoral angle

Mean values reported using clinical methods represent a more valgus alignment compared to radiographic measurements. This can be partially explained by the difference in which each method defined the femoral axis. While both

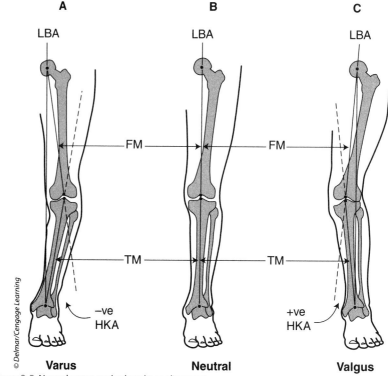

Figure 2-5 Neutral, varus, and valgus knee alignment.

of the clinical methods used landmarks that more closely represented the anatomical axis of the femur,[20, 102] the radiographic studies, with the exception of one, used the mechanical axis of the femur and reported mean values of varus alignment.[26, 80, 111] The radiographic study that used the anatomical axis of the femur reported a mean valgus alignment, which was closer to the values obtained with clinical measurement methods.[58]

There have been conflicting reports regarding sex differences in tibiofemoral angle, with some showing greater valgus angle in females,[58, 113] and others showing no difference between sex.[26, 111] While reported means between adults and older adults are similar, there appear to be no studies that examined differences between the adult population and the adolescent population. However, like femoral anteversion, tibiofemoral angle follows a pattern of development from infancy to adulthood.[50, 93, 116] A varus deformity is present during infancy which changes into valgus at two to three years of age.[93] Developmental changes during adolescence may differentially influence tibiofemoral angles in males and females. For example, one study reported a significant decrease of valgus angle in boys after the age 14, whereas the valgus angle of girls remained stable.[20] Future research is needed to examine tibiofemoral angle differences between males and females in both the adult and adolescent populations. This would contribute to the understanding of how tibiofemoral angle changes with age.

Clinical Implications: Tibiofemoral angle

Increase tibiofemoral angle has been related to abnormal contact pressures at the knee and possibly increasing the chances of osteoarthritis at the knee.[24, 58] The relationship to other lower extremity malalignments is still unclear. Abduction of the tibia due to increased valgus at the knee would seem to increase Q-angle due to a laterally directed tibial tuberosity. There may also be a relationship with increased tibiofemoral angle and excessive foot pronation, as the tibia is abducted in this posture, increasing the stress on the medial aspect of the foot.[109]

Genu Recurvatum

Genu recurvatum, or hyperextension of the knee (Figure 2-6), is defined as sagittal alignment of the knee beyond the zero position of extension.[68] This represents the sagittal alignment of the midline of the femur and the lateral midline of the lower leg at the tibofemoral joint. Genu recurvatum is influenced by capsule-ligamentous laxity and joint geometry.

Sex Differences: Genu recurvatum

It has been suggested that females have higher incidence of genu recurvatum than males,[54, 77] with 0°–5° of hyperextension considered to be the normal range.[76] Limited empirical data supports this clinically defined normal range,[32, 102, 113] however, two of these studies had relatively small sample sizes. Trimble et al.[113] reported sex differences in genu recurvatum, with mean values for males within the suggested normal range and mean values for females greater than 5°. Further, females have been shown to have greater general joint laxity than males, of which genu recurvatum (greater than 10°) is one of the criteria, and has been reported to be more prevalent in females.[63] Further research is

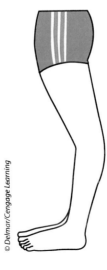

© Delmar/Cengage Learning

Figure 2-6 Genu recurvatum.

needed to clarify possible sex differences and establish a normal range on a healthy population.

Clinical Implications: Genu recurvatum

As previously noted, genu recurvatum can be a secondary compensation due to excessive anterior pelvic tilt. An increase in anterior tilt of the pelvis creates a flexion moment at the hip that is counteracted with an extension moment at the knee resulting in hyperextension at the knee joint.[68] The result of this relationship further influences other segments of the lower extremity. Hyperextension of the knee can also occur in combination with medial rotation of the femur and pronation of the foot, reflecting a "postural bowleg." Conversely, when genu recurvatum occurs in combination with lateral rotation of the femur and supination of the foot, a "postural knock-knee" results.[68]

Upper Extremity Posture

Differences between males and females of the upper extremity are not as prevalent compared to the lower extremity. This could possibly be explained by the influence of weight bearing on the lower extremity, whereas, the upper extremity does not commonly function in this fashion. Sex differences that are commonly identified to be different during clinical evaluation of the upper extremity are postures of the shoulder and the elbow. Females tend to have more rounded shoulders and greater frontal plane angle of the elbow, or carrying angle.

Rounded Shoulders

Increased prevalence of rounded shoulders in females has been hypothesized to be acquired due to poor postural habits. As females mature through puberty, they may adopt poor postural habits as a manner of hiding the beginning development of breasts. The presence of rounded shoulders is usually observed during posterior and lateral postural observations (Figure 2-7). During a posterior postural observation, rounded shoulders are characterized by abducted, or protracted, scapulae. Downward rotation of the scapulae and internal rotation of the humerus are also characteristic of this posture. This posture is associated with tightness of the pectoral muscles and weakness of the rhomboid and middle trapezius muscles. Scapular winging in association with rounded shoulder usually indicates weakness of the serratus anterior muscles. During lateral postural observations, rounded shoulders are often observed along with increased kyphosis of the thoracic spine, and a forward head posture.

It is commonly known that a rounded shoulder posture has been suggested to predispose individuals to overuse conditions of the shoulder, such as impingement syndrome and thoracic outlet syndrome. Muscle imbalances

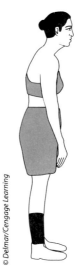

Figure 2-7 Forward head posture with rounded shoulders.

at the shoulder girdle may cause changes in neuromuscular control resulting in abnormal movement patterns during upper extremity motion.[44] In turn, these abnormal movement patterns can decrease the space under the cora-coacromial arch causing compression of structures located in the subacromial arch (supraspinatus tendon, subacromial bursa, long head of the biceps). Compression of neurovascular bundle (brachial plexus, subclavian artery, and subclavian vein) between the clavicle and first rib are also common, leading to thoracic outlet compression syndrome. Common management strategies are to correct the abnormal posture with stretching of tight structures and strengthening of the posterior shoulder muscles.

Carrying Angle of the Elbow

Carrying angle of the elbow is described as the angle formed by the long axis of the humerus and the long axis of the ulna with the elbow in extension and the forearm supinated. A slight valgus at the elbow in both males and females is normal with values for males between 5° and 10°, and females between 10° and 15° (Figure 2-8 a and b). Sex differences in carrying angles, also known as cubital valgus, appear to decrease with age, with the greater differences observed during adolescence compared to adults.[85] Hormonal influences may explain this sex difference in carrying angle since there appears to be no differences between males and females during childhood, while obvious differences are observed during puberty and continue into adulthood.[85] Injuries resulting from an excessive carrying angle commonly occur with overuse activities resulting from abnormal stress or friction of the elbow structure, specifically the ulnar nerve. This deformity places the medial humeral condyle in a more prominent position where the ulnar nerve can be impinged, irritated, or dislocated.

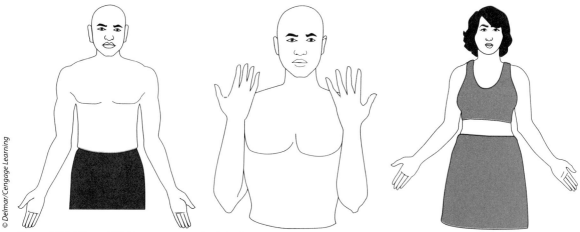

© Delmar/Cengage Learning

Figure 2-8 (a) Normal (b) Valgus carrying angle of the elbow.

Summary

With the onset of puberty, marked changes in endocrinology occurs in females and males, with females secreting more estrogen and males secreting more testosterone. In response to these hormonal changes, structural differences between males and females begin to emerge, with males having greater overall stature, greater muscle and bone mass, and lesser fat mass compared to females. These sex differences are further manifested in differences in body composition, where females have a higher relative percentage of body fat compared to males. While females and males are of equal strength per unit of muscle, the increased relative body fat in females requiring them to support and move similar amounts of body weight with less available muscle and potentially, smaller ligaments. Concomitant with these structural changes are sex differences in upper and lower extremity posture, with females having a tendency to stand with more rounded shoulders, and greater amounts of anterior pelvic tilt, internal femoral rotation, quadriceps angle, and genu recurvatum. Many of these sex differences in anatomy have important clinical implications, and should be considered during injury examinations, and when developing training and injury prevention strategies.

References

1. Abubaker AO, Hebda PC, and Gunsolley JN. Effects of sex hormones on protein and collagen content of the temporomandibular joint disc of the rat. *Journal of Oral and Maxillofacial Surgery.* 1996;54:721-727.

2. Acasuso-Diaz M, Collantes-Esteves E, and Sanchez-Guijo P. Joint hyperlaxity and musculoligamentous lesions: study of a population

of homogeneous age, sex and physical exertion. *British Journal of Rheumatology.* 1993;32:120-122.

3. Aglietti P, Insall JN, and Cerulli G. Patellar pain and incongruence, I: measurements of incongruence. *Clinical Orthopaedics and Related Research.* 1983;176:217-224.

4. Alviso DJ, Dong GT, and Lentell GL. Intertester reliability for measuring pelvic tilt in standing. *Physical Therapy.* 1988;68(9):1347-1351.

5. Alway SE, Grumbt WH, Gonyea WJ, and Stray-Gundersen J. Contrasts in muscle and myofibers of elite male and female bodybuilders. *Journal of Applied Physiology.* 1989;67(1):24-31.

6. American Orthopaedic Association. Manual of Orthopaedic Surgery. Chicago; 1979.

7. Anderson AF, Dome DC, Gautam S, Awh MH, and Rennirt GW. Correlation of anthropometric measurements, strength, anterior cruciate ligament size, and intercondylar notch characteristics to sex differences in anterior cruciate ligament tear rates. *American Journal of Sports Medicine.* 2001a; 29(1):58-66.

8. Anderson LA, McTernan PG, Barnett AH, and Kumar S. The effects of androgens and estrogens on preadipocyte proliferation in human adipose tissue: influence of gender and site. *Journal of Clinical Endocrinology and Metabolism.* 2001b;86(10):5045-5051.

9. Arabi A, Tamim H, Nabulsi M, et al. Sex differences in the effect of body-composition variables on bone mass in healthy children and adolescents. *American Journal of Clinical Nutrition.* 2004;80:1428 –1435.

10. Astrom M, and Arvidson T. Alignment and joint motion in the normal foot. *Journal of Orthopaedic & Sports Physical Therapy.* 1995;22(5): 216-222.

11. Beckett ME, Massie DL, Bowers KD, and Stoll DA. Incidence of hyperpronation in the ACL injured knee: A clinical perspective. *Journal of Athletic Training.* 1992;27(1):58-60.

12. Beighton P, and Horan F. Orthopaedic aspects of the Ehlers-Danlos syndrome. *Journal of Bone and Joint Surgery; British volume.* 1969;51: 444-453.

13. Beighton P, Solomon L, and Soskolne CL. Articular mobility in an African population. *Annals of Rheumatic Diseases.* 1973;32:413-418.

14. Bell DG, and Jacobs I. Electro-Mechanical response times and rate of force development in males and females. *Medicine and Science in Sport and Exercise.* 1986;18(1):31-36.

15.   Berardesca E, Gabba P, Farinelli N, Borroni G, and Rabbiosi G. Skin extensibility time in women: changes in relation to sex hormones. *Acta Dermato-Venereologica.* 1989;69(5):431-433.

16.   Beynnon BD, Bernstein I, Belisle A, et al. The Effect of Estradiol and Progesterone on Knee and Ankle Joint Laxity. *American Journal of Sports Medicine.* 2005;33(9):1298-1304.

17.   Birrell FN, Adebajo AO, Hazleman BL, and Silman AJ. High prevalence of joint laxity in West Africans. *British Journal of Rheumatology.* 1994;33(1):56-59.

18.   Borsa PA, Sauers EL, and Herling DE. Patterns of glenohumeral joint laxity and stiffness in healthy men and women. *Medicine and Science in Sport and Exercise.* 2000;32(10):1685-1690.

19.   Braten M, Terjesen T, and Rossvoll I. Femoral anteversion in normal adults. Ultrasound measurements in 50 men and 50 women. *Acta Orthopædica Scandinavica.* 1992;63(1): 29-32.

20.   Cahuzac JP, Vardon D, and Sales de Gauzy J. Development of the clinical tibiofemoral angle in normal adolescents. A study of 427 normal subjects from 10 to 16 years of age. *Journal of Bone and Joint Surgery; British volume.* 1995;77-B(5):729-732.

21.   Carter C, and Wilkinson J. Persistent joint laxity and congential dislocation of the hip. *Journal of Bone and Joint Surgery; British volume.* 1964;46:40-45.

22.   Cavanaugh PR, and Komi PV. Electromechanical delay in human skeletal muscle under concentric and eccentric contractions. *European Journal of Applied Physiology.* 1979;42:159-163.

23.   Chaitow L, and DeLany JW. The Pelvis. *Clinical Application of Neuromuscular Techniques.* New York, Churchill Livingstone; 2000;2: 301-386.

24.   Chao EYS, Neluheni EVD, Hsu RWW, and Paley D. Biomechanics of malalignment. *The Orthopedic Clinics of North America.* 1994;25(3): 379-386.

25.   Compston JE. Sex Steroids and Bone. *Physiological Reviews.* 2001;81(1):419-447.

26.   Cooke ID, Scudamore A, Li J, Wyss U, Bryant T, and Costigan P. Axial lower-limb alignment: comparison of knee geometry in normal volunteers and osteoarthritis patients. *Osteoarthritis and Cartilage.* 1997;5:39-47.

27. Crane L. Femoral torsion and its relation to toeing-in and toeing-out. *Journal of Bone and Joint Surgery; American volume.* 1959;41-A(3): 421-428.

28. D'Amico JC, and M Rubin. The influence of foot orthoses on the quadriceps angle. *Journal of the American Podiatric Medical Association.* 1986;76(6):337-340.

29. Day JW, Smidt GL, and Lehmann T. Effect of pelvic tilt on standing posture. *Physical Therapy.* 1984;64(4):510-516.

30. Decoster LC, Bernier JN, Lindsay RH, and Vailas JC. Generalized joint hypermobility and its relationship to injury patterns among NCAA lacrosse players. *Journal of Athletic Training.* 1999;34(2):99-105.

31. Deie M, Sakamaki Y, Sumen Y, Urabe Y, and Ikuta Y. Anterior knee laxity in young women varies with their menstrual cycle. *International Orthopaedics.* 2002;26:154-156.

32. Devan MR, Pescatello LS, Faghri P, and Anderson J. A prospective study of overuse knee injuries among female athletes with muscle imbalances and structural abnormalities. *Journal of Athletic Training.* 2004;39(3):263-267.

33. Dieudonne MN, Pecquery R, Leneveu MC, and Guiudicelli Y. Op-positive effects of androgens and estrogens on adipogenesis in rat preadipocytes: evidence for sex and site-related specificities and possible involvement of insulin-like growth factor 1 receptor and peroxisome proliferator-activated receptor y2. *Endocrinology.* 2000;141(2):649-656.

34. Dubey RK, Gillespie DG, Jackson EK, and Keller PJ. 17B-Estradiol, its metabolites, and progesterone inhibit cardiac fibroblast growth. *Hypertension.* 1998;31(2):522-528.

35. During J, Goudfrooij H, Keessen W, Beeker TW, and Crowe A. Toward standards for posture. Postural characteristics of the lower back system in normal and pathologic conditions. *Spine.* 1985;10(1):83-87.

36. Dyer R, Sodek J, and Heersche JM. The effect of 17 B-Estradiol on collagen and noncollagenous protein synthesis in the uterus and some periodontal tissues. *Endocrinology.* 1980;107:1014-1021.

37. Fabry G, MacEwen GD, and Shands ARJ. Torsion of the femur. A follow-up study in normal and abnormal conditions. *Journal of Bone and Joint Surgery; American volume.* 1973;55(8):1726-1738.

38. Fischer GM. Comparison of collagen dynamics in different tissues under the influence of estradiol. *Endocrinology.* 1973;93:1216-1218.

39. Gajdosik R, Simpson R, Smith R, and DonTigny RL. Pelvic tilt. Intratester reliability of measuring the standing position and range of motion. *Physical Therapy.* 1985;65(2):169-174.

40. Gilliam J, Brunt D, MacMillan M, Kinard RE, and Montgomery WJ. Relationship of the pelvic angle to the sacral angle: measurement of clinical reliability and validity. *Journal of Orthopaedic and Sports Physical Therapy.* 1994;20(4):193-199.

41. Gower BA, and Nyman L. Associations among oral estrogen use, free testosterone concentration, and lean body mass among post menopausal women. *Journal of Clinical Endocrinology and Metabolism.* 2000;85(12):4476-4480.

42. Grahame R. Joint hypermobility and genetic collagen disorders: are they related? *Archives of Disease in Childhood.* 1999;80:188-191.

43. Grana WA, and Moretz JA. Ligamentous laxity in secondary school athletes. *Journal of the American Medicine Association.* 1978;240: 1975-1976.

44. Greenfield B, Catlin PA, Coats PW, Green E, McDonald JJ, and North C. Posture in patients with shoulder overuse injuries and health individuals. *Journal of Orthopaedic and Sports Physical Therapy.* 1995;21(5):287-295.

45. Griffin LY, Albohm MJ, Arendt EA, et al. Update on ACL prevention: theoretical and practical guidelines. *American Journal of Sports Medicine.* In Press.

46. Guerra JP, Arnold MJ, and Gajdosik RL. Q angle: effects of isometric quadriceps contraction and body position. *The Journal of Orthopaedic and Sports Physical Therapy.* 1994;19(4):200-204.

47. Gulan G, Matovinovic D, Nemec B, Rubinic D, and Ravlic-Gulan J. Femoral neck anteversion: values, development, measurement, common problems. *Collegium Antropologicum.* 2000;24(2):521-527.

48. Hama H, Yamamuro T, and Takeda T. Experimental studies on connective tissue of the capsular ligament. Influences of aging and sex hormones. *Acta Orthopaedica Scandinavica.* 1976;47:473-479.

49. Hassager C, Jensen LT, Podenphant J, Riis BJ, and Christiansen C. Collage synthesis in postmenopausal women during therapy with anabolic steroid or female sex hormones. *Metabolism.* 1990;39: 1167-1169.

50. Heath CH, and Staheli LT. Normal limits of knee angle in white children—genu varum and genu valgum. *Journal of Pediatric Orthopaedics.* 1993;13(2).

51. Heitz NA. Hormonal changes throughout the menstrual cycle and increased anterior cruciate ligament laxity in females. *Journal of Athletic Training.* 1999;343(2):144-149.

52. Hertel JN, Dorfman JH, and Braham RA. Lower Extremity Malalignments and Anterior Cruciate Ligament Injury History. *Journal of Sports Science and Medicine.* 2004;3:220-225.

53. Ho KKY, and Weissberger AJ. Impact of short-term estrogen administration on growth hormone secretion and action: distinct route-dependent effects on connective and bone tissue metabolism. *Journal of Bone and Mineral Research.* 1992;7:821-827.

54. Hoppenfeld S. Physical Examination of the Spine and Extremities. Norwalk, Appleton-Century-Crofts; 1976:165-166.

55. Horton MG, and Hall TL. Quadriceps femoris angle: normal values and relationship with gender and selected skeletal measures. *Physical Therapy.* 1989;69:897-901.

56. Hosokawa M, Ishii M, Inoue K, Yao CS, and Takeda T. Estrogen induces different responses in dermal and lung fibroblasts: special reference to collagen. *Connective Tissue Research.* 1981;9:115-120.

57. Hruska R. Pelvic stability influences lower extremity kinematics. *Biomechanics* 1998;6:23-29.

58. Hsu RW, Himeno S, Coventry MB, and Chao EY. Normal axial alignment of the lower extremity and load-bearing distribution at the knee. *Clinical Orthopaedics and Related Research.* 1990;255:215-227.

59. Hungerford D, and Barry M. Biomechanics of the patellofemoral joint. *Clinical Orthopaedics.* 1979;144:9-15.

60. Hvid I, Andersen LI, and Schmidt H. Chondromalacia patellae. The relation to abnormal patellofemoral joint mechanics. *Acta Orthopædica Scandinavica.* 1981;52(6):661-666.

61. Hvid I, and Andersen LI. The quadriceps angle and its relation to femoral torsion. *Acta Orthopaedica Scandinavica.* 1982;53(4):577-579.

62. Ireland ML, Gaudette M, and Crook S. ACL injuries in the female athlete. *Journal of Sport Rehabilitation.* 1997;6:97-110.

63. Jansson A, Saartok T, Werner S, and Renstrom P. General joint laxity in 1845 Swedish school children of different ages: age- and gender specific distributions. 2004;93(9):1202-1206.

64. Jonson SR, and Gross MT. Intraexaminer reliability, interexaminer reliability, and mean values for nine lower extremity skeletal measures in healthy naval midshipment. *Journal of Orthopaedic & Sports Physical Therapy.* 1997;25(4):253-263.

65.   Kanehisa H, Muraoka Y, Kawakami Y, and Fukunaga T. Fascicle arrangements of vastus lateralis and gastrocnemius muscles in highly trained soccer players and swimmers of both genders. *International Journal of Sports Medicine.* 2003;24:90-95.

66.   Karageanes, SJ, Blackburn K, and Vangelos ZA. The association of the menstrual cycle with the laxity of the anterior cruciate ligament in adolescent female athletes. *Clinical Journal of Sports Medicine.* 2000;10(3):162-168.

67.   Kendall FP, and EK McCreary. *Muscles: Testing And Function.* Baltimore, Williams and Wilkins; 1983.

68.   Kendall FP, McCreary EK, and Provance PG. *Muscles Testing and Function.* Philadelphia, Lippincott Williams & Wilkins; 1993:72-98.

69.   Kernozek TW, and NL Greer. Quadriceps angle and rearfoot motion: relationships in walking. *Archives of Physical Medicine and Rehabilitation.* 1993;74(4):407-410.

70.   Kisner C, and Colby LA. *Therapeutic Exercise: Foundations and Techniques.* Philadelphia, F.A. Davis Co.; 1996:388.

71.   Kubo K, Kanehisa H, Azuma K, et al. Muscle architectural characteristics in young and elderly men and women. *International Journal of Sports Medicine.* 2003;24:125-130.

72.   Larsson LG, Baum J, and Mudholkar GS. Hypermobility: features and differential incidence between the sexes. *Arthritis and Rheumatism.* 1987;30:1426-1430.

73.   Levine D and MW Whittle. The effects of pelvic movement on lumbar lordosis in the standing position. *Journal of Orthopedic and Sports Physical Therapy.* 1996;24(3):130-135.

74.   Lin YC, Lyle RM, Weaver CM, McCabe LD, McCabe GP, Johnston CC, and Teegardena D. Peak spine and femoral neck bone mass in young women. *Bone.* 2003;32:546-553.

75.   Livingston LA, and Mandigo JL. Bilateral within-subject Q angle assymetry in young adult females and males. *Biom Sci Instrument* 1997;33:112-117.

76.   Loudon JK, Jenkins W, and Loudon KL. The relationship between static posture and ACL injury in female athletes. *Journal of Orthopedic and Sports Physical Therapy.* 1996;24(2):91-97.

77.   Loudon JK, Goist HL, and Loudon KL. Genu Recurvatum Syndrome. *Journal of Orthopedic and Sports Physical Therapy.* 1998;27(5):361-367.

78.   McDonough MW. Angular and axial deformities of the legs of children. *Clinical Podiatry.* 1984;1(3):601-620.

79. Mercado-Simmen RC, Bryant-Greenwood GD, and Greenwood FC. Relaxin receptor in the rat myometrium: regulation by estrogen and relaxin. *Endocrinology*. 1982;110:220-226.

80. Moreland JR, Bassett LW, and Hanker GJ. Radiographic analysis of the axial alignment of the lower extremity. *Journal of Bone and Joint Surgery; American volume*. 1987;69(5):745-749.

81. Moul JL. Differences in selected predictors of anterior cruciate ligament tears between male and female NCAA Div I college bastketball players. *Journal of Athletic Training*. 1998;33:118-121.

82. Nicholas JA. Injuries to knee ligaments: relationship to looseness and tightness in football players. *Journal of the American Medical Association*. 1970;212:2236-2239.

83. Norkin CC, and Levangie PK. *Joint Structure & Function: A Comprehensive Analysis*. Philadelphia, F.A. Davis Co.; 1992:312-313.

84. Oswald MH, Jakob RP, Schneider E, and Hoogewoud HM. Radiological analysis of normal axial alignment of femur and tibia in view of total knee arthroplasty. *Journal of Arthroplasty*. 1993;8(4):419-426.

85. Paraskevas G, Papadopoulos A, Papaziogas B, Spainidou S, Argiriadou H, and Gigis J. Study of the carrying angle of the human elbow joint in full extension: a morphometric analysis. *Surgical and Radiologic Anatomy*. 2004;26:19-23.

86. Pasciak M, Stoll TM, and Hefti F. Relation of femoral to tibial torsion in children measured by ultrasound. *Journal of Pediatric Orthopaedics*. 1996;5(4):268-272.

87. Prasad R, Vettivel S, Isaac B, Jeyaseelan L, and Chandi G. Angle of torsion of the femur and its correlates. *Clinical Anatomy* 1996;9(2):109-117.

88. Ramesh R, VonArx O, Azzopardi T, and Schranz PJ. The risk of anterior cruciate ligament rupture with generalised joint laxity. *Journal of Bone and Joint Surgery; British volume*. 2005;87-B:800-803.

89. Reikeras O, and Bjerkreim I. Idiopathic increased anteversion of the femoral neck: radiological and clinical study in non-operated and operated patients. *Acta Orthopædica Scandinavica*. 1982;53(6):839-845.

90. Rizzo M, Holler SB, and Bassett FH. Comparison of males' and females' ratios of anterior-cruciate-ligament width to femoral-intercondylar-notch width: a cadaveric study. *American Journal of Orthopaedics* 2001;30(8):660-664.

91. Rosene JM, and Fogarty TD. Anterior tibial translation in collegiate athletes with normal anterior cruciate ligament integrity. *Journal of Athletic Training*. 1999;34(2):93-98.

92.   Rozzi SL, Lephart SM, Gear WS, and Fu FH. Knee joint laxity and neuromuscular characteristics of male and female soccer and basketball players. *American Journal of Sports Medicine.* 1999;27(3):312-319.

93.   Salenius P, and Vankka E. The development of the tibiofemoral angle in children. *Journal of Bone and Joint Surgery; American volume.* 1975;57(2):259-261.

94.   Sanders G, and Stavrakas P. A technique for measuring pelvic tilt. *Physical Therapy.* 1981;61(1):49-50.

95.   Schneider B, Laubenberger J, Jemlich S, Groene K, Weber HM, and Langer M. Measurement of femoral antetorsion and tibial torsion by magnetic resonance imaging. *British Journal of Radiology.* 1997; 70(834):575-9.

96.   Schulthies SS, Francis RS, Fisher AG, and Van de Graaff KM. Does the Q angle reflect the force on the patella in the frontal plane? *Physical Therapy.* 1995;75(1):24-30.

97.   Seber S, Hazer B, Kose N, Gokturk E, Gunal I, and Turgut A. Rotational profile of the lower extremity and foot progression angle: computerized tomographic examination of 50 male adults. *Arch Orthop Trauma Surg* 2000;120(5-6):255-258.

98.   Sharma L, Lou C, Felson DT, et al. Laxity in health and osteoarthritic knees. *Arthritis and Rheumatism.* 1999;42(5):861-870.

99.   Shikata J, Sanda H, Yamamuro T, and Takeda T. Experimental studies of the elastic fiber of the capsular ligament: influence of aging and sex hormones on the hip joint capsule of rats. *Connective Tissue Research.* 1979;7:21-27.

100. Shultz SJ, Sander TC, Kirk SE, Johnson M, and Perrin DH. Relationship between sex hormones and anterior knee laxity across the menstrual cycle. *Medicine & Science in Sports & Exercise.* 2004;36(7):1165-1174.

101. Shultz SJ, Kirk SE, Sander TC, and Perrin DH. Sex differences in knee laxity change across the female menstrual cycle. *Journal of Sports Medicine and Physical Fitness.* In Press-a.

102. Shultz SJ, Nguyen A, Windley TC, Kulas AS, Botic TL, and Beynnon BD. Intratester and Intertester Reliability of Clinical Measures of Lower Extremity Anatomical Alignment; Implications for Multi-center Studies. *Clinical Biomechanics.* In Press-b.

103. Simoneau JA, and Boucher C. Human variation in skeletal muscle fiber-type proportion and enzyme activities. *American Journal of Physiology.* 1989;257(4):567-572.

104. Sobel E, Levitz S, Caselli M, Brentnall Z, and Tran MQ. Natural history of the rearfoot angle: preliminary values in 150 children. *Foot & Ankle International.* 1999;20(2):119-125.

105. Staeubli HU, Adam O, Becker W, and Burgkart R. Anterior cruciate ligament and intercondylar notch in the coronal oblique plane: anatomy complemented by magnetic resonance imaging in cruciate ligament-intact knees. *Arthroscopy.* 1999;15(4):349-359.

106. Staheli LT. Torsional deformity. *Pediatric Clinics of North America.* 1977;24(4):799-811.

107. Staheli LT, Corbett M, Wyss C, and King H. Lower extremity rotational problems in children. Normal values to guide management. *Journal of Bone and Joint Surgery [Br].* 1985;67A(1):39-47.

108. Staron R, F Hagerman, R Hikida, et al. Fiber type composition of the vastus lateralis muscle of young men and women. *J of Histochemistry and Cytochemistry*;48(5):623-629.

109. Subotnick SI. Podiatric aspects of children in sports. *Journal of the American Podiatry Association.* 1979;69(7):443-454.

110. Svenningsen S, Apalset K, Terjesen T, and Anda S. Regression of femoral anteversion. A prospective study of intoeing children. *Acta Orthopædica Scandinavica.* 1989;60(2):170-173.

111. Tang WM, Zhu YH, and Chiu KY. Axial alignment of the lower extremity in Chinese adults. *Journal of Bone and Joint Surgery American.* 2000;82-A(11):1603-1608.

112. Tiberio D. The effect of excessive subtalar joint pronation on patellofemoral mechanics: a theoretical model. *The Journal of Orthopedic and Sports Physical Therapy.* 1987;9(4):160-165.

113. Trimble MH, Bishop MD, Buckley BD, Fields LC, and Rozea GD. The relationship between clinical measurements of lower extremity posture and tibial translation. *Clinical Biomechanics.* 2002;17:286-290.

114. Uhorchak JM, Scoville CR, Williams GN, Arciero RA, StPierre P, and Taylor DC. Risk factors associated with non-contact injury of the anterior cruciate ligament. *American Journal of Sports Medicine.* 2003;31(6):831-842.

115. Van Lunen BL, Roberts J, Branch D, and Dowling EA. Association of menstrual cycle hormone changes with anterior cruciate ligament laxity measurements. *Journal of Athletic Training.* 2003;38(4):298-303.

116. Vankka E, and Salenius P. Spontaneous correction of severe tibiofemoral deformity in growing children. *Acta Orthopaedica Scandinavica.* 1982;3(4):567-570.

117. Wilkerson RD, and MA Mason. Differences in Men's and Women's mean ankle ligamentous laxity. *Iowa Orthopaedic Journal.* 2000;20: 46-48.

118. Wilmore JH, and Costill DL. *Physiology of Sport and Exercise.* Champaign, IL: Human Kinetics; 1999.

119. Winter EM, and Brookes FBC. Electromechanical response times and muscle elasticity in men and women. *European Journal of Applied Physiology.* 1991;63:124-128.

120. Woodland LH, and Francis RS. Parameters and comparisons of the quadriceps angle of college-aged men and women in the supine and standing positions. *American Journal of Sports Medicine.* 1992;20(2): 208-211.

121. Wu XP, Yang Y, Zhang H, et al. Gender differences in bone density at different skeletal sites of acquisition with age in Chinese children and adolescents. *Journal of Bone and Mineral Metabolism.* 2005;23: 253-260.

122. Zhou S, Lawson DL, Morrison WE, and Fairweather I. Electrome-chanical delay of knee extensors: the normal range and the effects of age and gender. *Journal of Human Movement Studies.* 1995;28:127-146.

CHAPTER 3

Performance Eating for the Female Athlete

Dawn Weahterwax-Fall, RD, CSSD, LC, ATC, CSCS

Introduction

Sports nutrition has important benefits for all active people, but it plays an even more important role when it comes to active women. Women, of course, have different builds than men. However, they have physiological differences that go beyond this. As a rule, they carry more fat and less muscle than men do. This extra fat both protects the sex organs and plays a role in nurturing the fetus during pregnancy. Being equipped for childbearing plays a huge rule in how a woman's body functions throughout her life and in her nutritional needs. When a woman is active, it's vital that her nutrition is adequate in both arenas.

The Unique Nutritional Needs of the Female Athlete

Just like men, active women usually need to increase their energy intake to fuel optimal performance. However, they often resist doing so because of concerns over their appearance and their size, concerns that are often a result of the sports they compete in or the social pressures that surround them.

In general, women tend to excel at sports that are high on the aesthetic scale[8]—activities like gymnastics, ballet, and other forms of dance, figure skating, diving, rowing, and running. These sports put a high premium on appearance. Some are actually referred to as "weight-dependent" sports, because what a woman weighs can make a huge difference in her performance. To be competitive, in these sports, women often restrict their calories to the point where they don't eat enough to keep themselves healthy, much less provide themselves enough fuel for good performance.

The demands of competing at the top levels in these sports put female athletes at risk for developing eating disorders, such as anorexia nervosa, anorexia athletica (exercising to excess to keep body weight down), and bulimia nervosa. However, it's not just elite athletes who are at risk for these disorders. Sadly, the number of women (active or not) who suffer from eating disorders is steadily increasing. Despite the amount of available information considering nutrition's role in preventing disease and maintaining good health, more women than ever before are putting their health in danger by eating inadequate diets. And, these problems aren't related to women who are starving themselves to stay thin. Normal-sized and overweight women suffer from nutritional deficiencies as well. This is often caused by conflicting advice as to what they should be eating. Consequently the diet of the week often turns into the eating disorder of the year.

Missing Minerals

All women the risk of lower-than-optimal levels of two important micro-nutrients: calcium and iron. Women between 19-50 years old need at least

1,000 mg of calcium[7] and 15 mg of iron daily just to meet their minimum requirements of these important minerals. However, many women don't come close to these levels. The lack of calcium, of course, can lead to osteoporosis.

More About Calcium

All minerals are important for good health, but calcium deserves some special attention. As the most abundant mineral in the body, it combines with phosphorus to build bones and teeth. The calcium in the blood enables muscles to contract to allow movement and workout weights. It also aids in preventing blood clotting, transmitting nerve impulses, and moving fluids in and out of cells. Calcium is needed throughout our lives to keep the bones strong, but most adults don't get nearly enough of this important mineral on a daily basis. Part of the problem is that we don't eat enough foods that are high in calcium. There are also a number of factors that can keep our bodies from absorbing the calcium we do eat including the following:

- eating too much protein
- repetitive alcohol use
- high sugary foods
- oxalic acids
- eating too much sodium
- phosphorus (soft drinks and meat)
- caffeine
- aluminum hydroxide (found in some antacids)
- cigarette smoking
- non weight-bearing exercises

Vitamin D increases calcium absorption, which is why milk is fortified with this vitamin.[10] The protein in the milk also stirs up the acid in the stomach and creates a higher amount of calcium absorption.

Dark green leafy vegetables also contain calcium, but a lot of these foods need to be eaten to get enough calcium to meet the daily requirement. Other ways to boost calcium intake are:

- adding powdered milk to baked goods or to milk "double strength milk"
- using yogurt as a base for salad dressings and dips
- eating a diet rich in dark leafy greens, broccoli, berries, soybeans, beans, flaxseeds and whole grains
- eating sardines and other fish with edible bones
- eating nuts and seeds that are rich in calcium, such as almonds, brazil nuts, macadamias, pecans, pistachios, sesame seeds, and sunflower seeds

- drinking orange and vegetable juices that are calcium-enriched
- tofu made with calcium sulphate

Calcium supplementation is often necessary, especially for women, to meet the minimum recommended daily intake (RDA) for this important micronutrient or if they have been diagnosed with bone loss. However, it is very important to recommend the right calcium supplement because not all of these supplements provide the right ingredients to maximize bone growth. Women should take a calcium supplement that has:

- calcium in carbonate and/or citrate form (must be in elemental form)
- 2mg of calcium to 1mg of magnesium
- 2mg of calcium to at least 1 International Unit (IU) of Vitamin D3 in cholecalciferol form
- boron, Silcon, and Vitamin K included and to decrease urination of calcium and magnesium and to strengthen connective tissue matrix and synthesis of osteocalcin
- been taken with food
- been taken throughout the day
- been taken in 200-500mg calcium increments
- 1200-1500mg/calcium a day (if showing bone loss, bone fracture)

Note that women should continue to supplement with calcium post fracture if bone loss is evident and that Viactive chews and Tums do not fit these guidelines.

More About Iron

Iron is the other important nutrient that many women are deficient in. According to the National Institutes of Health, approximately 20% of all women are believed to be iron deficient or anemic. These rates are higher in adolescent females, pregnant women, and female athletes. Studies show that 1/3-1/2 of athletic women have low iron stores.

Not having enough iron in the body is a problem when it comes to athletic performance. When iron levels are low, the blood's ability to carry oxygen to the cells falls along with it. As oxygen levels diminish, the muscles literally begin to suffocate. In technical terms, they lose their aerobic capacity. In other words, they can't function like they should.

As previously discussed, iron comes in two forms: plant-based and animal-based. Because many female athletes don't eat enough calories to start with, they don't get enough dietary iron from either source. But there's an even greater problem when it comes to iron, because the body doesn't absorb both forms equally.

The most easily absorbed form of iron is heme iron, which is found in animal protein and particularly in red meat. Nonheme iron comes with some baggage—fiber—that makes it harder to absorb. Because of this, it is necessary to eat more foods that contain nonheme iron to get the same amount of iron obtained by eating meat. It is possible to boost absorption of nonheme iron by eating a little meat along with veggies and grains.

The problem is, many female athletes don't eat meat. Even if they do, they often don't eat enough of it to supply the amount of iron they need. When iron levels get low, both health and athletic performance can be compromised. Athletes who are low in iron can suffer from the following problems:

- shortness of breath
- headache
- decreased appetite
- loss of endurance
- chronic fatigue

The cure is to increase the consumption of foods that contain iron and if necessary, to take supplemental iron. Unfortunately, most women who are iron deficient aren't aware of the problem, so they don't do anything about it. Also, some physicians are not aware that hemoglobin needs for female athletes can be as high as 16-18 grams per deciliter (g/dl) (Non Female athletes 12-16 g/dl), which can result in serious problems for the atehlete. Table 3-1 outlines various sources of iron.

An athlete must also check their ferritin levels. Ferritin is a marker of total body iron stores and might be low even when the hemoglobin is normal. A normal ferritin level is between 20-160 ug/dl and varies from lab to lab. An athlete should aim for 20-30 ug/dl ferritin. Higher levels have not been proven to excel performance.

If an athlete cannot reach their iron levels through food they should consider supplementing with ferrous sulfate. It is the most common and the most well absorbed iron supplement and is recommended 1-3 times a day. If the athlete is experiencing stomach discomfort and nausea she should first take the supplement with food. If this does not reduce the side effects, she should switch to ferrous gluconate. This ferrous gluconate is not as well absorbed as ferrous sulphate, but is often tolerated better.

The athelete should not take calcium or fiber supplements at the same time because, they interfere with the iron's absorption. Iron also absorbs better in an acidic environment which is why it is recommended that the athlete take iron with foods high in vitamin C. Never take iron supplements until the proper labs have been completed to validate its usage and when to stop taking them. Iron can be very toxic so an athlete should not exceed the recommended iron levels.

TABLE 3-1 • **Sources of Iron**

BEST SOURCES OF IRON	GOOD SOURCES OF IRON	FAIR SOURCES OF IRON
Liver, any kind	Lean beef	Turkey
Pork loin	Shrimp	Chicken
Oysters	Tuna	Salmon
Clams	Raisins	Haddock
Sardines	Prunes	Cod
Molasses	Dried apricots	Tofu
Raisin bran	Figs	Sesame seeds
	Kidney beans	Nuts
	Pinto beans	Peanut butter
	Navy beans	Eggs
	Lentils	Strawberry
	Split green peas	Banana
	Enriched cereals	Raspberries
	Enriched macaroni	Blueberries
	Spinach	Tomatoes
	Greens	
	Broccoli	
	Lima beans	
	Avocado	

Basic Nutrition for Active Women

Many female athletes do not take in enough calories to support their nutritional needs, even when they play sports that enable them to maintain a healthy weight.

Sedentary women can generally eat around 1,600 kilocalories (kcalories) to 2000 kcalories a day to maintain their weight. Active women, those women who work out on a regular basis and in general lead an active lifestyle usually need at least another 600 calories to keep them feeling right. Extremely active women and competitive athletes can eat as much as 3,000 kcalories a day or more, depending on their size and activity level.[3]

Some women who lead active lifestyles may eat enough calories, but they don't eat food that provides optimum nutrition. Therefore, all active women should take good multivitamin/multimineral nutritional supplementation. It doesn't make up for eating right, but it does add a layer of insurance against nutritional deficiencies.

The following guidelines will also help increase nutrient levels up and improve performance of the female athelete:

- Eat 45%-60% percent of calories from complex carbohydrates (vegetables, grains, fruit, dairy)
- High-quality protein should comprise 15%-30% percent of calories. If building muscle, the athlete will need to eat at the higher end of this range. Women in their 30s and beyond should consider getting some of their protein in the form of soy products, as they can help cushion the hormonal changes associated with perimenopause
- Eat 20%-30% of total calories from fat. 7%-10% or less should come from saturated fat
- Calcium intake should be between 1000 mg and 1300 mg a day. If experiencing menstrual irregularities, boost intake to 1500 mg a day. If the athlete does not consume dairy products, take supplements to reach these levels. Please follow the guidelines in this chapter for selecting or recommending a proper calcium supplement
- Iron intake should be 15 mg-18mg a day. The best sources are animal protein
- If iron deficiency is a concern, supplementation may be necessary but first have blood drawn to check hemoglobin (16-18g/dl) and ferritin levels (20-30 ug/dl). Ferrous sulfate is the best absorbed iron supplement. If athlete has nausea and GI distress switch to ferrous gluconate. Vitamin C also boosts iron absorption
- Drink 8-10 glasses of water a day or 30 ml per kg body weight
- Minimize intake of foods that are high in saturated/trans fat, sodium, and sugar
- Take a high quality multivitamin/mineral supplement that does not exceed upper limits
- Consider taking 1-2 teaspoons or 2-8 capsules of a high quality Omega-3 supplement if not getting this nutrient through food

Nutrition for the Pregnant Athlete

Pregnancy used to mean hanging up the athletic shoes for nine months, plus some time afterward to take care of the new little one. Times have definitely changed for the better. Not only do many women continue to stay active and compete for at least part of their pregnancies, the general wisdom today is that it's good to exercise as long as mother and child are in good health.

Pregnant athletes are the food supply for the baby. If the athlete doesn't eat right the baby won't get the nutrients it needs to thrive. It takes about 80,000 calories throughout the pregnancy for baby development. This means an athlete will consume on average 2200-2400 kcals a day. [6]

According to the March of Dimes, pregnant women should increase their daily food portions to include the following:

- 6-11 servings of bread and other whole grains
- 3-5 servings of vegetables
- 2-4 servings of fruit
- 4-6 servings of milk and milk products
- 3-5 servings of meat and protein foods

If the athlete is maintaining anything close to their usual activity level, they should eat on the high side of these recommendations. Appropriate weight gain during pregnancy is associated with increased infant birth weight. A woman's average weight gain during pregnancy is 24-28 pounds.

Protein needs increase to 60 grams of protein per day during pregnancy. Exercise may also increase the protein requirement. The intake of increased calories during this time should meet these requirements.

In addition, athletes drink at least 6-8 glasses of water a day. Studies have shown that dehydration increases the risk of premature contractions and early delivery.

It was once thought that if a woman did not eat well during pregnancy, her fetus would draw on her reserves to meet its needs. This is true with calcium, but research has shown that babies born to mothers who didn't follow good nutritional practices are more likely to be premature, small, and unhealthy.

Some pregnant women with low carbohydrate intake find it difficult to stay active. Not only does their body burn carbohydrates faster when they are pregnant, exercise also burns carbs. Combine the two and woman are under the risk of having low blood sugar levels when they work out and of developing harmful ketones which can cause fetal ketosis. Taking in enough carbs will prevent this problem.

As previously mentioned, anemia is another problem for many pregnant women. Since it hampers the blood's ability to carry oxygen, it also can have a big impact on their ability to exercise and how you feel when you do. While pregnant an athlete will need double amount of iron a day (30 mg a day) because the extra amount of iron is used for the fetus and delivery. Iron needs may also need to be increased even more so for endurance athletes. A measurement of serum ferritin is needed to see if this increase is required. It is important to eat an iron rich diet, take extra vitamin C with meals to increase iron absorption, and take iron supplements if your doctor prescribes them.

Calcium demands increase during pregnancy because the mineral is needed for hardening of the bones and teeth of the fetus and preparing for lactation. The average calcium intake is 1200 mg a day during pregnancy. If the athlete does not intake enough calcium the baby will take the calcium from the mother which could lead to osteoporosis to the athlete in future years. Also low calcium levels can lead to eclampsia. This is a rare but serious complication that involves fluid retention, loss of protein in the urine, high blood pressure and can lead to convulsions and coma.

Magnesium is important for tissue growth and proper muscle functioning. It is also important that there is a balance between magnesium and calcium. If these two are out of balance it could lead to irregular muscle contractions, spasms and heart palpitations. The level of magnesium needed during pregnancy is between 300 mg-600mg a day.

Folic acid and vitamin B12 are two very important vitamins before and during pregnancy. Folate needs vitamin B12 to be present in order for folate to function properly. These nutrients create red blood cells and the growth of the fetus and maternal tissues and are very important for the synthesis of RNA and DNA. Deficiency can impair fetal development, lead to malformations such as spina bifida and anencephaly (brain does not fully develop) and anemias. In addition to supplementation, the athlete should focus on eating raw green leafy vegetables, lima beans, cauliflower, liver, meats, fish, eggs, dairy products, and nuts.

A woman's vitamin B6 needs slightly increase during pregnancy because of the vitamin's role in making red blood cells and genetic material. Vitamin B6 is in whole grains and meats. A slight increase is also needed from vitamins D, E, C, thiamin, riboflavin, and niacin. Be careful of too much vitamins A and K. Too much vitamin A has been linked to birth defects.

The nerves, eyes, and the brain consist mostly of lipids, or fatty acids. Because of the development of the fetus's nervous system, it is important that the athlete take adequate amounts before getting pregnant. Fatty acids continue to be important because the brain develops throughout pregnancy and after birth.

The Least You Need to Know

A woman should consult a physician first before applying the following nutrition suggestions:

- Consume at least 2200 kcalories-2400 kcalories a day not including activity
- Consume at least 64 fl. oz. of water a day not including activity
- Consume/supplement with 30 mg/Fe a day
- Consume/supplement with 1200 mg/Ca a day
- Consume/supplement with 800 micrograms/folate a day
- Consume/supplement with 4 micrograms/B12 a day
- Consume/supplement with 2.2 mg/B6 a day

- Consume/supplement with 300-600 mg/Mg a day
- Take a high quality multivitamin/mineral supplement
- Consume/supplement with 4000 mg/fish oil (make sure contains EPA and DHA) a day (2 teaspoons or 2-4 capsules). Please make sure they guarantee no contaminates

Nutrition for the Young Athlete

Anyone with children, already knows that their nutritional needs are different from an adult. Making sure an active child's nutritional needs are met will not only support their growth, it will also help them perform better in sports. Like the pregnant athlete, children of both sexes have unique demands when it comes to nutrition.

Children vs. Food

Children are notoriously quirky and fussy about food, which can make it a real challenge for parents to ensure that their offspring eat the things they need to keep them healthy and support their growth. Young children have sensitive taste buds and are often not very adventuresome about eating. Others have aversions to specific foods, such as vegetables.

Some children have such limited palates that their food choices are narrowed down to a few favorites. The result is a diet that is almost guaranteed to be lacking important nutrients.

Poor eating habits often get worse as children get older. As they approach puberty, many young people begin skipping meals. Boys and girls are both guilty of this, although girls tend to be the worst offenders, as concerns over appearance and body size begin to surface. Unfortunately, this bad habit often kicks in at about the same time that children's nutritional needs are at their highest. Puberty is a time of rapid growth, and optimal nutrition is also needed to support the hormonal changes that mark the beginning of adolescence. When kids are active, and especially if they play sports, it is even more important to make sure that they eat right and that they know how to make good food choices on their own if the parent is not there to supervise them.

Starting Right, Right Away

The best time to start good nutritional practices for children is when they are very young. To ensure the best success, it's a good idea for the parents to have their own eating and exercise habits in proper order. Parents are usually the earliest and best role models that children have when it comes to understanding what a healthy lifestyle is all about. Parents who eat the right foods and exercise on a regular basis, send a positive message to their children. Supporting an active lifestyle for the children, even if it is just tossing a football in the backyard or driving them to and from practices and events, is another great way to drive home the message that staying fit is important.

Starting children off with good nutrition and good exercise narrows the chances of them developing bad habits that are tougher to break as they get older. As children mature, the parent will have less control over their schedules and less oversight regarding what they put in their bodies. However, it is not impossible and it is never too late to start.

Having young athletes in the house also necessitates teaching them how their eating choices can affect their performance and endurance. If the parent starts this education when the child is young, there is less of a chance of the child developing harmful eating habits later on. Children who participate in sports like gymnastics, ballet and other forms of dance, wrestling, running, and figure skating are especially vulnerable to the lure of unhealthy eating, as they often feel pressure, real or imaginary to be painfully thin in order to be competitive.

Beginning with the Basics

A basic diet for young athletes is based on the same sound nutritional principles that of any good diet and should:

- provide sufficient calories
- be high in complex carbohydrates and especially nutrient dense carbs
- provide a variety of different foods in each food group
- have a moderate amount (30% less) of fat (10% or less) of saturated fat, and cholesterol
- contain moderate amounts of protein, sodium, salt, and sugars

Children, like adults, need to eat throughout the day to keep their energy levels up. From the time that they are able to understand the concept of meal times, they should be coached on the importance of eating regular meals.

To ensure the best chance of getting all the nutrients young bodies need for optimum health, growth, and performance, children should also be taught about the five essential food groups and encouraged to eat foods from all of them every day.

The United States Department of Agriculture food pyramid might not be the best model for adult athletes when it comes to optimal nutrition, but it works pretty well for younger athletes. Not only that, it is colorful, and lots of food companies include it on their labeling and packaging, which makes it an ideal tool for some great on the spot lessons.

Nutritional Needs of Sporting Children

As previously mentioned, active children and those who participate in sports have nutritional needs that go beyond those of children who are less active. For starters, they need more calories. In fact, they might need as much, or more than their parents do. How much more they need largely depends on their age and how active they are. Table 3-2 is based on the USDA food pyramid and is a good starting point for determining calorie levels and servings for children ages 6-12, teenage boys and teenage girls.

As always, food choices from the meat group should emphasize healthy, lean cuts of meat. Milk group choices should be low in fat. There are no recommended servings from the fat, oils, and sweets group at the top of the list. As a reminder, these foods add little nutritional value to the diet. As such, they should be eaten sparingly and not as a substitute for any of the foods that are lower on the nutritional pyramid.

Pumping up Calorie Counts

Depending on the frequency, intensity, and duration of exercise, young athletes can need as much as an extra 500 calories-1,000 calories a day to meet their energy requirements. Some parents will boost calorie counts simply by serving larger portions at meals. This is not a good idea, because it can lead to problems with portion control as children get older. A better approach is to encourage children to eat snacks between meals; snacks should contain high quality, nutrient dense carbohydrates from the bread, fruit, milk, and vegetable groups. Possible choices include the following:

- veggies with hummus
- pita chips and hummus
- natural peanut butter and jelly sandwich
- Baby Bel Lite Cheese and low fat crackers

TABLE 3-2 · **Recommended Calories and Servings for Youth Athletes**

	TEENAGE GIRLS	TEENAGE BOYS
Calorie Level	About 2,200	About 2,800
Servings		
Bread Group	9	11
Vegetable Group	4	5
Fruit Group	3	4
Milk Group	2-3	2-3
Meat Group	2	3
	(for a total of 6 ounces)	(for a total of 7 ounces)

- trail mixes (Choose products that are low in fat and sodium and don't have added sugar or candy)
- cottage cheese and fruit
- yogurt with fruit
- smoothies
- fruit leather
- cereals that have 5 g of fiber per serving and 7 g-9 g of protein per serving

Make it convenient for children to get the extra calories they need by stocking healthy snack choices in their pantry. Take along snacks in their backpacks for after school practice sessions or away games. Give them boxes of power bars to store in their locker at school. The easier a parent makes it for them to make healthy choices, the less likely they will be to grab for high fat, high sugar foods from school vending machines or fast food restaurants when hunger overtakes them.

If the child is a finicky eater, it might be tough to get them to choose healthy food to augment their calorie intake. While high quality carbs are always going to deliver the best nutritional bang per calorie, it is okay to let young athletes have some simple carbohydrates to boost their nutrient intake once in a while. An occasional soft drink or candy bar will not only help supply part of their calorie needs, but it will keep kids from feeling deprived, especially when their friends are enjoying these treats.

To tell if the child is eating enough calories, track his or her height and weight. If he or she is gaining weight, but not height, it might be time to cut back on the serving sizes of snacks, or substitute some lower-calorie alternatives. Don't eliminate them completely, and never cut back on the food choices at main meals. It is important to get children into the habit of eating enough food for these meals as doing so will help them eat right as adults.

The child's athletic performance is another way to gauge adequate nutrient intake. If he or she is doing well while competing or working out, then it is a good indication that he or she is eating right. However, if he or she is feeling fatigued, draggy, or irritable, then he or she probably needs more to eat and drink.

Young female athletes, especially those who are highly competitive in physically challenging sports, also run the risk of developing serious long term health problems if they don't take in enough food to meet their energy needs. It is important to keep an eye on what children eat regardless of the reason, but especially so when it comes to children in this at risk population. A parent's good counsel might cause some temper tantrums, especially if their daughter is feeling pressured into maintaining a low body weight in order to compete at top form. Remember, though, that any fights that may erupt are well worth the long term benefits of such intervention.

More about Young Athletes and Carbohydrates

Young athletes need carbohydrates to fuel their performance just like adults do. They need to eat enough carbs on a regular basis and especially after exercise to keep their glycogen levels where they should be for optimal performance.

Like adults, many young athletes tend to take in more fat than they really need, which means their carbohydrate levels are lower than they should be. Active children should eat 50%-55% of their total calories as carbohydrates, or about 2.7 g of carbohydrates per pound of body weight. As an example, if the young athlete weighs 120 pounds, he or she would need to eat around 324 g of carbohydrates per day.

To meet their carbohydrate needs, encourage children to eat complex carbohydrates—vegetables, whole grain breads, pasta, cereals, brown rice, and so on, instead of the simple carbohydrates contained in candy, soda and sugary items. Choosing complex carbohydrates will also give them better supplies of some essential nutrients, such as B vitamins, iron, dietary fiber and other important vitamins and minerals.

Young Athletes and Protein

All young athletes need protein in order to grow well and build strong muscles. If they eat balanced meals, most children get enough protein in their diets. However, adequate protein intake can be a problem for athletic children. Active children need between 0.5 g-1 g of protein daily per pound of body weight, depending on activity level. This equates to 50 g-100 g of protein for a child who weighs 100 pounds. Hitting the mark for dairy intake can provide most of the protein that young athletes need. Small servings of protein at lunch and dinner should get levels to where they need to be.

Children who don't drink much milk are at a greater risk for protein deficiency. If a parent has a young one at home who doesn't care for cow's milk, try them on other dairy products like yogurt and low-fat cheeses. Another way to boost dairy intake is to add powdered milk to baked goods and smoothies. Doing so will increase both protein and calcium intake. Although it is not a good idea to give children too much fruit juice, some juices are now fortified with calcium.

Young Athletes and Fat

All of the warnings about fat that have surfaced in recent years are directed mostly at adults, but we tend to forget that moderate fat intake for children is just as important. As a result, adults sometimes allow their children to eat too much fat, especially saturated and trans fats. Children generally need to get about 30% of their calories from fat (10% or less from saturated fat) for optimum nutrition.

The Right Stuff at the Right Times

When young athletes eat it is just as important as what they eat. As is the case with adult athletes, timing is everything when it comes to fueling performance.

Pregame Nutrition Strategies

Eating a healthy meal before a game or practice is important for maintaining energy levels both during the activity and after it. Making sure children eat right before a game is fairly easy if a parent is able to sit them down for a pregame meal at home, but this often isn't possible. When young athletes travel to an away event it is hard for a parent to make sure they get what they need before competition.

One of the best ways to ensure proper nutrition when you can't be there to provide it is to map out a pregame eating strategy with your children. Go through their training and competition schedules and determine what they should be eating and drinking as well as when. To make sure they get what they need, load a backpack or athletic bag with take along foods such as snack bars, bagels, fruit, fruit or vegetable juice, or sandwiches.

The biggest thing to remember is that less is more when you get closer to the event. Also, pre-event food choices must emphasize carbohydrates and be lower in fat and protein. Peanut butter is a bad choice right before a game as it's hard to digest. The best way to find out what works for your young athletes is through experimentation. Make sure to limit your experiments to practices, though. The day of the big game is not the time to be trying new foods that may not be tolerated well.

Postgame Eating

Postgame eating is important as well to replenish the glycogen levels in the muscles and liver. Try to get your children to eat a carbohydrate snack within 30 minutes after their activity. This snack should contain between 15 g-30 g of carbs and 3 g-5 g of protein, the amount found in the following snacks:

- a glass of milk and 1 cup carrots
- a smoothie made with a dairy source or added protein powder
- ½ whole grain bagel and 1 T peanut butter
- a yogurt and fruit

Follow this up with a well-balanced meal within two hours of the practice or event.

Water Woes

Active children also have special fluid needs that have to be met. Like adults, they need to drink before, during, and after practice sessions or competition and they need to do so whether they feel thirsty or not. Parents should emphasize the importance of staying hydrated and in terms of health and performance.

Children, like adults, tend to go by their feelings of thirst to determine when they should drink water. However, by the time the "I am thirsty" signal kicks in, their bodies are already dehydrated.

Dehydration might be the culprit if your young athlete gets tired easily at practice or fades during competition. Other indications of low hydration levels in children include:

- crankiness or irritability
- dark colored urine that has a strong odor
- sunken eyes
- dry tongue and lips
- infrequent urination
- reduced urine volume

Dehydration is dangerous for children and adults alike, but it can be especially dangerous for young athletes. Kids do not cool off as efficiently as adults do. They over heat and can become dehydrated more easily. This can cause a significant decrease in performance. Teenagers need just as much water as adults do, at least eight, 8-ounce glasses of water a day. Younger athletes should drink between five-eight 8-ounce glasses a day. Before strenuous activity, children should drink 4-8 ounces of fluids. During activity, fluid intake should be at least 4 ounces of fluids for every 15 minutes. Teenagers need to up their intake to 6 ounces-8 ounces every 15-20 minutes.

If there are times when your child isn't thrilled about drinking water, sports drinks are a good substitute. Sports drinks also stimulate thirst, which means your children will end up drinking more fluids.

Sports drinks are absorbed just as quickly as water. They are a good source of carbohydrates for working muscles during exercise and especially for workouts or practices that last an hour or more. They are also good for days when more than one workout or exercise period is scheduled.

The best sports drink selections are those that contain between 4%-8% carbohydrates, anything more than this can delay fluid absorption when young athletes need it most. Children are big fans of carbonated drinks. It is okay to occasionally let them have a soft drink; just remind them that moderation is important when it comes to carbonated or sugary beverages, because those kinds of drinks can interfere with training and competition schedules. These drinks are absorbed slowly and they contain high fructose corn syrup, which can cause stomach cramps, nausea, and diarrhea. Therefore, water as always is the best beverage choice for young athletes and adults.

The Least You Need to Know

- Young athletes need more calories than their more sedentary counterparts. When adding calories to the diet, it is best to give children nutrient dense between meal snacks instead of increasing main meal portion sizes.
- 50%-55% total calories come from carbohydrates (fruit, vegetables, dairy, grains) or about 2.7 g of carbohydrates per pound of body weight

- 15%-25% total calories come from protein or 0.5 g-1 g of protein per pound of body weight
- 20%-30% total calories from fat (only 10% or less from saturated and trans fats)
- A young athlete should eat regularly (every 2-4 hours)
- It is okay to let your children have an occasional sweet treat or soft drink. However, they should only be eaten in addition to, not in place of, more nutritious foods from other food groups. Recommend only seven "Freebies" a week
- Recommend a high quality, age specific daily multivitamin/multimineral supplement
- A young athlete should hydrate with 4 oz-8 oz glasses of water a day
- A young athlete should eat 3 g-5 g of protein and 15 g-30 g of carbohydrates after activities that last longer than 90 minutes

The Female Athlete Triad

An inadequate diet—one that lacks important nutrients and calories—is an early indicator of the "female athlete triad"—a syndrome of disordered eating, amenorrhea (the absence of menstruation that lasts for longer than six months, or a decrease in the frequency of menstrual periods), and osteoporosis that is occurring with increased frequency among physically active girls and women.

Recognizing the Syndrome

The female athlete triad typically begins when females control body weight by adopting one or more of the following behaviors:

- eating erratically—skipping meals and/or avoiding certain foods
- reducing food intake
- not eating as many calories as they are expending
- making poor food choices
- using appetite suppressants and diet pills
- using laxatives, diuretics, or enemas
- vomiting after meals
- high-intensity exercise beyond what is called for by their particular sport or activity

As previously mentioned, the decrease in calories often leads to nutritional deficiencies and especially deficiencies in calcium and iron. Performance levels often decline because these women simply don't get enough energy and nutrients. Their health declines as well, with gastrointestinal problems and hypothermia, or lower-than-normal body temperatures, being common. As this pattern of poor eating and excessive exercise continues, estrogen levels decline, causing menstrual periods to either become less frequent or stop completely. Lower estrogen levels can also reduce calcium levels in the bones, as the body needs normal levels of this hormone for optimal calcium absorption. As calcium levels drop, bones lose thickness and strength, resulting in low bone mass and osteoporosis.[1]

Although these habits are a concern for all women, they're a particular problem for young female athletes. Lower-than-normal estrogen and calcium levels disrupt the growing process of the bones, which means that they might never develop as they should. Bringing estrogen and calcium levels back up can halt bone loss and eventually rebuild it, although some experts believe that bone strength and density will always be somewhat less than what they should be in these women.

Women who are most likely to be at risk for developing the female athlete triad syndrome include these groups:

- High school and intercollegiate athletes who are highly competitive in endurance sports, such as distance running, race-walking, bicycling, rowing, etc.

- Girls and women who participate in activities that emphasize appearance and leanness, such as gymnastics, ballet, figure skating, diving, rowing, horseback riding, cycling, and track and field; or sports like rowing which involve weight classifications.

- Noncompetitive but still physically active girls and women who diet and exercise to excess.

If allowed to continue, the female athletic triad behaviors can have serious consequences. Not being able to compete at optimal levels are the least of the problems that these women face. They also run the risk of having difficulties bearing children and of suffering crippling bone fractures.

While awareness of the female athlete triad has increased substantially since the syndrome was identified, it remains a problem as the symptoms can be difficult to detect. Most of the girls and women who are at the highest risk for developing these problems look perfectly healthy, in fact, they are often the envy of their friends because they look so fit and lean. An x-ray of their spine, however, would tell another story. The spinal bone density of a young athlete who has stopped or never started having menstrual periods can resemble that of a 70-year-old woman.

According to researchers, the incidence of eating disorders in female athletes ranges from 16%-72%, compared to 5%-10% in the general population. Menstrual irregularities are also more prevalent among women who participate in varsity athletics, with 28% of them experiencing no or few periods.[2]

Preventing the Syndrome

Unfortunately, as long as there are sports that place a high premium on appearance and weight, there will be women running the risk of damaging their health when they compete in them. For the women who do enjoy these activities, it is essential to develop good nutritional habits and proper education early on to avoid long-term health problems. The food they eat needs to be as nutrient-packed as possible. If eating continues to be a problem, it's a good idea to consult with a sports nutritionist who can assess current food habits and needs, and develop an eating program based on them.

The following sidebar provides the appropriate guidelines physicians, athletic trainers, and dietitians should follow when treating female athletes with certain conditions.

Recommended Protocols When Treating Female Athletes

Recommended Protocol for an Athlete with a Stress Fracture/Female Athletic Triad

Physician:

1. Order a bone scan to eliminate any chance of bone loss

2. Ask, if the female athlete has an irregular menstrual cycle or if it has been absent

3. Recommend a high quality calcium supplement (follow the guidelines discussed earlier in the chapter)

4. Refer to a dietitian to rule out a possible eating disorder, female athletic triad, too low in body fat and/or a deficiency in calories, calcium, magnesium, and vitamin D3

5. May consider birth control pills.[9] Advise waiting to do this until athlete has worked with dietitian over a 2-3 month time to naturally get menstrual cycle back if not due to hormonal or ovary issues.

Athletic Trainer:

1. For prevention purposes, each year ask female athlete if she has a normal menstrual cycle. Advise athlete to let you know this is ever disrupted. Any absence should be taken seriously and referred to a dietitian to address any dietary issues and refer to a OBGYN to rule out any hormonal issues. An Orthopedic or Sports Medicine doctor may order a bone scan for prevention. Consider recommending a calcium supplement.

2. Follow protocol set by your school/organization

3. May need to set up a contract with athlete and health professionals involved if suspect athlete will not follow through and jeopardize their health

Dietitian:

1. Perform a body composition analysis on the three dietitian sections using a Bod Pod, Hydrostatic weighing, or Lange Skinfolds

2. Measure Resting Metabolic Rate (RMR) using a MedGem or Metabolic Cart and calculate what burning everyday with activity. Note any deficits.

3. Have the athlete complete a 24-hour recall or a 7-day food log

4. Analyze the 24-hour recall or 7-day food log and look for deficiencies in calories, calcium, magnesium, and vitamin D3

5. Look for signs of disordered eating, dangerous weight control behaviors, the female athletic triad and mineral deficiencies. May need to set up a contract with health professionals and staff if needed.

6. Recommend a high quality calcium supplement

7. May need to recommend a high quality multivitamin/mineral supplement

8. Design an optimal menu for the athlete based on the information you collected. Female athletes respond well to this step because it helps them take out the "guess work." Make sure increase calories to meet expenditure. You may need to add the calories in increments over weeks/months if the deficit is too large.

9. Other Facts to consider: Is the athlete getting enough vitamin D3. More research is indicating people are deficient.[4]

Strength Trainer:

1. Add over the head training to put pressure on the spine

2. Add weight bearing exercises

Recommended Protocol for an Athlete with an Eating Disorder

Physician:

1. Order any lab work to detect any abnormalities in electrolytes, blood work, etc.

2. May order a bone scan to check if there is any bone loss

3. Ask if she has an irregular menstrual cycle or if the cycle is absent

4. Refer to a dietitian to rule out a possible eating disorder, female athletic triad, too low in body fat and/or a deficiency in calories or nutrients

5. May need to admit into an eating disorder treatment center or set up a contract with other health professionals

Athletic Trainer:

1. Observe any change in behavior, interaction with athletes and performance

2. Research what other athletes observe

3. Research what the coaching staff observes

4. Follow protocol set by your school/organization

5. Set up a contract with the athlete and have all health professionals involved if athlete has an eating disorder. Athlete must see a psychologist.

Dietitian:

1. Do a body composition analysis using a Bod Pod, Hydrostatic weighing or Lange Skinfolds

2. Measure RMR using a MedGem or Metabolic Cart and calculate what burning everyday with activity. Note any deficits.

3. Have the athlete complete a 24-hour recall or a 7-day food log

4. Analyze the 24-hour recall or 7-day food log and look for deficiencies in calories and nutrients

5. Look for signs of disordered eating, dangerous weight control behaviors, the female athletic triad and mineral deficiencies. May need to set up a contract with health professionals and staff if needed. May need to decrease or cease activity.

6. May need to recommend a high quality calcium supplement

7. May need to recommend a high quality multivitamin/mineral supplement

8. Design an optimal menu for the athlete based on the information you collected. Female athletes respond well to this step because it helps them take out the "guess work." Make sure you increase calories to meet expenditure. You may need to add the calories in increments over weeks/months if the deficit is too large. If the athlete does not follow through, her lack of action is a sign on how bad her eating issue really is.

9. If signs of an eating disorder exist the athlete MUST see a psychologist in conjunction with all other health professionals

10. Work as a team and always communicate. Recommend monthly meetings to discuss all eating disorder cases. Athletes with eating disorders are very good at manipulating health professionals against each other.

Strength Trainer:

1. May need to decrease activity all together

Recommended Protocol for an Athlete with Fatigue/Anemia

Physician:

1. Order labs to rule out anemia (remember female athlete's hemoglobin can be as high as 16-18 g/dl and ferritin 20 ug/dl-30 ug/dl)

2. Ask if there is a family history of anemia

3. Ask if she is a vegetarian

4. Ask if she has a heavy menstrual cycle and how long they last

5. Refer to a dietitian to rule out a possible eating disorder, female athletic triad, too low in body fat and/or a deficiency in calories, calcium, magnesium, and vitamin D3, vitamin B12, and iron.

Athletic Trainer:

1. For prevention purposes ask female athlete if she has any family history of anemia, a heavy menstrual cycle, how long it lasts and if they are vegan? Possibly refer out then or make a note to observe for signs.

2. Refer to physician to run labs on iron status and any other issues for fatigue (example: mononucleosis)

3. Refer to a dietitian to rule out a possible eating disorder, female athletic triad, too low in body fat and/or a deficiency in calories, calcium, magnesium, and vitamin D3, vitamin B12, and iron.

4. Follow protocol set by your school/organization

5. May need to set up a contract with athlete and health professionals involved if fatigue is caused by an eating disorder, female athletic triad or overtraining.

Dietitian:

1. Do a body composition analysis using a Bod Pod, Hydrostatic weighing, or Lange Skinfolds

2. Measure RMR using a Med Gem or Metabolic Cart

3. Have the athlete complete a 24 hour recall or a 7 day food log

4. Analyze the 24 hour recall or 7 day food log and look for deficiencies in calories, calcium, magnesium, Vitamin D3, B12, Iron, and Zinc

5. Look for signs of an eating disorder, female athletic triad, and mineral deficiencies. May need to set up a contract with health professionals and staff if needed.

6. Recommend they have labs done to rule out anemia or review the labs they have had drawn

7. May need to recommend a high quality multivitamin/mineral supplement

8. May need to recommend supplementing with iron[5]

9. May need to design an optimal menu for the athlete based on the information you collected

10. May need to show athlete how to get more iron in her diet through food

Strength Trainer:

1. Keep track of their workouts and note any decrease in performance

2. Look for signs of overtraining, not taking enough days off, or adding more workouts than you prescribe

3. Make adjustments in workouts if needed

Summary

Just as a women's physical characteristics are different than men's nutritional needs are different. As well these needs support the unique characteristics of the women's body and functions of the body. Nutritional needs will vary at life stages as well, the pregnancy athlete will need a different approach to nutritional objectives than the non-pregnant athlete or the child athlete. Understanding the characteristics unique to women at various stages of growth and development will help support a women's overall nutritional status and health, allowing the women improved participation in sports.

References

1. Birch, Karen. Female Athlete Triad. *BMJ*. 2005; 330:244-246.

2. Cobb KL, Bachrach LK, Greendale G et al. Disordered eating, Menstrual irregularities, and bone mineral density in female runners. *Med Sci Sports Exer*. 2003; 35:711-719.

3. Economos CD, Bortz SS, and Nelson ME. Nutritional practices of elite athletes. Practical recommendations. *Sports Med*. December 1993;16(6): 381-99.

4. Karen K Miller. Mechanisms by which nutritional disorders cause reduced bone mass in adults. *Journal of Women's Health*. February 1, 2003; 12(2): 145-150.

5. Manuela Di Santolo, Giuliana Stel, Giuseppe Banfi, Fabio Gonano, and Sabina Cauci. Anemia and iron status in young fertile non-professional female athletes. *Eur J Appl Physiol*. April 2008;102(6): 703-9.2007 Dec 19.

6. Nancy F Butte, William W Wong, Margarita S Treuth, Kenneth J Ellis, and E O'Brian Smith. Energy requirements during pregnancy based on total energy expenditure and energy deposition. *American Journal of Clinical Nutrition*. June 2004; 79(6): 1078-1087.

7. National Institute of Health – Office of Dietary Supplements. Accessed at: http://dietary-supplements.info.nih.gov/.

8. Reinking, Mark F, and Alexander, Laura E. Prevalence of Disordered Eating Behaviors in Undergrad Female Collegiate Athletics & Non-Athletes. *Journal of Athletic Training*. 2005; 40(1): 47-51.

9. Warren MP, and Shantha S. The female athlete. *Baillieres Best Pract Res Clin Endocrinol Metab*. March, 2000; 14(1): 37-53.

10. Weaver CM, and Fleet JC. Vitamin D requirements: current and future. *Am J Clin Nutr*. December 2004; 80(6 Suppl): 1735S-9S.

Understanding the Female Athlete Triad

CHAPTER 4

The Female Athlete Triad

Mike Brunet, PhD, ATC, CPT, STS

Introduction

The term "Female Athlete Triad" was originally coined in 1992 by the American College of Sports Medicine (ACSM) as a focus from a consensus conference called by The Task Force on Women's Issues of the ACSM.[22] In terms of how much people knew about the Triad at that time, the American College of Sports Medicine spokesman stated that there was a limited understanding.[22] At that conference it was also stated that although silently observed for decades by coaches, parents, and athletes, only recently has (the triad) been described in the medical literature.[17] Since that time, an explosion in the research of the Female Athlete Triad has occurred.

The Three Interrelated Pathologies

The Female Athlete Triad (Triad) is a complex condition comprised of three interrelated pathologies: disordered eating, amenorrhea, and osteoporosis (Figure 4-1). Since the three pathologies are interrelated in pathogenesis, etiology, and consequences, it is difficult to recognize which is the most influential. Although the prevalence of the Triad is believed to be high due to the abundance of eating disorders in young women, the documented cases of amenorrhea in female athletes, and the pressures athletes feel regarding being thin or lean in order to conform to an appearance standard characteristic of their sport or to perform better athletically. The Triad affects female athletes at virtually all ages and all levels of competition. An athlete with signs or symptoms of one of the Triad components should be assessed with respect to the other two.

The Triad usually begins with unhealthy or inadequate caloric intake. This may occur inadvertently when the athlete simply does not adequately fuel her body or when the athlete willfully restricts her caloric intake for the purpose of creating a negative energy balance to lose weight. This inadequate intake can disrupt the reproductive cycle and result in amenorrhea.[11,12] The combination of decreased estrogen and inadequate nutrition can lead to low bone mass and osteoporosis.[3,7,23]

The athlete does not have a clinical eating disorder to produce amenorrhea and osteoporosis. Certainly, eating disorders can have a deleterious effect on reproductive and bone health.

Disordered Eating

Though the classic definition of the Triad includes disordered eating which was broad in scope, some authors have incorrectly published eating disorders as a component of the triad instead as it is more defined. Most athletes are not anorexic or bulimic by strict definition, but the majority of them practice unhealthy dietary practices for the purpose of weight loss, which has lead to much research on the Triad.

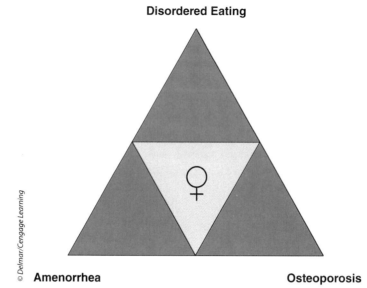

Figure 4-1 The Female Athlete Triad.

Over the decade, the term "Disordered Eating" has been deemed a more appropriate clinical term as it describes potentially pathological behaviors instead of diagnosing someone with an eating disorder. Specifically, the American Psychological Association describes eating disorders as anorexia nervosa (AN), bulimia nervosa (BN), and eating disorders not otherwise specified (EDNOS)[2] whereas disordered eating simply describes "bad" eating habits. Though these bad eating habits can encompass just about anything, when taken to the extreme it does include AN, BN, and the EDNOS eating disorders categories.

In the realm of athletics, the majority of the athletic training rooms across the United States do not have a clinical psychologist on staff to diagnose athletes with eating disorders. This leaves much of the responsibility in the Certified Athletic Trainer's (ATC) hands to pick up on these poor dietary habits. If eating disorders are used instead of disordered eating, the ATC has a difficult challenge in terms of labeling someone with all three components of the Triad. Only a clinical psychologist can diagnose an eating disorder. Although an ATC cannot diagnose someone with this psychological disorder, using the current definition of disordered eating to describe poor dietary habits the ATC can recognize an athlete at risk. Using the correct terminology of disordered eating allows the ATC or health care professional to better identify and deal with at risk athletes.

Ammenorrhea

Ammenorrhea is the loss of menstrual periods. Ammenorrhea may signal a change in the body's hormonal system. Hormonal imbalance can occur from underfeuling the body which can in turn result in decreases in estrogen levels. Diminished estrogen levels in the body can have many effects the most immediate however being bone loss or osteoporosis. Bone loss can occur after just a few months of missed menstrual periods.

Osteoporosis

Changes in the criteria for osteoporosis also impact the ATC's ability to identify at risk athletes.[8] Traditionally, osteoporosis was diagnosed as an individual's bone mineral density consisting of at least 2.5 standard deviations from aged matched individuals using T-scores.[21] Recently the International Society for Clinical Densitometry (ISCD) 22,[9, 10] stated that the World Health Organization's (WHO) osteoporosis criteria should not be used for healthy women 20 years of age to menopause. The WHO's diagnostic criteria included the use of T-scores, where as the ISCD's diagnostic criteria uses Z-scores as well as diagnosing those with osteoporosis if there is low bone mineral density with secondary causes. They also go on to state the diagnosis of osteoporosis in premenopause which should not be made on the basis of densitometry alone. This change affects the inclusion criteria because more individuals are now be included in the osteoporotic category and it is more age and physiologically applicable when compared to the original criteria.

High-Risk Sports

According to the ACSM, there are some sports that are at greater risk for developing one or more components of the triad, especially eating disorders.[1, 14, 23] Such sport disciplines include:

- sports in which performance is subjectively scored (dance, figure skating, gymnastics)

- endurance sports favoring participants with a low body weight (distance running, cycling, and cross country skiing)

- sports in which body contour-revealing clothing is worn for competition (volleyball, swimming, diving, and running)

- sports using weight categories for participation (wrestling, horse racing, martial arts, and rowing)

- sports in which prepubertal body habitus favors success (figure skating, gymnastics, and diving)

Weight class and aesthetic athletes have all reported higher scores (more at risk) on the two questionnaires, the Eating Attitudes Test (EAT)[5] and the Eating Disorder Inventory (EDI)[6] when compared to untrained individuals

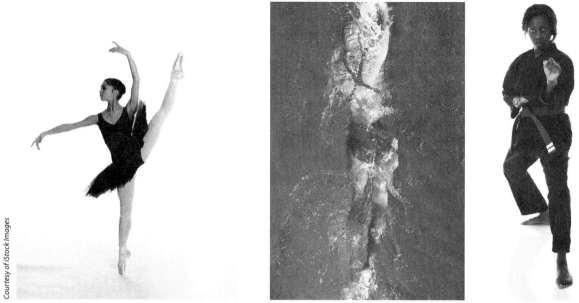

Courtesy of iStock Images

Figure 4-2 Women competing in sports that emphasize specific body types, size, and weight are at risk for developing conditions associated with the Female Athlete Triad.

(Figure 4-2 A-C.).[4,18,20] Though the majority of the literature supports this theory, other authors have different conclusions.[13,19]

Rosen et al.[15] showed that in 182 female collegiate athletes, 32% had been using laxatives, vomiting, or using diuretics/diet pills every day for at least 1 month. Interesting enough, the athletes thought of these practices as being harmless, and that losing weight by any means possible will enhance performance. In another study by Rosen et al.[16] conducted on female gymnasts, they revealed that 62% were using at least 1 method of disordered eating, two times a week for over three or more months. Twenty six percent of the gymnasts reported diet pill use, 24% reported that they regularly fasted while 12% reported using diuretics and 7% used laxatives. Though all of these statistics are staggering, it appears that they have become widely accepted as components of sport.

Summary

With increased participation of women in sports and an emphasis on weight and physical size appropriate to sports participation, the Female Athlete Triad is increasing in prevalence. Certified athletic trainers need to be aware of the elements of the triad as well as the factors that may but an athlete at risk for developing these conditions.

References

1. American College of Sports Medicine (ACSM). Position stand: The Female Athlete Triad. *Medicine & Science in Sports & Exercise.* 1997; 29:i-ix.

2. American Psychological Association. Diagnostic and Statistical Manual of Mental Disorders IV-TR; 2004.

3. Drinkwater BL, Nilson K, Chesnut CH, III, Bremner WJ, Shainholtz S, and Southworth MB. Bone mineral content of amenorrheic and eumenorrheic athletes. *New England Journal of Medicine.* 1984; 311: 277-281.

4. Frusztajer NT, Dhuper S, Warren MP, Brooks-Gunn J, and Fox RP. Nutrition and the incidence of stress fractures in ballet dancers. *American Journal of Clinical Nutrition.* 1990; 51: 779-783.

5. Garner DM, and Garfikel PE. The eating attitudes test: An index of the symptoms of anorexia nervosa. *Psychological Medicine.* 1979; 9: 273-279.

6. Garner DM, Garner MV, and Rosen LR. Anorexia nervosa "restrictors" who purge: implications for sub-typing anorexia nervosa. *International Journal of Eating Disorders.* 1993; 13: 171-185.

7. Ilhe R, and Loucks AB. Dose-response relationships between energy availability and bone turnover in young exercising women. *Journal of Bone Mineral Research.* 2004; 19: 1231-1240.

8. International Society for Clinical Densitometry position statement for the diagnosis of osteoporosis. *Journal of Clinical Densitometry.* 2004; 7:1.

9. Lewiecki EM, Kendler DL, Kiebzak GM, et al. Special report on the official positions of the International Society for Clinical Densitometry. *Osteoporosis International.* 2004; 15(10): 779-84.

10. Lewiecki EM, Watts NB, McClung MR, et al. International Society for Clinical Densitometry. Official positions of the international society for clinical densitometry. *Journal of Clinical Endocrinology & Metabolism.* 2004; 89(8): 3651-3655.

11. Loucks AB, Verdun M, and Heath EM. Low energy availability, not stress of exercise, alters LH pulsatility in exercising women. *Journal of Applied Physiology.* 1998; 84: 37-46.

12. Manore MM. Dietary recommendations and athletic menstrual dysfunction. *Sports Medicine.* 2002; 32: 887-901.

13. Nattiv A, Loucks AB, Manore MM, et al. The American College of Sports Medicine. Position Statement on the Female Athlete Triad. *Medicine & Science in Sports & Exercise*. October 2007; 39(10):1867-1882.

14. O'Connor PJ, Lewis RD, and Kirchner EM. Eating disorder symptoms in female college gymnasts. *Medicine & Science in Sports & Exercise*. 1995; 27: 550-555.

15. Otis C, Drinkwater B, Johnson M, Loucks A, and Wilmore J. Position stand on the female athlete triad. *Medicine & Science in Sports & Exercise*. 1997; 29: i-ix.

16. Rosen LW, and Hough DO. Pathogenic weight-control behaviors of female college gymnasts. *Physician and Sportsmedicine*. 1988; 16: 141-146.

17. Rosen LW, McKeag DB, Hough DO, and Curley V. Pathogenic weight-control behavior in female athletes. *Physician Sportsmedicine*. 1986; 14(1): 79-86.

18. Skolnick A. Female Athlete Triad risk for women. *Journal of the American Medical Association*. August 1993; 270(8): 921-923.

19. Sundgot-Borgen J. Nutrient intake of female elite athletes suffering from eating disorders. *International Journal of Sport Nutrition*. 1993; 3(4): 431-42.

20. Walberg JL, and Johnston CS. Menstrual function and eating behavior in female recreational weight lifters and competitive body builders. *Medicine & Science in Sports & Exercise*. 1991; 23:30-36.

21. Weight LM, and Noakes TD. Is running an analogue of anorexia?: a survey of the incidence of eating disorders in female distance runners. *Medicine & Science in Sports & Exercise*. 1987; 19: 213-217.

22. World Health Organization (WHO). The ICD-10 classification of mental and behavioral disorders: Clinical descriptions and diagnostic guidelines; 1992.

23. Yeager KK, Agostini R, Nattiv A, and Drinkwater B. The female athlete triad: disordered eating, amenorrhea, osteoporosis. *Medicine & Science in Sports & Exercise*. 1993; 25(7): 775-777.

CHAPTER 5

Eating Disorders and Disordered Eating

Mike Brunet, PhD, ATC, CPT, STS

Ron A. Thompson, PhD, FAED

Roberta Trattner Sherman, PhD, FAED

Introduction

"Eating disorders" represent a significant problem for many individuals, especially girls and young women. The prevalence of anorexia nervosa and bulimia nervosa is reported to be approximately 0.8% and 1%-3%, respectively, in the female population.[6] Although these percentages appear small, they represent at least 8 million women in the United States at any one time. There isn't currently enough epidemiological data from methodologically strong studies to reliably attest to the prevalence of such disorders in athletes. Some studies have found a higher prevalence among athletes than the general population.[134,159] If viewing athletics as a microcosm of the world at large, one would expect similar prevalences in athletes. However, athletes may be more at risk for eating disorders based on additional risk factors. But, does more risk translate into more disorders?

"Disordered eating" is a term that has become increasingly popular since the American College of Sports Medicine's Position Stand on the Female Athlete Triad.[2] The term is broader than "eating disorder," and it includes the spectrum of unhealthy eating behaviors ranging from restricting food intake to clinical eating disorders. Although the prevalence of disordered eating is obviously higher than that of eating disorders, necessary studies are lacking to make definitive statements about its prevalence.

This chapter describes and discusses the etiology, signs, symptoms, and special issues associated with eating disorders (ED) and disordered eating (DE), as well as how these problems affect the female athlete's health and performance. Additionally, common and related conditions that often co-exist with ED and DE will be covered. These include mood, anxiety, personality, and substance-related disorders.

Eating Disorders

Eating disorders are classified as a mental health diagnosis,[4] however there are serious health consequences that follow. Eating disorders have the highest rate of premature death of any mental health diagnosis (4%-20% if symptomatology associated with these conditions remains unresolved) and they have the highest rate of short-and long-term physiological complications.[78,61,89,4] More importantly, they affect young women more than any other population.[78]

Eating disorders include anorexia nervosa, bulimia nervosa, and eating disorder not otherwise specified (EDNOS).[3] Eating disorders are not simply disorders of eating. They are emotional disorders that manifest themselves in a variety of eating and weight-related symptoms. Theoretically, an eating disorder can involve virtually every aspect of the individual's life—certainly physical/medical and psychological/emotional, but also familial and social. For the athlete, the disorder could affect all aspects of her life including her sport performance.

Anorexia Nervosa

Anorexia nervosa, a psychiatric syndrome classified as an addiction,[97] is a chronic illness that effects close to 1% of young females. According to the Diagnostic and Statistical Manual of Mental Disorders (DSM-IV-TR),[3] diagnostic criteria for anorexia nervosa[5] includes:

- refusal to maintain body weight characterized by body weight less than 85% of expected body weight for age and height
- intense fear of gaining weight or becoming fat
- body image disturbance (the body is perceived as being larger than it actually is)
- amenorrhea

Refusal to Maintain Body Weight

The first criteria of anorexia, the refusal to maintain body weight at or above a minimally normal weight for age and height matched individuals, can be broken down into two different fundamental aspects. First, an individual needs to be "significantly" underweight. Though a strict definition does not exist, the DSM-IV-TR[3] offers guidelines of weighing less than 85% of that for age matched individuals. Different from the DSM-IV-TR,[3] the ICD-10 criterion[186] states that an individual has to have a body mass index (BMI) equal to or less than 17.5 kg/m^2 in order to be labeled as anorexic.[83] Second, the individual must consciously attempt to avoid gaining weight. Since anorexics normally exhibit an intense fear of gaining weight, they will avoid gaining weight by a number of methods. Garner and Garfinkel[60] state that anorexics will typically skip meals, and when eating, avoid foods that they view as high in fat. In other words, anorexics will avoid food that will result in largest weight gains, or they may avoid food all together.

Fear of Gaining Weight

The second criteria of anorexia is exhibition of an intense fear of gaining weight or becoming fat, even though underweight. Although anorexics typically are underweight, they are impressively concerned that they will become substantially overweight if they cease their vigorous efforts to remain in control of their eating and exercising.[60] The authors make a key distinction between what the word fat means to both the individual and the health care provider. They state that though the term "fat" does not actually mean obese, it may mean that the individual is fatter then they actually feel they can tolerate. This leads to individual interpretation of levels of fatness.

Body Image Disturbance

The third criterion for anorexia is a disturbance in the way in which one's body weight or shape is experienced. This means that an individual with anorexia may portray herself as or parts of her body as being too large (Figure 5-1). The authors

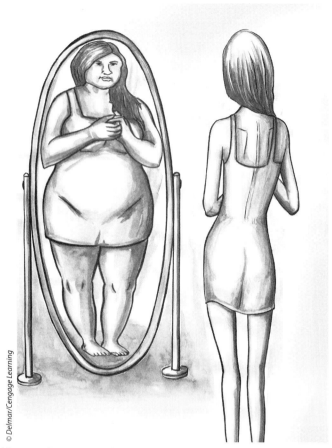

© Delmar/Cengage Learning

Figure 5-1 Women with anorexia see themselves as being overweight even though in reality they are excessively thin.

add that many anorexics will base their self-esteem on their weight and shape. If they gain weight, they may feel ashamed, frustrated, embarrassed, and frightened, whereas weight loss is accompanied by a feeling of deep accomplishment.

Amenorrhea

The last criteria for anorexia is related to amenorrhea. Women with anorexia do not menstruate or only menstruate with the aid of hormone replacement therapy. Although this criterion does not apply to men, male reproductive axis undergoes similar alterations in anorexia.[60] The International classification of Diseases-10 (ICD-10)[186] criteria require that men exhibit a loss of sexual interest and potency to be included in the anorexia category.

Subtypes of Anorexia Nervosa

Once an individual has been diagnosed with anorexia, he or she can be further classified into either a restricting type or a binge-eating purging type. What differentiates the two is the Restrictor will not have participated in binge-eating or any purging behavior. Conversely, the binge-eating/purging individual will have regularly engaged in binge-eating or purging behaviors. Though these two subtypes may prove to be useful in terms of clinical classifications, many uncertainties surround a number of its details. Clear definitions for the frequency of binge eating and purging do not exist.[60] Therefore, careful consideration must be taken into account when using these guidelines for purposes of diagnosis. Table 5-1 presents an overview of the features often exhibited in individuals with an eating disorder.

Comorbidities

Accompanying symptoms of anorexia nervosa often include depressed mood, irritability, social withdrawal, obsessions and rituals related to food, and a decrease in concentration.[14] A more in depth discussion of comorbidities related to eating disorders occurs later in this chapter.

Two very important features of anorexia nervosa are the relationship between estrogen deficiency (with both primary and secondary amenorrhea) and a large reduction in body weight.[82] They both are important risk factors for

TABLE 5-1 • **Diagnostic Features of Eating Disorders**

SYMPTOMS	CLINICAL FINDINGS
Depression	Amenorrhea
Social withdrawal	Constipation
Irritability	Abdominal pain
Insomnia	Cold intolerance
Diminished interest in sex	Lethargy
Obsessive – compulsive behaviors (may be related to food)	Dryness of skin
Concerns about eating in public	Excess energy
Feelings of ineffectiveness	Lanugo (fine downy body hair)
Strong need to control their environment	
Inflexible thinking	
Limited social spontaneity	
Overly restrained initiative and emotional expression	

osteoporosis as amenorrhea is a byproduct of physical activity as well as anorexia nervosa.[40] Not only is there a precipitous decline in bone marrow depression (BMD) (4%-10% per year), but the recovery rate from anorexia nervosa is only 30%-50%, with an increased risk of fracture if it manifests for more than 7-10 years.[97] Hotta et al. (1998)[71] further state that it normally takes several years for anorexia nervosa patients to restore their body weight to 85% or more of their ideal body weight. This may occur even with the individual normally menstruating and depending on the female's age, irreversible damage could occur. For instance, if the individual is an adolescent with anorexia nervosa, the time it takes to restore weight back to normal levels may take up the critical years of bone formation. Furthermore, if the emaciation remains below a BMI of 15, there does appear to be an association with severe hypogonadism.[71] Since this illness can do such a great deal of harm, the time line for identifying anorexia is very important as research has shown eating disorders to begin as early as 10 years of age.[25]

Bulimia Nervosa

According to the Diagnostic and Statistical Manual of Mental Disorders,[3] diagnostic criteria for bulimia nervosa[3] includes:

- cycles of binge-eating characterized by eating within a specific time frame, eating an amount of food larger than average, and a sense of lack of control over eating
- compensatory behaviors designed to "undo" the effects of binge eating
- cycles of binging and compensatory behaviors occurring at least twice per week for at least a three month period
- self-evaluation significantly affected by body shape and weight
- symptoms do not occur exclusively during episodes of anorexia nervosa

Recurrent Episodes of Binge Eating

The first criteria for bulimia is, recurrent episodes of binge eating defined by the American Psychiatric Association (APA),[3] which appears to be the most common attribute of bulimia nervosa (Figure 5-2). Garner and Garfinkel[60] further state that the salient behavior of bulimia nervosa is the frequent occurrence of binge-eating episodes. Another discussion point with regards to the diagnostic criteria is the definition of "large." Again, the authors of the DSM-IV have struggled with this since many individuals with eating problems describe eating binges as not being objectively large.[174] Another factor to consider when deciphering this criterion of binge eating is the time frame of when they are eating the meal. For instance, the size meal eaten at noon is larger when compared to a midnight snack and should be dealt with differently. In the criteria, a "discrete period of time" leaves some room for error. Garner and Garfinkel[60] also state that if a person decides to eat all day long, that this

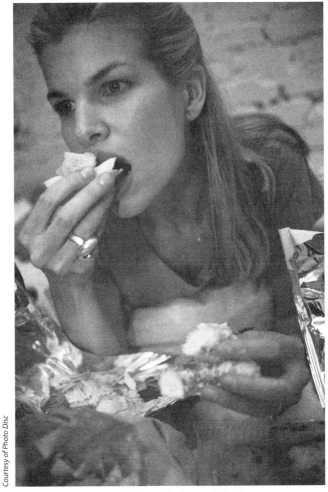

Courtesy of Photo Disc

Figure 5-2 The most dominant feature of bulimia is the binging behavior.

is not viewed as a binge-eating episode as it did not occur within a "discrete period of time."

Compensatory Behavior

The second criterion of bulimia nervosa is recurrent inappropriate compensatory behavior in order to prevent weight gain. Though different forms of inappropriate behaviors exist, self-induced vomiting remains the most frequent behavior.[60] Other individuals with bulimia nervosa do not use any purging methods, but instead do not eat anything for 24 hours or they might excessively exercise. Though fasting and excessive exercise are important compensatory methods, it has been difficult to provide explicit criteria for the two.[60] Some signs of purging behaviors may include swelling of the parotid glands, dental enamel erosion, esophagitis, and electrolyte disturbances.[28]

Time Period for Cycle of Behaviors

The third criteria states that the occurrences of binge-eating and inappropriate compensatory behaviors must occur on average twice a week for a duration of three months for a diagnosis of bulimia.

Self Evaluation of Body Shape and Weight

It is no secret that individuals who engage in pathological weight control behaviors cannot effectively or appropriately self evaluate their body shape and/or weight. No matter their current make-up, it will always fall short of an unreachable goal. Here lies one of the major problems as pathological individuals will most always view themselves as being too fat. This means that it is imperative for individuals to be sensitive to situations which include individuals who constantly are critiquing themselves and/or are having others do it. Furthermore, there is much evidence which exists in the literature to support the link between low self esteem and pathological weight control behaviors. This sets the stage for pathologies like bulimia.

Not Occurring Exclusively with Anorexia

The last criteria for bulimia states that the disturbance does not occur exclusively during episodes of anorexia. This was written for two reasons. First, anorexia nervosa appears to have more complications than bulimia nervosa does, therefore the authors take an aggressive approach to diagnosis by labeling someone as anorexic instead of bulimic if both characteristics are present. For instance, an individual who meets criteria for both disorders will be labeled as anorexic instead of bulimic. It also serves to emphasize that the individual has only one disorder and not two existing ones.

Subtypes of Bulimia

Once the individual is classified as bulimic, he or she can then further be labeled as a purging type or non-purging type. The purging type regularly engages in self-induced vomiting or the misuse of other inappropriate weight loss methods. The non-purging type participates in other compensatory inappropriate behaviors, such as fasting or excessive exercise, but has not regularly engaged in methods like self-induced vomiting.[60] Many bulimic patients use both purging and non-purging compensatory behaviors. Even though binge eating and compensatory behaviors characterize bulimia nervosa, the disorder begins with restrictive eating.

Differentiating Bulimia from Anorexia

What commonly differentiates bulimia nervosa from anorexia nervosa is that individuals exhibiting bulimia nervosa are normally within their normal weight range, though some may be slightly underweight or overweight. This makes identification of bulimia nervosa difficult, as bulimics may appear normal in weight. Anorexics are a bit easier to recognize as they may appear to be emaciated.

Eating Disorder Not Otherwise Specified

Eating disorder not otherwise specified (EDNOS) is the most prevalent eating disorder diagnosis.[66] This diagnosis is given when the individual has some of the criteria, but does not meet full criteria, for anorexia nervosa or bulimia nervosa. For example, an individual may have the other three criteria for anorexia nervosa but may be 90% of expected body weight. Or, for example, she may have all of the criteria for bulimia nervosa except she purges 1 time per week rather than 2. Fairburn and Walsh[52] suggested, however, that EDNOS not simply be thought of as extensions of anorexia nervosa or bulimia nervosa because of the range of eating problems contained in the diagnosis. They also recommend that EDNOS not be viewed as mild or subclinical in terms of severity of impairment. Included within this broad diagnostic category is Binge Eating Disorder (BED). Individuals with BED usually engage in binge eating like individuals with bulimia nervosa but do not purge as bulimic individuals do.

According to the Diagnostic and Statistical Manual of Mental Disorders,[3] diagnostic criteria for EDNOS[5] includes:

* all criteria for anorexia nervosa except: individual has regular menses and current weight is in normal range despite weight loss
* all criteria for bulimia nervosa except binging and compensatory periods occur less than twice a week within a three month period
* compensatory behavior after eating small amounts of food in a person of normal body weight
* repeatedly chewing and spitting out food, but not swallowing, large amounts of food

Additional Categories and Research

Though the EDNOS category now exists, other sub-clinical eating disorder categories have been researched. For instance, Sundgot-Borgen[162] first discussed the term anorexia athletica. It was concluded that some athletes do participate in severe caloric restriction and exercise due to a fear of becoming fat, but do not fit the classical criteria of an eating disorder. The criteria for anorexia athletica are as follows:

* weight loss >5% of expected body weight
* restriction of energy intake (<1,200 kcalories a day)
* excessive fear of weight gain or becoming obese
* absence of medical illness or affective disorder to explain the weight loss

Since this category of eating disorder is new in the literature, little or no research exists regarding athletes. This does not mean that research in this area is not warranted, though. Recently, the authors who made up the framework of the EDNOS category[138] profiled college women for EDNOS. They found that this new category is warranted, since many women do fit some but not all of the criteria for either anorexia nervosa or bulimia nervosa.[138]

The Continuum of Eating Disorders

Eating disorders have been described as distinct categories, but it is probably more helpful to think of these disorders as occurring on a continuum with considerable overlap. Many eating disorder patients move back and forth between and among the different diagnoses. For example, it is not uncommon for some bulimic patients to have also been diagnosed with anorexia nervosa at previous times and anorexic patients having experienced times when bulimia nervosa was probably a more accurate diagnosis. Certainly, many patients eventually diagnosed with anorexia nervosa or bulimia nervosa probably would have been diagnosed as EDNOS early in the development of their disorders. Even though diagnosis is important, a general rule of thumb regarding eating disorders (or disordered eating) is that if the eating behavior compromises physical or psychological health and/or interferes with normal everyday activities (i.e. job, school, relationships, etc.) treatment is warranted, regardless of diagnosis.

Diagnostic information related to anorexia nervosa, bulimia nervosa, and EDNOS in this chapter is derived primarily from the *Diagnostic and Statistical Manual of Mental Disorders* (4th ed.).[3] Preliminary discussions regarding possible changes in diagnostic criteria for eating disorders for the next DSM include the elimination of amenorrhea as a criterion for anorexia nervosa, modification or elimination of EDNOS, the inclusion of BED as a separate disorder, and the use of a dimensional rather than categorical system of classification.

Disordered Eating

Eating problems do not need to meet criteria for an eating disorder in order for the eating to create problems that warrant intervention. As mentioned previously, "disordered eating" includes the spectrum of unhealthy eating from simple dieting to clinical eating disorders. "Disordered eating" rather than eating disorders was chosen for inclusion in the initial position stand on the Female Athlete Triad because the athlete's eating does not have to be disordered to the extent of a frank eating disorder in order to play a role in amenorrhea and bone loss in athletes.

Other terms such as "subclinical" or "subthreshold" problems have sometimes been used to characterize disordered eating, and research suggests that the prevalence of such eating problems is higher than actual clinical disorders in athletes.[116] Although Johnson, Powers, and Dick[79] found the prevalence of frank eating disorders to be low in female collegiate athletes, 13% were assessed to have clinically significant symptoms, while 34.5% and 38% were judged to be at risk for anorexia nervosa and bulimia nervosa, respectively. Similarly,

Sanford-Martens, Davidson, Yakushko, Martens, Hinton, and Beck[134] found that 20% of their female collegiate athletes were "symptomatic" for an eating disorder. For information regarding the management of disordered eating and the Female Athlete Triad, the reader is directed to NCAA (2005).

Low Energy Availability

A more recent term "energy availability" has been associated with disordered eating in athletes.[188] Energy availability is defined as dietary energy intake minus exercise energy expenditure,[90] or energy that remains after the energy cost of exercise has been spent. Low energy availability occurs when the athlete either inadvertently or willfully ingests insufficient calories to adequately fuel her physical activity and the caloric needs for normal health, growth, and development. Low energy availability may or may not involve an eating disorder or disordered eating. If the problem is severe and persistent, amenorrhea can result. In theory, low energy availability would appear to be relatively simple to overcome. It usually requires an increase in caloric intake and/or a decrease in energy expenditure. The process of recovery is apt to be made more difficult as the athlete's eating becomes more disordered due to possible resistance by the athlete to either increase her intake or decrease her output.

Related Comorbid Conditions

Individuals with eating disorders often have multiple "comorbidities" or conditions that occur at the same time with the eating disorder.[188] Sometimes the comorbid condition begins before the eating disorder, but its onset can also follow that of the eating disorder. These comorbid conditions can negatively affect the eating disorder and its treatment. Generally, it is recommended to try to restore the patient's weight and/or decrease binge/purge behaviors before focusing on the treatment of the comorbid conditions, unless they are severe.[6] The decision in this regard must be made based on the risk or danger to the patient. For example, if an eating disorder patient becomes so depressed that she is suicidal, the focus of treatment must be on alleviating the depression. Regarding the effect of comorbidity on eating disorder treatment, Milos, Spindler, Buddenberg, and Crameri[99] reported that eating disorder patients with higher levels of comorbidity required more intensive treatment.

Eating disorders (and disordered eating) are not only affected by the comorbid conditions; these conditions can also be negatively affected by the eating disorder. In fact, they may at times be attributable to the eating disorder. "Starvation effects" of the eating disorder often include such symptoms as a preoccupation with food (i.e. food and eating rituals, increased sensitivity to food, etc.), depression, anxiety, social withdrawal, decreased concentration, and sleep difficulty.[87] "Starvation effects" may be a bit of a misnomer. In their landmark study Keys, and his colleagues did not really starve their subjects. Rather, they were placed on half of their usual daily intake (about 1500 calories-1600 calories). In essence, these "starvation effects" were produced with dietary restriction. "Semistarvation" might be a more accurate term. Because many of these symptoms can be produced with the restrictive dieting that is characteristic of eating disorders and many forms of disordered eating, any of these symptoms may improve or remit with adequate nutrition.

Mood Disorders

Mood disorders have sometimes been referred to as "affective disorders" or more commonly as "depression." Typically, mood disorders are characterized by some if not most of the following symptoms: low mood, decreased energy, activity, and motivation, decreased interest and concentration, negative thoughts that may include suicidal ideation, social withdrawal, disturbance in sleep and appetite or eating, and feelings of helplessness, hopelessness, and worthlessness. Mood disorders are common disorders as approximately 10% of the American population suffers from a mood disorder during any one-year period and the National Institute of Mental Health reports that 20% of the population will suffer from a "major depression" at some time during their lifetime. Women more often present for treatment with mood disorders than their male counterparts. Again, if viewing the sport world as being a microcosm of the larger world, one would expect a similar incidence in the female athlete population.

The *Diagnostic and Statistical Manual of Mental Disorders (4th ed.)*[3] lists several mood disorders. A thorough discussion of each of these disorders is well beyond the scope of this chapter. Our primary focus here will be more generally on depression and eating disorders and how these are manifested in female athletes. For this reason, we will mention one of the more common ones, major depressive disorder (MDD; one or more major depressive episodes of at least two weeks of depressed mood or loss of interest in addition to at least four other depressive symptoms), which also frequently co-exists with eating disorders. Suffice it to say that estimates of the percentage of anorexic women who reported at least one episode of major depression range as high as 80% and that major depression is the most common comorbid condition found in bulimic women.[23] A caution in this regard, however, is that a combination of severe weight loss and depression is not always indicative of an eating disorder per se. Severe weight loss can occur in MDD without an eating disorder with the critical differential diagnostic criterion being that MDD patients would have no desire for weight loss or no fear of weight gain.[3]

The relationship between eating disorders and mood disorders is a complex one. A mood disorder or depressive symptoms can occur prior to or after the onset of anorexia nervosa or bulimia nervosa and can persist even following recovery from the eating disorder. Interestingly, eating disorder symptoms are often associated with depression, even in women with no history of eating disorder symptoms.[180] It appears that there is a genetic component to both depression and eating disorders, and although each has its own specific set of genes, there may also be shared genetic factors between the two disorders.[23]

Given the usual symptoms of depression (i.e. low mood, decreased energy, concentration, and motivation, negative thinking, etc.), one would expect to see athletic performance decrease with depression, even without the complicating factor of an eating problem. Certainly, adding the common symptoms of an eating disorder (i.e. dehydration, malnutrition, muscle weakness, etc.) will only further decrease performance. Unfortunately, such a decrease in performance can increase the athlete's depression and need for the eating disorder. This often sets up a vicious cycle in which the eating disorder decreases performance while increasing depression. The athlete's attempt to deal with decreasing performance and increasing depression is usually through the eating disorder.

Depression is a common symptom for overtrained or stale athletes. Related to this, research with some endurance athletes has indicated that increases in training volume can increase mood disturbance.[123] With these athletes, a decrease in training volume can decrease mood disturbance.

As discussed previously, several symptoms manifested by an individual can be a result of semistarvation. Depressed mood, decreased concentration, social withdrawal, and sleep difficulty are just some of the possible effects. For this reason, more "normal" eating might need to be restored in order to adequately assess the athlete's depression. That is, it may result from the disordered eating, or it may in fact be a separate disorder, requiring additional treatment. But again, if the depression is severe, it must be dealt with early in the treatment process, primarily because the patient (athlete) may be a suicide risk, but also because depression is apt to complicate treatment and recovery.

Anxiety Disorders

Anxiety disorders are very common. An estimated 19 million Americans experience anxiety disorders. More women than men suffer from such disorders.[3] Some of the more common anxiety disorders listed in DSM-IV include:

- agoraphobia (anxiety about/avoidance of, situations/places from which escape might be difficult)
- generalized anxiety disorder (persistent and excessive anxiety/worry)
- obsessive compulsive disorder (obsessions causing anxiety/distress and/or compulsions which serve to neutralize anxiety)
- panic disorder (recurrent, unexpected panic attacks)
- posttraumatic stress disorder (reexperiencing of a traumatic event with symptoms associated with the trauma)
- specific phobia (anxiety evoked a specific feared object/situation)
- social phobia (anxiety evoked by certain social/performance situations)

Anxiety disorders frequently co-exist with eating disorders. Over half of those diagnosed with anorexia nervosa and bulimia nervosa have a lifetime presence of an anxiety disorder (most often generalized anxiety disorder, obsessive compulsive disorder, or social phobia) and the anxiety disorder usually precedes the eating disorder.[23] Regarding the effect of an anxiety disorder on the prognosis for eating disorder patients, at least one study found that obsessive-compulsive disorder was associated not only with an earlier onset of the eating disorder but also a longer duration of illness.[99]

We previously discussed mood disorders occurring with eating disorders and now anxiety disorders with eating disorders. Mood disorders and anxiety disorders also occur frequently within the same individual. For example, major depressive disorder occurs in 50%–65% of individuals with Panic Disorder.[3] Additionally, comorbidity with other anxiety disorders is also common.[3]

It is expected that athletes with anxiety disorders show difficulties in concentration, focus, and decision-making. "Choking" (failing to meet the challenge of competition demand due to pressure), which is often attributed to anxiety, would probably be more likely to occur in an athlete with an anxiety disorder. The "obsessiveness" that is often associated with eating disorders, not to mention the effect of semistarvation on cognitive function, would only increase the athlete's difficulty.

As discussed with depression, symptoms of anxiety can also be produced through semistarvation. Thus, some of these symptoms may remit with adequate nutrition, and a focus on the eating disorder rather than the anxiety symptoms would appear to be prudent. Two things to keep in mind, however, are that anxiety disorders usually predate the eating disorder, and anxiety symptoms, especially obsessiveness, often remain even after recovery from the eating disorder.

Personality Disorders

Personality disorders involve enduring patterns of inner experience and behavior that deviate from cultural expectations, and/or are inflexible and pervasive, and/or lead to significant distress or impairment in important areas of functioning.[3] The DSM-IV[3] lists 10 personality disorders. For the purpose of this discussion only those that occur more frequently with eating disorders will be addressed:

• antisocial (disregard for, and violation of, the rights of others)
• avoidant (social inhibition, feelings of inadequacy, and hypersensitivity to negative criticism)
• borderline (instability of relationships and affect and impulsivity)
• dependent (submissive, clinging behavior, and a need to be cared for)
• histrionic (excessive emotionality and attention seeking)

- obsessive-compulsive (preoccupation with orderliness, perfection, and control) borderline, dependent, and histrionic personality disorders are diagnosed more often in women.

Personality disorders occur frequently in eating disorder patients as evidenced by a range of prevalence rates of 27%–93% having been reported for any personality disorder with any eating disorder.[149,171] Apparently, different relationships can exist between personality disorders and eating disorders. Any personality trait may be a precipitant, consequence, or a correlate of an eating disorder and some, such as perfectionism and obsessiveness, often remain following successful eating disorder treatment.[184]

Personality disorders are probably "normal" personality traits carried to an extreme. Some traits, such as perfectionism, that are often associated with eating disorders, may help athletes perform better. A potential problem with identification of a symptomatic athlete occurs when such a trait is perceived positively in the athletic environment but may be an eating disorder symptom.[168] Another such example might involve an athlete with a dependent personality disorder. She might be apt to be overly compliant and try to do whatever her coach wanted her to do in order to please (or at least not displease) him/her. Again, this might be (mis)perceived as the athlete being very "coachable," which would likely be viewed as a positive trait rather than a potential problem.

Personality disorders often complicate or interfere with treatment of an eating disorder or the personality disorder itself. Similarly, it could be anticipated that personality disorders will negatively impact athletic performance. Remember that personality disorders deviate from cultural expectations and create stress or impairment in important areas of functioning. Again, if the sport world is viewed as a microcosm of the larger world, it would be expected for such disorders in athletes to create difficulty for self, coaches, and teammates.

Substance Related Disorders

Substances as defined by the DSM-IV include drugs of abuse, medications, and toxins.[3] This section will deal primarily with drugs of abuse (i.e. alcohol, amphetamines, caffeine, cocaine, and marijuana) and their relationship to eating disorders in female athletes, but we will also examine the abuse of substances used for the purposes of weight loss or to "undo" the effects of eating (i.e. diet pills, diuretics, enemas, emetics, and laxatives). Regarding drug use among athletes, a recent NCAA study of substance use by collegiate athletes[65] reported of the eight substance categories surveyed, only alcohol and amphetamines were used more often by female athletes than male athletes. The authors suggested that the drive for weight loss might in part explain the amphetamine use.

Lifetime substance abuse rates are higher for individuals with anorexia nervosa and bulimia nervosa than for individuals without eating disorders, and eating disorders usually precede the substance abuse.[182] Although substance abuse (especially alcohol and stimulants) occurs in approximately ⅓ of individuals with bulimia nervosa, and within anorexia nervosa, individuals with binge-eating/purging type are more apt to abuse alcohol and other drugs than the restricting type anorexic individuals.[3]

As mentioned previously, a general guideline regarding eating disorders and comorbid conditions is to treat the eating problem first, unless the comorbid condition is severe. When eating and substance disorders co-exist, there are reasons why it might be prudent to treat the substance abuse before the eating disorder or at least concurrently, especially if the substance abuse is severe. First, as discussed previously, many individuals with eating disorders are depressed, and some need to take antidepressant medication as part of their treatment. Some substances may run counter to antidepressant medications (i.e. alcohol), or may increase depressive symptoms, thereby worsening the eating disorder and negatively affecting treatment. Second, some substances may be used as a "substitute" for eating disorder symptoms. That is, they may be used to manage whatever emotion or condition the eating disorder might be managing. Third, some bulimic patients will need to establish therapeutic controls (those without the diseases), and some substances can loosen those controls.

Alcohol

It may seem counterintuitive for an eating disorder patient to use alcohol because of the ingestion of calories. Interesting, some eating disorder patients seem to allow for the calories associated with alcohol. In fact, some patients will avoid eating in order to "save" calories for alcohol consumption. Some patients will sometimes allow themselves to ingest (more) food after having drunk alcohol.[6]

Stimulants

Stimulants may be the drugs of choice for some eating disorder patients for several reasons. First, many stimulants suppress appetite. Some bulimic patients use methamphetamines or cocaine to avoid urges to binge-eat.[6] Second, stimulants provide a "boost" (drug effect) for malnourished individuals who need energy. Some patients use large amounts of caffeine for "energy," in addition to suppressing appetite. Additionally, some eating disorder patients also use caffeine in the form of diet sodas to fill their stomachs to avoid eating and to give themselves a taste of sweetness without ingesting calories. Another stimulant, nicotine, has also been used by females who smoke to suppress appetite.[32,185] Third, stimulants provide some mood elevation for some depressed patients.

Nonmedical Substance Use for Weight Loss, Purging, or Performance Enhancement

Included in this group of substances are ones that have traditionally been used for weight loss and for compensatory behaviors in eating disorders, such as over the counter (OTC) diet pills, diuretics, laxatives, enemas, and emetics. Also included here are less traditional substances such as ephedrine and anabolic steroids.

The DSM-IV[6] lists the misuse of diuretics, laxatives, and enemas as compensatory behaviors. All of the substances are designed to control weight, primarily through dehydration. Diuretics are frequently used by bulimic women as a means to lose weight.[101] Similarly, laxative use is common in women with eating disorders[104] and may indicate more severe disturbance.[24] Another class of substances that have been used as purgatives or compensation for eating would be emetics, or drugs that have been used to induce vomiting. The most popular (and dangerous) of these has been syrup of Ipecac. Its use has been associated with cardiomyopathy and cardiac toxicity leading to death in some eating disorder patients.[124] With regard to the effect on athlete performance, all of these substances are apt to have a negative affect on performance, given the fact that they cause dehydration.

Another class of substances that has sometimes been associated with athletic performance is anabolic steroids, but usually it has been discussed with regard to male athletes. However, a study by Yesalis, Barsukiewicz, Kopstein, and Bahrke[189] found that steroid use by adolescent girls has increased and that adolescent girls were using steroids to become thinner or leaner in addition to improving athletic performance.

Substance Use by Athletes and Female Athlete Triad Symptoms

The concerns regarding substance use as it relates to the physical and psychological health of the athlete should be obvious, especially with respect to drugs such as alcohol, cocaine, methamphetamine, and the substances typically used by eating disorder patients for the purpose of purging or weight loss. A less obvious but nonetheless significant concern involves the effect of substances as they relate to the Female Athlete Triad. Anabolic steroid use can result in amenorrhea.[111] The excessive use of alcohol, nicotine, and caffeine can negatively affect bone mass.[102] The use of such substances in combination with the malnutrition often associated with disordered eating can place the athlete at considerable risk. Thus, in assessing the female athlete regarding Triad symptoms, it is important to inquire about the use of these substances.

NOTE:

Comorbid conditions have been presented with respect to disordered eating and eating disorders. This should not be misconstrued to suggest that the comorbid conditions discussed in this chapter are not serious disorders that warrant treatment even when existing without eating difficulties. For more information on these conditions, the reader is directed to the Diagnostic and Statistical Manual of Mental Disorders (4th ed.)[3] *and for more information on comorbid conditions in athletes, the reader is directed to NCAA (2007).*

Risks for ED/DE in the Athletic Environment

As healthy as sport participation can be for most girls and young women, there are aspects of the athletic environment that likely increase an athlete's risk for developing disordered eating or an eating disorder. These risks fall into two major categories. The first involves aspects of the sport environment that encourage a focus on weight and weight loss and includes an emphasis on thinness and performance, revealing uniforms with issues of competitive thinness, and the presumption of health with good performance. The second major category involves conditions in the sport environment that increase the difficulty in identifying symptomatic or at-risk athletes. These include sport body stereotypes and possible eating disorder symptoms that may be misperceived as "normal" or even desirable.

Emphasis on Thinness and Performance

For several years, a prevailing notion in the sport world suggests that a decrease in weight or body fat can enhance athletic performance.[179] The research in this area is equivocal. Some athletes in some sports do perform better some of the time following such a decrement. However, the issue is not really whether such a decrement produces better performance. Dieting and the pursuit of thinness are related to the development of eating disorders.[58,72,119] Thus, attempts to lose weight or body fat can increase the risk of developing an eating disorder.

Revealing Uniforms

Many girls and young women feel uncomfortable or self-conscious about their bodies. If this is the case for an athlete, she may feel that her body is too "exposed" in a uniform that shows too much of her body (Figure 5-3). As a consequence, she may attempt to lose weight or body fat, believing that she will look better and feel better if she is thinner. Again, any situation or issue that increases the likelihood of dieting, increases the risk of developing disordered eating or an eating disorder.

Related to revealing uniforms is *competitive thinness*. Many girls and young women engage in competitive thinness if they are tempted to try to lose weight when encountering others who they believe to be thinner. Most athletes tend to be competitive people. This competitiveness may lead them to be competitive with teammates or other athletes in terms of thinness and sport performance. This competitiveness often involves body comparisons. If an athlete notices that a competitor or teammate, who is performing better than she, looks thinner, she may consider trying to improve performance through weight loss. Revealing uniforms facilitate these unhealthy comparisons and competitions and thus the dieting that often accompanies them.[75]

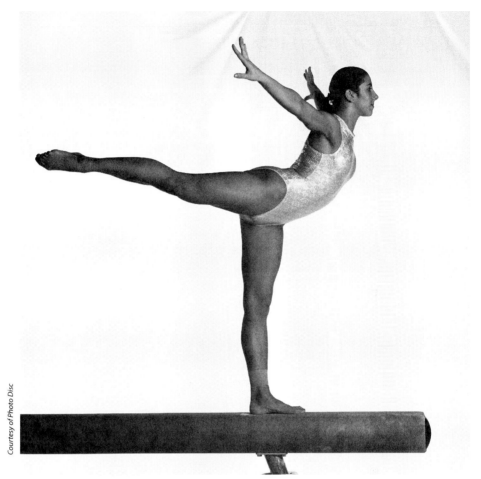

Courtesy of Photo Disc

Figure 5-3 Uniforms in many women's sports are very tight fitting and figure revealing, often making the athlete acutely aware of the shape of her body and her weight.

Presumption of Health with Good Performance

Although an eating disorder will eventually take its toll on the athlete physically and psychologically, many athletes with such disorders can perform well for extended periods. It is sometimes difficult for coaches, athletes, and parents to believe that the athlete has a serious problem when she performs well athletically. Thus, identification and treatment can be delayed.

Sport Body Stereotypes

A sport body stereotype (expectation of how a typical body looks within a particular sport) that includes a small or thin body size or shape can increase the likelihood of attempted weight or body fat loss by the athlete. That process

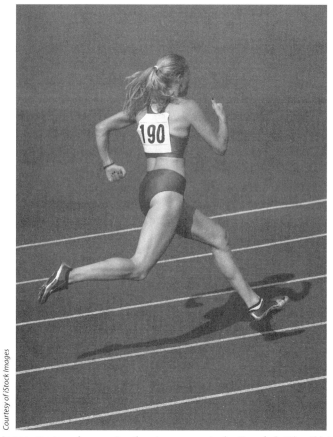

Courtesy of iStock Images

Figure 5-4 In many sports, such as running, there is a preconceived notion of what the athletes body type should look like.

in turn increases the risk of disordered eating and eating disorders. For example, the sport body stereotype for distance running is one of thinness (Figure 5-4). That is, many distance runners are thin and the expectation of many people, both within and outside sport, is that distance runners are (should be) thin. Thus, a thin distance runner fits the stereotype and may be less noticeable than a heavier runner, who does not fit the stereotype. For this reason, a distance runner who might be too thin and even anorexic may be overlooked because she is a distance runner and a thin body shape is consistent with the body stereotype for distance running.

A sport body stereotype of thinness can also complicate the eating disorder/disordered eating identification process for sport personnel. When identification is delayed, treatment is delayed, thereby putting the athlete at greater risk.

Misperception

Anything that complicates the identification of disordered eating or an eating disorder can delay treatment, thereby placing the athlete at increased risk for physical and psychological complications related to her eating difficulties. For example, amenorrhea (loss of menses) is a diagnostic criterion for anorexia nervosa.[3] Although amenorrhea occurs in only 2%-5% of nonathletes, it has been reported to be as high as 66% in some athlete groups.[188] In fact, it is so common, that it is sometimes viewed as being "normal".[145] Amenorrhea is a diagnostic criterion for anorexia nervosa, it is often the first symptom of the Female Athlete Triad that is identified.[2,144] When it is viewed as "normal," treatment is delayed.

Another complication in identification for the athlete, as well as for sport personnel, involves the fact that accepted or even desired traits in athletes may be characteristics of individuals who have eating disorders,[169] for example, excessive exercise and overtraining syndrome. Table 5-2 shows a list of "good athlete traits" and their corresponding "anorexic characteristics." Looking at all these traits exemplifies an athlete who is willing to train very hard, play despite pain or injury, comply with all coaching instructions, be a selfless team player, and be willing to lose weight in order to enhance performance. She sounds like a coach's dream. Is this a "good athlete," an anorexic athlete, or both?

NOTE:

It is not the intent of the authors to suggest that good athletes are "pathological;" nor that the personalities of good athletes are similar to anorexic patients. The intent is to alert the Athletic Trainer Certified (ATC) to the possibility that some characteristics of anorexic individuals are not only present in some "good athletes," they may in part play a role in successful athletic performance.

Excessive Exercise

Excessive exercise is a common symptom in anorexia nervosa.[85] Even though it is common with anorexia and other eating difficulties, it can be difficult to identify in non-athletes and even more so in athletes. What is excessive exercise for an athlete? When an athlete is training (exercising) harder and longer than

TABLE 5-2 • **Triat Comparison of a Good Athlete and an Anorexic Patient**

GOOD ATHLETE	ANOREXIC PATIENT
Mental toughness	Aceticism
Commitment to training	Excessive exercise
Pursuit of excellence	Perfectionism
Coachability	Overcompliance
Unselfishness	Selflessness
Performance despite pain	Denial of discomfort

her teammates, her exercise is apt to be viewed by coaches and sport personnel as a willingness to work hard—an attribute that coaches would admire and desire in their athletes. Although this may be an attribute of a "good athlete," it may also be a symptom of an eating disorder.[166]

Part of the difficulty with identifying excessive exercise in an athlete (or non-athlete) is that the term "excessive exercise" implies a "quantity" of exercise. Another part of the difficulty is that several other terms have been used in the literature synonymously or interchangeably with excessive exercise—terms such as "compulsive exercise," "obligatory exercise," "exercise abuse," and "exercise addiction." The issue is further complicated by the fact that the *Diagnostic and Statistical Manual of Mental Disorders*[3] is not clear what constitutes excessive exercise in eating disorder patients. It avoided quantifying the term; rather, it defined excessive exercise with the "qualitative" factor of "appropriateness." Specifically, it defined exercise as excessive when it "significantly interferes with important activities, when it occurs at inappropriate times or in inappropriate setting, or when the individual continues to exercise despite injury or other medical complications.[3] Interestingly, DSM-IV does not include excessive exercise as a diagnostic criterion for anorexia nervosa, despite the fact that many if not most anorexic patients engage in excessive physical activity. DSM-IV does list excessive exercise as a "compensatory behavior" for bulimia nervosa.

Identification of excessive exercise in an athlete is also complicated by aspects of the sport environment. To coaches and other sport personnel, the athlete who is training harder and longer than her teammates and more than is being required by her sport and her coach may look like a "good athlete." As mentioned previously, eating disorder symptoms (i.e. excessive exercise) not only may not be identified as problematic, they may be encouraged, desired, and rewarded.[166] At the same time, excessive exercise in terms of quantity of exercise may not indicate an eating disorder. A study by Seigel and Hetta[141] suggested that eating disorder symptoms were related more to obligatory attitudes regarding exercise than the quantity of exercise. In a related study, Adkins and Keel (2005) found that the compulsive quality of exercise rather than the excessive quantity better characterized the exercise associated with eating disorders. For these reasons, it has been suggested by Powers and Thompson (2008) that the term "excessive exercise" would be more appropriately termed "unhealthy" or "unbalanced," and they have provided a list of signs and symptoms that can be used to identify such exercise in competitive athletes.

Overtraining Syndrome

A complication of excessive training that occurs in some athletes has been the term "overtraining syndrome" or "staleness".[125] These individuals often experience physical and psychological difficulties that include fatigue, weight loss, amenorrhea, sleep disturbance, and depression, as well as a decrement in athletic performance. As a result of decrease in performance, athletes with overtraining syndrome will often train harder, only to exacerbate their difficulties. Stale, overtrained athletes need just the opposite—rest and time away from their sport.

Incidence of Eating Disorders in Athletes

In a pivotal study by Johnson et al.,[79] the researchers reported on the NCAA national eating disorder project. They surveyed 883 men and 562 women from 11 NCAA Division I schools. The survey they used was a conglomeration of three different tools. The first was the Eating Disorder Inventory-2 (EDI-2) with the three subscales of body dissatisfaction, drive for thinness, and bulimia. The remaining two tools used were the Rosenberg Self-Esteem Scale[132] and the Body Cathexis Scale.[139] All three questionnaires were given at the same time to NCAA Division I athletes. They found that 1.1% of the females met the DSM-IV criteria for bulimia nervosa and 0% for males. None of the athletes met the criteria for anorexia nervosa. Binge eating was reported in more than one quarter of both male and female athletes, but female athletes were much more likely to feel out of control during an episode of overeating (81% in females vs 45% in males). Therefore, when the full criteria for a binge were used, more female athletes (22.68%) than male athletes (11.97%) binge ate.

The researchers also found that more females vomited to lose weight than males, and they were more likely to have vomited monthly, weekly, or daily in the preceding three months. What was interesting was that 2% of the females and 0% of the males self-reported that they had anorexia nervosa, while 6% of females and .005% of males self-reported that they had bulimia nervosa. Unfortunately, the researchers did not report if the self-labeled individuals with eating disorders were the same ones that had elevated questionnaire scores.

Johnson et al.[79] also stated that their results were lower than other previous reported studies, but offered two explanations. First, the more rigorous sampling procedure, larger sample size, and stringent criteria might have resulted in a more accurate estimate. The second reason might be related to the caliber athletes studied. It could be possible that the risk factors for disturbed eating behavior may be higher among lower tier athletes. Though these results show a lower incidence at the D-1 level, they are still quite high. Female athletes consistently reported significantly higher rates of disordered eating attitudes and behaviors, and also reported lower on self-esteem than male athletes. The authors also reported that the female's goal was to achieve a body fat content that resulted in amenorrhea.

The new ACSM position statement on the female athlete triad[103] sites studies with statistics comparing athletes to non-athletes. One study[76] found 31% of the "thin-build" athletes had an eating disorder versus 5.5% of the non-athletes and the other study[191] found 25% of the female elite athletes, those in endurance sports, aesthetic sports had clinical eating disorders compared to 9% in the general population. Therefore, it is evident that eating disorders exist in athletics at an alarmingly high rate.

Predisposition to Eating Disorders

There are many predispositions to eating disorders.[103] Spurrell et al.[153] showed that 45% of the subjects reported that dieting preceded their first binge episode and 55% reported that binge eating preceded the first diet. They further found that the age of onset differs between eating disorders and individuals who binge first may be at greater risk for psychiatric disturbance. Patton et al.[115] showed that dieting was a predisposing factor for eating disorders in adolescents and concluded that exercise should be used as a mode of weight loss instead of dieting. This may be due to the fact that adolescent girls gain almost double the amount of fat mass when compared to boys of the same age.[95] Consequently, this could cause adolescent girls to diet well before boys and therefore increase the number of eating disorder cases in females than in males.

Therefore, it appears that age and early dietary habits are associated with eating disorders. Other predisposing factors include the following: depression, anxiety, personality disorders, cognitive and emotional deficits, and psychological or physical trauma, prolonged periods of dieting, frequent weight fluctuations, a sudden increase in training volume, and traumatic events such as injury or loss of a coach[62,160] as well as a possible genetic link.[142]

Psychological or Physical Trauma

Sex abuse has been positively linked with patients with anorexia nervosa,[113,185] but Palmer et al.[112] later showed that it might be a more general vulnerability to psychiatric illness. Wonderlich[182] showed a history of childhood sexual abuse is associated with weight and body dissatisfaction along with purging and dietary restriction. More specifically, they were able to show that the sexually abused children were more likely to express weight dissatisfaction, food restriction when emotionally upset, pursuit of thin body ideals, and heightened purging behavior versus controls. One idea that might be plausible is that the children who were abused may have been more likely to diet in an effort to overcome dissatisfaction with body size, shape, and weight. Wonderlich[182] also revealed lower perfectionism scores in the abused group. Another idea that Wonderlich offers is the idea that childhood sexual abuse results in pervasive psychobiological dysregulation. This might then increase the risk of different forms of psychopathology, which may include eating disorders.[182] Garner further suggests that psychological or physical trauma is not causal; they can be associated with symptom severity and should be considered central to management.

Genetic and Familial Predisposition

Two twin studies[69,175] found that a genetic component might exist, but hard evidence is lacking due to a lack of research. What might be genetic is the vulnerability to a specific trait which might cause anorexia nervosa or obesity. Wade et al.[172] concluded that the most likely influences determining individual variation in disordered eating are additive genetic and non-shared environment influences. Familial description has the mother as being dominant, intrusive, and ambivalent, while the father is portrayed as passive and ineffectual. What is interesting is the higher risk of female first-degree relatives developing an eating disorder versus controls.[67,156]

Body Image Dissatisfaction

Though one would think that an athlete should be satisfied with their body, researchers have discovered subgroups of physically active individuals that have body image concerns and participate in disordered eating habits.[79] Like the general population, athletes are also negatively influenced by socio-cultural pressures to be thin and to obtain an unrealistic body shape. Not that this is bad enough by itself, the female athlete also has the pressure to be thin in order to maximize performance.[79,129,163] Together, these pressures make a dangerous combination and could easily predispose someone with an eating disorder.

Eating Disorders and Athletics

Important to note is that there remains no specific eating disorder criteria for athletes, only the non-athletic population. In other words, the current DSM-IV clinical criteria for eating disorders were developed for the non-athletic population, but over time an adoption of these criteria has occurred in the athletic realm. Realistically, athletes will less frequently present with a frank eating disorder, but will more than likely show signs that better represent variations of sub-clinical eating disorders.[150,9]

In terms of the prevalence of eating disorders in athletics, it is known that they occur, at an alarmingly high rate,[37,163,103,17] however the prevalence rates have been reported at an inconsistent basis throughout the literature. For instance, frequencies of 1% and up to 66% have been reported by some researchers.[150,26,21,90,151,163] One reason may include dishonest answers when given questionnaires. Another reason may be due to the fact that the EDNOS eating disorder category did not exist in earlier studies. Only a label of "sub-clinical eating disorder" group was given to athletes who did not fit the eating disorder criteria, but were not necessarily removed from the eating disorder numbers. Also, and probably most important, was a lack of standardization existed between research studies. In other words, this high prevalence incorporates athletes that practice pathogenic weight loss practices, but do not fit the criteria for an eating disorder.

Three earlier studies by Rosen and Hough,[130] Rosen and McKeag et al.,[131] and Sundgot Borgen and Corbin[161] all discuss the prevalence of pathogenic weight control behaviors. Unfortunately, the papers that followed used their data to describe the prevalence of eating disorders rather than discuss the weight loss practices of athletes. This was done even though specific criteria were not met with regards to eating disorders. What these papers do show is the high prevalence of pathogenic weight loss practices in athletes, but not necessarily a high prevalence of eating disorders. With the use of this new category (EDNOS), a more realistic prevalence of eating disorders and those who practice unhealthy weight loss practices may now be unraveled.

Fogelholm and Hilloskorpi[54] looked at weight and diet concerns of male and female Finnish athletes aged 18-20 years. They found that regarding weight and diet concerns, the type of athletic event was the largest dependent variable. When compared to male subjects, female subjects were less satisfied with their present weight. There also were lower Eating Disorder Inventory (EDI)[63] scores in athletes when compared to controls. What was interesting was that these researchers asked the athletes to fill in their names when taking the survey. This could have resulted in lower than truthful scores since anonymity was not kept.

Regarding weight reduction, Fogelholm and Hilloskorpi[54] also found that the prevalence of athletes reporting weight reduction was much higher (51% and 55% among female and male athletes, respectively) than the 31% previously reported.[158] Even without the sports with weight-classes, their prevalence was 44% and 33% in female and male athletes, and most of the weight class athletes used rapid weight reduction techniques.

Regarding menstrual disorders, the prevalence was highest in athlete groups characterized by a lean body (aesthetic), heavy training by volume, or intensity or frequent weight reduction attempts. Therefore, they concluded that the risk for eating disorders is dependent on the type of sport.

Dale and Landers[36] reported on the dietary habits of wrestlers. They wanted to see if some of the poor dietary habits were of a disordered eating nature, or if they were eating disorders. To do this, the researchers administered the EDI to in season and off-season wrestlers. The subjects were younger (junior high school and high school), but this identified an important point. Eating disorders normally start at younger ages. The DSM-IV[3] reports that the mean age of onset for an eating disorder is 17 years of age, with bimodal peaks at ages 14 and 18. Therefore, this study was relevant in terms of addressing younger populations. They found that the wrestlers concerns with weight were due entirely to the demands of wrestling, and did not meet the severity level required for a diagnosis of bulimia nervosa.

Eating Disorders and Performance

Although most athletes believe that disordered eating habits do aid in performance, literature states the opposite.[17] In a book by Thompson and Sherman,[167] they discuss the different effects of anorexia nervosa to the athlete. First, anorexia nervosa can negatively impact sport performance, and the magnitude is often related to the severity of the disease. Anorexia nervosa can effect different systems, or effect the overall health of the athlete. This could result in a diminished level or performance. They also state that anorexia nervosa may have different effects on different types of athletes. For instance, anorexia nervosa will probably have a much greater impact on a runner or wrestler (endurance athlete) versus a diver who is much less active during competition. The endurance athletes depend much more on their energy systems to perform well versus other athletes who depend on correct form.

Physiological Effects

Though numerous physiological effects do exist,[17] the depletion of muscle glycogen stores ranks as one of the top. During normal training, glycogen is the primary source of energy, replenished by a healthy diet. This is no different in individuals with anorexia nervosa. Most anorexics participate in rigorous exercise and need adequate glycogen stores. When not enough carbohydrates are ingested possibly due to the fear of weight gain, this may cause premature fatigue from low glycogen stores.[165] This is when performance may be sacrificed.

Dehydration can also cause many different complications. Bergstrom and Hultman[13] showed that a fluid loss of 5% of the athlete's body weight could result in a 20%-30% decrease in performance. It is also known that fluid loss due to purging can disrupt the electrolyte and acid-base balance of the body which is needed for normal nerve and muscle function.[10] These dehydration effects may be experienced for up to one week after a purging episode.[110] Other side effects may include fatigue, muscle spasms, dizziness, loss of consciousness, irritability, swelling of the hands, generalized bloating, heart palpitations, and decreased coordination and balance.[135]

Other physiological consequences include cardiac arrhythmias. For instance, starvation normally causes hypotrophy of the heart, but pumping performance is retained in all but the most severe inanition.[165] What does occur is electrocardiogram changes (ECG). Swenne and Larsson[165] showed patients with eating disorders had bradycardia, diminished amplitudes of the QRS complex, T wave, and prolongation of the QT interval on the printout of the electrocardiogram, which is in agreement with other studies.[45, 148] Other research has shown that ventricular arrhythmias and cardiac death may be heralded by increased QT duration and QT dispersion[37,154] and these changes have been observed in individuals with eating disorders.[45,43,30, 77] In a follow up study, Swenne[164] looked at the effects of re-feeding. The author found that QT prolongation and dispersion normalized within three days of re-feeding and there were no complications with re-feeding syndrome or electrolyte aberrations in the first two weeks. Other complications include arrhythmia related sudden death, ipecac-induced cardiomyopathy, and coronary artery disease.[57,81]

In addition to the electrolyte and acid-base imbalances due to purging behaviors, aerobic power will likely be affected, as will oxygen consumption. This could stress the circulatory system. As for the skeletal system, anorexic female athletes who also exhibit amenorrhea, increase the likelihood of suffering from stress fractures, due mostly from depleted adipose tissue. It is within this adipose tissue that the body will store most of its estrogen. Without this estrogen, the skeletal system can become osteoporotic. For instance, Siemers et al.[147] showed that in non-athletes aged 20-43 who met the DSM – IIIR for anorexia nervosa, all exhibited decreased lumbar and total body bone mineral density (BMD) versus controls. In relationship to bone loss, Maugars et al.[97] reported that anorexic individuals lose bone as rapidly. They showed bone loss as much as 4%-10% per year, and they were positively associated with osteoporotic fractures when the eating disorder lasted longer than 7-10 years.[97] They further state that young people could have increased BMD if *mild* anorexia nervosa is treated. The question then rises, what happens to BMD when anorexia nervosa is treated? Hotta et al.[71] showed that BMD does not increase to normal range even several years post-recovery from eating disorders. They also still remain a high-risk group for osteoporosis in the future.

Therefore it is crucial to catch the warning signs of eating disorders and disordered eating patterns as soon as possible.

Men and Eating Disorders

Though this book focuses primarily on female sports and athletes, it is still appropriate to touch on men and eating disorders. Different from female athletes, men may tend to suppress their disorder due to the perception that eating disorders are a "female illness".[136,154,128,50,55] Other studies have also shown that males are more satisfied with both the shape and appearance of their bodies and therefore are less likely to develop compensatory eating disorders.[55] Contrary to the belief that eating disorders are strictly a female problem, studies have shown that males have elevated scores (more problematic) on both eating disorder questionnaires versus controls.[47,166,157]

In a retrospective study, Andersen et al.[5] showed that male anorectics and bulimics not only had deficient BMD when compared to normals, but their depressed BMD were lower than aged matched females with eating disorders. They also found that they had lowered testosterone levels in both anorexia nervosa and bulimia nervosa, which would be indicative of lower than normal BMDs. Until this study, only case studies were published with regards to BMD deficiencies in men with eating disorders.[128]

In the last few years, research has surfaced other correlated eating disorder terms which are more associated with men than women. These terms are reverse anorexia, body dysmorphic disorder and muscle dysmorphia.[120,121] Though closely related to eating disorders,[123] they are different. Eating disorders lead individuals to become leaner or smaller, where as the previous three discussed drive the individual to become larger in terms of muscle mass, but overtly lean. This is why the target population for these disorders are body builders.

Though these studies support the notion that males do have eating disorders, they affect females up to 10 times as much as males.[187] Given these reasons, this might be why little information is found with regards to males and eating disorders.

PERSONAL ENCOUNTER:

Before every athletic season begins, a pre-participation physical examination is conducted. In association with physical findings, a detailed history is conducted in the form of a questionnaire. This particular year, I had an athlete who we found out had a history of depression/suicide in her family and that she herself had been treated before coming to my institution. She also indicated that she occasionally drank. Just by looking at and talking to her, you would think she had things all together, but given these answers, and my institutional policy, we referred her along to a psychologist just to serve as a point person if that athlete felt she needed someone to talk to. After the initial visits, the psychologist felt they did not have to meet face to face and a scheduled phone conversation was initiated. Though nothing happened to her through the years that she attended my institution, it is important to note that our institution had a policy in place where we were able to refer this athlete to a specialist from the beginning.

Summary

It is evident that eating disorders do occur in athletics, but a more common occurrence is disordered eating. It remains difficult to perform athletics at high levels when your body is being starved of the nutrition which it needs for fuel. This may be the reason why bulimia is more common in the athletic realm versus frank anorexia. Exercise can also be a purging method just like vomiting and/or laxative usage and over time this can develop into a psychological issue. Therefore it is imperative to recognize the risk factors, signs, and symptoms of both eating disorders and disordered eating.[188,17] When taken to extremes, they can be fatal.

The National Athletic Trainer's Association recently published a position statement on preventing, defecting, and managing disordered eating in Athletes. It gives a plethora of information about disordered eating as well as gives a "heads-up" to the reader on what to look for in athletes who are suspects for this pathology. For instance, two important tables which they included in this manuscript show signs and symptoms of eating disordered athletes. While this information was covered in this chapter, these tables do a great job of putting it all together. They also highlight 6 points on prevention and they are as follows:

1. There needs to be mandatory educational programs for athletes, coaches, certified athletic training, and other athletics should be implemented on an annual basis.

2. All athletes should be educated on the importance of proper nutritional practices to reduce the risk of medical and performance problems associated with prolonged energy and nutrient deprovation.

3. Female athletes should be educated on the health and performance consequences of menstrual irregularities the importance of seeking timely medical intervention at the first sigh if abnormalities.

4. The educational program should be routinely evaluated.

5. Certified Athletic Trainers should be familiar with reputable websites (discussed in a later chapter) that provide factual information on disordered eating, healthy eating, weight-reputation practices.

6. Certified athletic trainers should be familiar with disreputable sites such as pro-am (anoreria) and pro-mia (bulimia), consisting of harmful information devoted to the continuation, promotion, and support of eating disorders that glamorize the deadly disorder.

References

1. Adkins E C, and Keel P K. Does "excessive" or "compulsive" best describe exercise as a symptom of bulimia nervosa? *International Journal of Eating.*

2. American College of Sports Medicine (ACSM). Position stand: The female athlete triad. *Medicine and Science in Sports and Exercise.* 1997;29, i-ix.

3. American Psychiatric Association (APA). *Diagnostic and statistical manual of mental disorders* (4th ed.). Washington, DC: Author; 1994.

4. American Psychiatric Association. *Diagnostic and statistical manual of mental disorders* (4th ed., TR). Washington, DC: American Psychiatric Association; 2000.

5. Andersen AE, Watson T, and Schlechte J. Osteoporosis and osteopenia in men with eating disorders. *The Lancet.* 2000;355(9219):1967-1968.

6. Andersen AE. The diagnosis and treatment of eating disorders in primary care medicine. In: Mehler PS, and Andersen AE (Eds.), *Eating Disorders: A Guide to Medical Care and Complications.* Baltimore, MD: The John Hopkins University Press; 1-26.

7. Baker ER, Mathur RS, Kirk RF, et al. Plasma gonadotrophins, prolactin and steroid hormone concentrations in female runners after along distance run. *Fertility Steril.* 1982;38:38-41.

8. Bates GW, Bates SR, Whitworth NS. Reproductive failure in women who practice weight control. *Fertility Steril.* 1982;37:373-378.

9. Beals KA. Disordered eating among athletes. *A Comprehensive Guide for Health Professionals.* Champaign, IL: Human Kinetics; 2004.

10. Becker AE, Ginsspoon SK, Kilbanski A, and Herzog DB. Eating disorders. *New England Journal of Medicine.* 1999;340:1092-1098.

11. Beitins IZ, McArthur JW, Trunbull BA, Skrinar GS, and Bullen BA. Exercise induces two types of human luteal dysfunction: confirmation by urinary free progesterone. *J Clinical Endorinol Metabolism.* 1991;72: 1350-1358.

12. Bergen H, and Leung PCK. Norepinephrine inhibition of pulsatile LH release: receptor specificity. *American Journal of Physiology.* 1986;<u>250.</u>

13. Bergstrom J, and Hultman E. Nutrition for maximal sports performance. *Journal of the American Medical Association.* 1972;221:999-1006.

14. Beumont, PJV. Clinical presentation of anorexia nervosa and bulimia nervosa. In Fairburn CG, and Brownell KD (Eds.), *Eating Disorders and Obesity: A Comprehensive Handbook* (2nd ed.). New York: The Guilford Press. 2002;162-170.

15. Black DW, Noyes R, Goldstein RB, and Blum N. A family study of obsessive-compulsive disorder. *Archives of General Psychiatry*. 1992;49:362-368.

16. Black DW, Goldstein RB, Noyes R Jr., and Blum N. Compulsive behaviors and obsessive-compulsive disorder (OCD): lack of a relationship between OCD, eating disorders, and gambling. *Comprehensive Psychiatry*. 1994;35(2):145-8.

17. Bonci CM, Bonci LK, Granger LR et al. National Athletic Trainer's Association position statement: preventing, detecting and managing disordered eating in athletics. *Journal of Athletic Training*. 2008;43(1): 80-108.

18. Bonen A, and Keizer HA. Pituitary, ovarian and adrenal hormone responses to marathon running. *International Journal of Sports Medicine*. 1987;8:161-167.

21. Bonen A, Haynes JF, Watson-Wright W, et al. Effects of menstrual cycle on metabolic responses to exercise. *Journal of Applied Physiology*. 1983;55:1506-1513.

22. Boyden TW, Pamenter RW, Stanforth P, et al. Impaired gonadotropin response to gonadotropin releasing hormone stimulation in endurance-trained women. *Fertility Steril*. 1984;41:359-363.

23. Bulik CM. Anxiety, depression, and eating disorders. In Fairburn, CG, and Brownell, KD (Eds.), *Eating Disorders and Obesity: A Comprehensive Handbook* (2nd ed.). New York: The Guilford Press. 2002;193-198.

24. Bulik CM, Sullivan PF, Joyce PR, and Carter FA. Temperament, character, and personality disorder in bulimia nervosa. *Journal of Nervous and Mental Disease*. 1995;183:593-598.

25. Bulik CM, Sullivan PF, Joyce PR, and Carter FA. Initial manifestations of disordered eating behavior: dieting versus bingeing. *International Journal of Eating Disorders*. 1997;22:195-201.

26. Burrows M, and Bird S. The physiology of the highly trained female endurance runner. *Sports Medicine*. 2000;30(4):281-300.

28. Carlat DJ, Camargo CA Jr., Herzog DB. Eating disorders in males: a report on 135 patients. *American Journal of Psychiatry*. 1997;154: 1127-1132.

29.   Casper R. Personality features of women with good outcome from restricting anorexia nervosa. *Psychosom Med.* 1990;52:156-170.

30.   Cooke RA, Chambers JB, Singh R et al. QT interval in anorexia nervosa. *British Heart Journal.* 1994;72: 69-73.

31.   Creatsas G, Salakos N, Averkiou M, Miras K, and Aravantinos D. Endocrinological profile of oligomenorrheic strenuously exercising adolescents. *Journal Gynecol Obstet.* 1992;38:215-221.

32.   Crisp A, Sedgwick P, Halek C, Joughin N, and Humphrey H. Why may teenage girls persist in smoking? *Journal of Adolescence.* 1999;22: 657-672.

33.   Crist AH, Callender JS, Halek C, and George-HSU LK. Long term mortality in anorexia vervosa; a 20 yr follow-up of the St George's and Aberdeen Cohorts. *British Journal of Psychiatry.* 1992;161:104-107.

34.   Cumming DC, Vickovic MM, Wall SR, et al. Defects of pulsatile LH release in normally menstruating runners. *Journal of Clinical Endocrine Metabolism.* 1985;60:810-812.

35.   Cumming DC, Vickovic MM, Wall SR, et al. The effect of acute exercise on pulsatile release of luteinizing hormone in women runners. *American Journal of Obstetics Gynecology.* 1985;153:482-485.

36.   Dale KS, and Landers DM. Weight control in wrestling: eating disorders or disordered eating? *Med. Sci. Sport and Ex.* 1999;31(10):1382-1389.

37.   Day CP, McComb JM, and Campbell WF. QT dispersion: an indication of arrhythmia risk in patients with long QT intervals. *British Heart Journal.* 1990;63:342-344.

38.   De Souza MJ, Miller BE, Loucks AB, et al. High frequency of luteal phase deficiency and anovulation in recreational women runners: blunted elevation in follicle-stimulating hormone observed during luteal-follicular transition. *Journal of Clinical Endocrinol Metabolism.*1988;83: 4220-4232.

      a.   *Disorders, 38, 24-29.*

39.   Dolan B, Evans C, and Norton K. Disordered eating behavior and attitudes in female and male patients with personality disorders. *Journal of Personaliyl Disorders.* 1994;8:17-27.

40.   Drinkwater BL, Loucks A, Sherman RT, Sundgot-Borgen J, and Thompson RA. International Olympic Committee (IOC) consensus statement on the Female Athlete Triad. 2005. Available at: www.olympic.org.

41. Drinkwater BL, Nilson K, Chesnut CH, III, Bremner WJ, Shainholtz S, and Southworth, MB. 1984. Bone mineral content of amenorrheic and eumenorrheic athletes. *New England Journal of Medicine.* 1984;311: 277-281.

42. Dumoulin SC, de Glisezinski I, Saint-Martin F, et al. Hormonal changes related to eating behavior in oligomenorrheic women. *European Journal of Endocrinology.* 1996;135(3):328-34.

43. Durakovic Z, Durakovic A, and Korsic M. Changes of the corrected Q-T interval in the electrocardiogram of patients with anorexia nervosa. *International Journal of Cardiology.* 1994;45:115-120.

44. Eckert Ed, Halmi KA, Marchi P, and Cohen J. Comparison of bulimic and non-bulimic anorexia nervosa patients during treatment. *Psychological Medicine.* 1987;17:891-898.

45. Ellis LB. Electrocardiographic abnormalities in severe malnutrition. *British Heart Journal.* 1946;8:53-61.

46. Ellison PT, and Lager C. Moderate recreational running is associated with lowered salivary progesterone profiles in women. *American Journal of Obstetics Gynecol.* 1986;154:1000-1003.

47. Enns MP, Drewnowski A, and Grinker JA. Body composition, body size estimation, and attitudes towards eating in male college athletes. *Psychosomatic Medicine,* 1987;49:56-64.

48. Epling WF, and Pierce WD (Eds). *Activity Anorexia: Theory, Research and Treatment.* Mahwah, NJ: Erlbaum; 1996.

49. Fabian LJ, and Thompson JK. Body image and eating disturbance in young females. *International Journal Eating Disorders.* 1989;8:63-74.

50. Fairburn and Beglin. Studies of the Epidemiology of Bulimia Nervosa. *American Journal of Psychiatry.* 1990;147(4):401-408.

51. Fairburn CG, and Cooper PJ. Self-induced vomiting and bulimia nervosa: an undetected problem. *British Medical Journal.* 1982;284:1153-1155.

52. Fairburn C G, and Walsh BT. Atypical eating disorders (eating disorders not otherwise specified). In Fairburn CG, and Brownell KD (Eds.). *Eating Disorders and Obesity: A Comprehensive Handbook* (2nd ed.). New York: The Guilford Press. 2002;171-177.

53. Fichter MM, Quadflieg N, and Hedlund S. Twelve year course and outcome predictors of anorexia nervosa. *International Journal of Eating Disorders.* 2006;39(2):87-100.

54. Fogelholm M, and Hilloskorpi H. Weight and diet concerns in Finnish female and male athletes. *Medicine and Science in Sports and Exercise.* 1990;31(2):229-235.

55. Franco KSN, Tambruuion MB, Carroll BT, and Bernal GA. Eating attitudes in college males. *International Journal of Eating Disorders.* 1988;7(2):285-288.

56. Frusztajer NT, Dhuper S, Warren MP, Brooks-Gunn J, and Fox RP. Nutrition and the incidence of stress fractures in ballet dancers. *American Journal of Clinical Nutrition.* 1990;5:779-783.

57. Garcia-Rubira JC, Hidalgo R, Bomez-Barrado JJ, Romero D, Cruz Fernandez J, Anorexia nervosa and myocardial infarction. *International Journal of Cardiology.* 1994;45:138-140.

58. Garfinkel PE, and Garner DM. *Anorexia nervosa: A multidimensional perspective.* New York: Brunner/Mazel; 1982.

59. Garner DM, and Bemis KM. A cognitive-behavioral approach to anorexia nervosa. *Cognitive Therapy and Research.* 1982;6:123-150.

61. Garner DM, and Garfinkel PE. *Handbook of Treatment for Eating Disorders.* NY: Guilford Press; 1997.

62. Garner DM, Garner MV, and Rosen LR. Anorexia nervosa "restrictors" who purge: implications for sub-typing anorexia nervosa. *International Journal of Eating Disorders.* 1993;13:171-185.

63. Garner DM, Olmsted MP, and Plivy. Development and validation of a multi-dimensional eating disorder inventory for anorexia nervosa and bulimia. *International Journal of Eating Disorders.* 1983;2:15-34.

64. Garner DM, Olmsted MP, Bohr Y, and Garfinkel PE. The eating attitudes test: psychometric features and clinical correlates. *Psychological Medicine.* 1982;12:871-878.

65. Green GA, Uryasz FD, Petr TA, and Bray CD. NCAA study of substance use and abuse habits of college student-athletes. *Clinical Journal of Sport Medicine.* 2001;11:51-56.

66. Grilo CM, Sanislow CA, Skodol AE et al. Do eating disorders co-occur with personality disorders? Comparison groups matter. *International Journal of Eating Disorders.* 2003;33:155-164.

67. Halmi KA, Eckert E, Marchi P, Sampugnaro V, Apple R, and Cohen J. Comorbidity of psychiatric diagnoses in anorexia nervosa. *Archives of Genral Psychiatry.* 1991;48:712-718.

68. Hewitt PL, Coren S, and Steel GD. Death from anorexia nervosa: age span and sex differences. Aging and mental Health. 2001;5(1):41-6.

69. Holland AJ, Sicotte N, and Treasure J. Anorexia nervosa: evidence for a genetic basis. *Journal of Psychosomatic Research.* 1998;32:561-571.

70. Hopkinson RA, and Lock J. Athletics, perfectionism, and disordered eating. *Eating & Weight Disorders.* 2004;9(2):99-106.

71. Hotta M, Shibasake T, Sato K, and Demura H. The importance of body weight history in the occurrence and recovery of osteoporosis in patients with anorexia nervosa: evaluation by dual X-ray absorptiometry and bone metabolic markers. *European Journal of Endocrinology.* 1998;139:276-283.

72. Hsu LKG. *Eating disorders.* New York: Guilford Press; 1990.

73. Hudson JI, Pope HG, Yurgelun-Todd D, Jonas JM, and Frankenburg FR. A controlled study of lifetime prevalence of affective and other psychiatric disorders in bulimic outpatients. *American Journal of Psychiatry.* 1987;144:1283-1287.

74. Ilhe R, and Loucks AB. Dose-response relationships between energy availability and bone turnover in young exercising women. *Journal of Bone Mineral Research,* 2004;19:1231-1240.

75. International Olympic Committee Medical Commission. Consensus statement on the female athlete triad. Available at: www.olympic.org. Accessed November 2005.

76. Byrne S, and McdLean N. Elite athletes: effects of the pressure to be thin. *Journal of Sports Science and Medicine.* 2002;5:80-94.

77. Isner JM, Roberts WC, Heymsfield SB, and Yager J. Anorexia nervosa and sudden death. *Annals of Internal Medicine.* 198;5102:49-52.

78. Johnson CJ. Current challenges in recognizing and treating eating disorders. *Minnesota Medicine.* 2003;86(11):34-39.

79. Johnson Cr, Crosby R, and Engel S et al. Gender, ethnicity, self-esteem and disordered eating among college athletes. *Eating Behaviors.* 2004;5:147-156.

81. Joy E. Cardiac concerns. In: Ireland ML, and Nattiv A (Eds.). *The Female Athlete.* Philadelphia, PA: Saunders; 2002:271-281.

82. Joyce JM, Warren DL, Humphries LL, Smith AJ, and Coon, JS. Osteoporosis in women with eating disorders: Comparison of physical

parameters, exercise, and menstrual status with SPA and DPA evaluation. *Journal of Nuclear Medicine*. 1990;31:325-331.

83. Kanis JA, Melton LJ, Christiansen C, Johnston CC, and Khattaev N. The diagnosis of osteoporosis. *Journal of Bone and Mineral Research*. 1994;9:1137-1141.

85. Katz JC. Clinical observation on the physical activity in anorexics. In: *Activity Anorexia* by Epling F, and Pierce D. Lawrence Erlbaum Associates; 1996.

87. Keys AJ, Brozek J, Henschel A, Mickelsen O, and Taylor HL. *The Biology of Human Starvation (vol.2)*. Minneapolis: University of Minnesota Press; 1950.

89. Kirk G, Singh K, and Getz H. Risk of eating disorders among female college athletes and nonathletes. *Journal of college counseling*; Fall, 2001;4(2):122.

90. Loucks, AB. Energy availability, not body fatness, regulates reproductive function in women. *Exercise and Sport Sciences Reviews*. 2003;31: 144-148.

91. Loucks AB, and Horvath SM. Athletic amenorrhea: a review. *Medicine and Science in Sport and Exercise*. 1985;17:56-72.

95. Malina RM, Bouchard C, and Bar-Or. Growth, Maturation, and Physical Activity (2nd ed.). Champaign, IL: Human Kinetics; 2004.

99. Milos G, Spindler A, Buddenberg C, and Crameri, A. Axis I and II comorbidity and treatment experiences in eating disorder subjects. *Psychotherapy and Psychosomatics*. 2003;72:276-285.

101. Mitchell JE, Hatsukami D, Eckert ED, and Pyle RL. Characteristics of 275 patients with bulimia. *American Journal of Psychiatry*. 1985;142:482-485.

102. National Collegiate Athletic Association (2005). *NCAA coaches handbook: Managing the female athlete triad*. Indianapolis, IN: The National Collegiate Athletic Association.

103. National Collegiate Athletic Association (2007). *Managing student-athlete's mental health issues*. Indianapolis, IN: The National Collegiate Athletic Association.

104. National Osteoporosis Foundation. (2003, February). *Disease statistics*. Retrieved October 7, 2005, from http://www.nof.org/osteoporosis/stats.html.

105. Nattiv A, Loucks AB, Manore MM, et al. The American College of Sports Medicine. Position Statement on the Female Athlete Triad. *Medicine and Science in Sports and Exercise.* October 2007;39(10):1867-1882.

106. Neims DM, McNeill J, Giles TR, and Todd F. Incidence of laxative misuse in community and bulimic populations: A descriptive review. *International Journal of Eating Disorders.* 1995;17:211-228.

112. Otis C, and Goldingay R. *Campus health Guide: The College Student's Handbook for Healthy Living.* New York: College Board; 1989.

113. Otis CL, and Goldingay R. *The Athletic Woman's Survival Guide.* Champaign, IL: Human Kinetics; 2000.

114. Palmer RL, and Oppenheimer R. Childhood sexual experiences with adults: a comparison of women with eating disorders and those with other diagnoses. *International Journal of Eating Disorders.* 1992;12(4):359.

115. Palmer RL, Oppenheimer R, Kignon A, Chaloner DA, and Howells K. Childhood sexual experiences with adults reported by women with eating disorders: an extended series. *British Journal of Psychiatry.* 1990;156:699-703.

117. Patton GC, Selzer R, Coffey C, Carlin JB, and Wolfe R. Onset of adolescent eating disorders: population based cohort study over 3 years. *British Medical Jorunal.* 1999;318(7186):765-768.

118. Petri TR. Disordered eating in female collegiate gymnasts: Prevalence and personality/attitudinal correlates. *Journal of Sport & Exercise Psychology.* 1993;15:424-436.

121. Polivy J, and Herman CP. Diagnosis and treatment of normal eating. *Journal of Consulting and Clinical Psychology.* 1987;55:635-644.

122. Pope HG, and Katz DL. Anorexia nervosa and "reverse anorexia" among 108 male body builders. *Comparative psychiatry.* 1993;34: 406-409.

123. Pope HG, and Katz DL. Psychiatric and medical effects of anabolic-androgenic steroid use: A controlled study of 160 athlete4s. *Archives of General Psychiatry.* 1994;51:375-382.

125. Pope HG, Gruber AJ, Mangweth B, et al. Body image perception among men in 3 countries. *A. J. Psychiatry.*August 2000;157(8): 1297-1301.

126. Powers PS. Eating disorders: Cardiovascular risks and management. In: Mehler PS, and Andersen AE (Eds.) *Eating Disorders: A Guide*

to Medical Care and Management. Baltimore: The Johns Hopkins University Press; 1999:100-117.

127.   Powers, P. S., & Thompson, R. A. (2008). *The exercise balance.* Carlsbad, CA: Gurze Books.

128.   Raglin JS, and Wilson GS. Overtraining in athletes. In: Hanin Y (Ed.) *Emotions in Sports.* Champaign, IL: Human Kinetics; 2000:191-207.

131.   Rigotti NA, Neer RM, and Jameson L. Osteopenia and bone fracture in a man with anorexia and hypogonadism. *Journal of the American Medical Association.* 1986;256:385-388.

132.   Rodin J, and Larson L. Social factors and the ideal body shape. In: Brownell KD, Rodin J, Wilmore JH, eds. Eating, body weight, and performance in athletes: disorders of Modern Society. Philadelphia, PA: Lea and Febiger; 1992:146-158.

133.   Rosen LW, and Hough DO. Pathogenic weight-control behaviors of female college gymnasts. *Physician and Sportsmedicine.* 1988;16:141-146.

134.   Rosen LW, McKeag DB, Hough DO, and Curley V. Pathogenic weight-control behavior in female athletes. *Physician Sportsmedicine.* 1986;14(1):79-86.

135.   Rosenberg M. *Society and the Adolescent Self-Image.* Princeton, NJ: Princeton University Press; 1965.

137.   Sanford-Martens, Davidson MM, Yakushko OF, Martens MP, Hinton P, and Beck N. Clinical and subclinical eating disorders: An examination of collegiate athletes. *Journal of Applied Sport Psychology,* 17:79-86.

138.   Sansone RA, and Sansone LA. Bulimia nervosa: medial complications. In: Alexander-Mott L, Lumsden DB (eds.) *Understanding Eating Disorders: Anoerxia Nervosa, Bulimia Nervosa and Obesity.* Washington, DC: Taylor and Francis; 1994:181-201.

139.   Schneider JA, and Agras WS. Bulimia in males: a matched comparison with females. *International Journal of Eating Disorders.* 1987;6(2): 235-242.

141.   Schwitzer AM, Rodriguez LE, Thomas C, and Salimi L. The Eating Disorder NOS diagnostic profile among college women. *Journal of American College Health.* 2001;49:157-166.

142.   Secord PF, and Jourard SM. The appraisal of body cathexis: Body cathexis and the self. *Journal of Consulting Psychology.* 1953;17:343-347.

144.   Seigel K, and Hetta J. Exercise and eating disorder symptoms among young females. *Eating and Weight Disorders.* 2001;6:32-39.

145.   Sher C. Possible genetic link between eating disorders and seasonal changes in mood and behavior. *Medical Hypotheses*. November 2001;57(5):609-611.

147.   Sherman RT, Thompson RA. The female athlete triad. *Journal of School Nursing*. August 2004;20(4):197-202.

148.   Sherman RT, DeHass D, Thompson RA (in press), and Wilfert M. (2005) NCAA coaches survey: The role of the coach in identifying and managing athletes with disordered eating. *Eating Disorders: The Journal of Treatment and Prevention*; *13*, 447-466.

150.   Siemers B, Chakmakjian Z, and Gench B. Bone density patterns in women with anorexia nervosa. *International Journal of Eating Disorders*. 1996;19(2):179-186.

151.   Simonson E, Henschel A, and Keys A. The electrocardiogram of man in semistarvation and subsequent rehabilitation. *American Heart Journal*, 1948;35:584-602.

152.   Skodol AE, Oldham JM, Hyler SE, Kellman, HD, Doidge N, and Davies M. Comorbidity of DSM-III-R eating disorders and personality disorders. *International Journal of Eating Disorders*. 1993;14:403-416.

153.   Smolack L, Murnen S, and Ruble AE. Female athletes and eating problems: a meta-analysis. *International Journal of Eating Disorders*. 2000;27:371-380.

154.   Snow-Harter CM. Bone health and prevention of osteoporosis in active and athletic women. *Clinics in Sports Medicine*. 1994;13:389-404.

156.   Spurrell BE, Wilfley DE, Tanofsky MB, and Brownell KD. Age of onset for binge eating: are there different pathways to binge eating? *International Journal of Eating Disorders*. 1996;21(1):55-65.

157.   Statters DJ, Mlik M, Wark DE, and Camm AJ. QT dispersion: problems of methodology and clinical significance. *Journal of Cardiovascular Electrophysiology*. 1994;5:672-685.

158.   Stice E, Killen JD, Hayward C, and Taylor CB. Age of onset for binge eating and purging during late adolescence: a 4-year survival analysis. *Journal of Abnormal Psychology*. 1998;107(4):671-675.

159.   Strober M, Lampert C, Morrell W, Burroughs J, and Jacobs C. A controlled family study of anorexia nervosa: evidence of familial aggression and lack of shared transmission with affective disorders. *International Journal of Eating Disorders*. 1990;9:239-253.

161. Sundgot-Borgen J. Nutrient intake of female elite athletes suffering from eating disorders. *International Journal of Sport Nutrition*. 1993;3(4):431-442.

162. Sundgot-Borgen J. Prevalence of eating disorders in elite female athletes. *International Journal of Sport Nutrition*. 1993;3:29-40.

163. Sundgot-Borgen J. Risk and trigger factors for the development of eating disorders in female elite athletes. *Medicine & Science in Sports & Exercise*. 1994;26(4):414-419.

164. Sundgot-Borgen J, and Corbin CB. Eating disorders among female athletes. *Physician and Sportsmedicine*. 1987;15(2):89-95.

165. Sundgot-Borgen J, and Larsen S. Pathogenic weight-control methods and self-reporting eating disorders in female elite athletes and controls. *Scand. J. Med. Sci Sports*. 1993;3:150-155.

166. Sundgot-Borgen J, and Torstveit MK. Prevalence of eating disorders in elite athletes is higher than in the general population. *Clinical Journal of Sport Medicine*. 2004;14(1):25-32.

167. Swenne I. Heart risk associated with weight loss in anorexia nervosa and eating disorders: electrocardiographic changes during the early phase of refeeding. *Acta Paediatrica*. 2000;89(4):447-452.

168. Swenne I. Larsson PT. Heart risk associated with weight loss in anorexia nervosa and eating disorders: risk factors for QTc interval prolongation and dispersion. Acta Paediatrica. 88(3):304-9, 1999.

169. Thiel AH, Gottfried H, and Hesse FW. Subclinical eating disorders in male athletes. *Acta Psychiatr. Scand*. 1993;88:259-265.

170. Thompson RA, and Sherman RT. *Helping Athletes with Eating Disorders*. Champaign, IL: Human Kinetics; 1993.

171. Thompson RA, and Sherman RT. Good athlete" traits and characteristics of anorexia nervosa: Are they similar? *Eating Disorders: The Journal of Treatment and Prevention*. 1999a;7:181-190.

172. Thompson RA, and Sherman RT. Athletes, athletic performance, and eating disorders: Healthier alternatives. *Journal of Social Issues*. 1999b; 55:317-337.

174. Vitousek K and Manke, F. Personality variables and disorders in anorexia nervosa and bulimia nervosa. *Journal of Abnormal Psychology*. 1994;103:137-147.

175. Wade T, Martin NG, Neale MC, et al. The structure of genetic and environmental risk factors for three measures of disordered eating. *Psychological Medicine*. 1999;29:925-934, 1990.

177. Walsh B T. Binge eating bulimia nervosa. In Fairburn CG, and Wilson CT (Eds.) *Binge Eating: Nature, Assessment, and Treatment*. New York: Guilford Press, 1993; 37-49.

178. Waters BGH, Beaumont PJV, Touyz S, and Kennedy M. Behavioral differences between twin and non-twin female sibling pairs discordant for anorexia nervosa. *Int J Eat Disord*. 1990;9:265-273.

179. Weight LM, and Noakes TD. Is running an analogue of anorexia? A survey of the incidence of eating disorders in female distance runners. *Medicine and Science in Sports and Exercise*. 1987;19:213-217.

180. Wells, CL. Women, sport and performance: a physiological perspective (2nd ed.). Champaign (IL): Human Kinetics; 1991.

183. Wildes JE, Simons AD, and Marcus MD. Bulimic symptoms, cognitions, and body dissatisfaction in women with major depressive disorder. *International Journal of Eating Disorders*. 2005;38:9-17.

184. Wilmore JH. Body weight standards and athletic performance. In: Brownell KD, Rodin J, and Wilmore J (Eds.) *Eating, Body Weight and Performance in Athletes: Disorders of Modern Society*. Philadelphia: Lea & Febiger. 1992;315-329.

185. Wilson GT. Eating disorders and addictive disorders. In: Fairburn CG, and Brownell KD (Eds.) *Eating Disorders and Obesity: A Comprehensive Handbook* (2nd ed.). New York: The Guilford Press. 2002;199-203.

186. Wiseman CV, Turco RM, Sunday SR, and Halmi KA. Smoking and body image concerns in adolescent girls. *International Journal of Eating Disorders*. 1998;24:429-433.

187. Wonderlich SA. Personality and eating disorders. In Fairburn CG, and Brownell KD (Eds.) *Eating disorders and obesity: A comprehensive handbook* (2nd ed.). New York: The Guilford Press; 204-209.

188. Wonderlich SA, Crosby RD, Mitchell JE, et al. Relationship of childhood sexual abuse and eating disturbance in children. *Journal of American Academy of Child Adolescent Psychiatry*. 2000;39(10):1277-1283.

189. World Health Organization (WHO). The ICD-10 classification of mental and behavioral disorders: Clinical descriptions and diagnostic guidelines. Geneva: Author; 1992.

190.   Yates A. Biologic consideration in the etiology of eating disorders. *Pediatric Annals*. 1992;21:739-744.

191.   Yeager KK, Agostini R, Nattiv A, and Drinkwater B. The female athlete triad. *Medicine and Science in Sports and Exercise*. 1993;25:775-777.

192.   Yesalis CE, Barsukiewicz CK, Kopstein AN, and Bahrke MS. Trends in anabolic-androgenic steroid use among adolescents. *Archives of Pediatrics and Adolescent Medicine*. 1997;151:1197-1206.

CHAPTER 6

Amenorrhea and the Physiology of the Menstrual Cycle

John Storment, MD, Mike Brunet, PhD, ATC, CPT, STS

Introduction

Historically, many societies viewed a woman's menstrual cycle in a positive ligh. For example:

- The ancient Greeks believed that the wisdom of men and gods was centered in the blood that came from his mother. Post-menopausal women were often considered the wisest because they retained their "wise blood."

- In many ancient societies, menstrual blood carried authority, transmitting lineage of the clan or tribe. Among the Ashanti tribe in Africa, female children are more prized than male because a girl is the "carrier of the blood."

- Chinese sages called menstrual blood the essence of Mother Earth, the principle of giving life to all things.

- Easter eggs, the classic womb symbol, were dyed red and laid on graves to strengthen the dead.

- A born-again ceremony from Australia shows the aborigines linked rebirth with the blood of the womb.

However, menstruation has not always been viewed positively in society:

- Between the 8th and 11th centuries, Christian churches refused communion to menstruating women.

- In the late 17th century, the psychological disturbance termed *hysteria* (the root word *hyster-* comes from the Greek word for "womb") was originally believed to be a disease of women and resulted from some disturbance in the uterus.

- In the 1600s, post-menopausal women were constantly persecuted for witchcraft because it was believed their menstrual blood remained in their veins.[54]

- The Torah prohibits Jewish men from having sexual relations with menstruating women and Orthodox Jewish tradition requires the physical separation of husband and wife during menstruation for a period lasting approximately 12 days.[82]

Today we know that the regulation of the menstrual cycle is a well-ordered series of events involving changes in hormones secreted by the hypothalamus gland, the pituitary gland, and the ovary. This chapter first reviews the hormonal changes and interaction between the brain and the ovary required to produce a mature oocyte, or egg. The chapter then reviews how these hormonal changes affect the uterine lining or endometrium. Finally, it discusses normal menses and different patterns of abnormal menstrual bleeding.

Regulation of the Menstrual Cycle

To best understand the menstrual cycle, it is helpful to divide it into three phases: the follicular phase, usually from cycle days 1–13; ovulation, which typically takes place on cycle day 13 or 14; and the luteal phase occurring on cycle days 14–28. Each phase is characterized by changes in hormonal secretions with the final goal of releasing a mature oocyte and creating a nurturing environment in the uterus for implantation of an embryo, or fertilized egg. The duration and timing of each phase can vary between women and even in the same woman.

The Follicular Phase

The follicular phase of the menstrual cycle begins with the onset of menstruation, cycle day 1, and continues through approximately cycle day 13. During this phase, the ovaries contain multiple immature oocytes (eggs) called *primordial follicles*. Each group of primordial follicles has been growing for approximately three months before the follicular phase begins. When the time comes for them to develop into more mature eggs, a series of hormonal changes occurs that allows only one dominant follicle to mature and be released.

The hypothalamus, a region of the brain which functions to regulate body temperature and some metabolic processes, releases a hormone called gonadotropin releasing hormone (GnRH) which then stimulates the pituitary gland to release two other hormones: follicle stimulating hormone (FSH), which stimulates the primordial follicles to develop, and luteinizing hormone (LH), which stimulates the dominant follicle to be released. In the first few days of the follicular phase of the menstrual cycle, the follicle destined to release the egg, or ovulate, is recruited. Although the other follicles may grow a little, it is this dominant follicle which will grow the most and release, usually by cycle day 14. During this follicular phase, the dominant follicle begins to produce estrogen, while the other follicles undergo a process called apoptosis, or programmed cell death. This complex interaction between the follicles occurs in order to prevent multiple eggs being released each month, potentially resulting in twins, triplets, or higher order gestation. The dominant follicle continues to be dependent on FSH as well as multiple other proteins called growth factors. In the presence of all of the growth factors, the estrogen level continues to increase peaking approximately 24–36 hours prior to ovulation.[63] When peak estrogen levels are achieved, LH begins to increase. This LH surge will then stimulate the mature (dominant) follicle to begin to release.

Ovulation

Ovulation typically occurs on cycle day 13 or 14 of the menstrual cycle, although considerable variation in timing exists from cycle to cycle, even in the same woman. Usually, ovulation occurs 10–12 hours after the LH peak and 24–36 hours after peak estrogen levels are attained.[90] The onset of the LH surge is the most reliable indicator of impending ovulation, occurring 34–36 hours prior to the release of the egg[40] and typically lasting 48–50 hours.[63]

The actual release of the egg is not an explosive event, but rather a series of changes which cause the final maturation of the egg and the breakdown of the follicular wall. The process by which the egg matures is called meiosis. Prior to the LH surge, the growth of the egg has been temporarily arrested. With the LH surge, meiosis resumes and will be completed only when fertilized by a sperm. Up until this point, estrogen has been the dominant hormone released by the ovary during the follicular phase. In fact, the follicular phase is sometimes called the estrogenic phase. As LH surges, estrogen levels begin to decrease and progesterone, the other main ovarian hormone, increases. Progesterone is useful in stimulating the follicular wall to become more elastic and fill with more fluid. When the wall becomes thin and stretched, multiple enzymes are released which disrupts the follicular wall. The fully developed preovulatory follicle is approximately 20 mm in diameter. The smooth muscle cells which surround the follicle begin to contract and the oocyte (egg) is then freed from the follicle. The release of the egg also requires prostaglandins[30,50] and patients who are attempting pregnancy should avoid drugs that inhibit prostaglandins, such as ibuprofen (Motrin) or aspirin.[62,68]

Luteal Phase

Before rupture of the follicle and release of the egg, the cells contained within the follicle (called granulosa cells) begin to enlarge and accumulate a yellow pigment called lutein. Once the egg is released, the dominant follicle then becomes the corpus luteum, which means "yellow body." The corpus luteum is the main source of progesterone which is the dominant hormone in the luteal phase (usually days 14–28). Progesterone levels rise sharply after ovulation reaching a peak approximately eight days after the LH surge.[32]

A negative feedback system prevents new follicles from growing at this time. The high levels of estrogen and progesterone signal the hypothalamus and the pituitary gland to reduce FSH and LH production prohibiting the growth of new follicles. This system is important to allow progesterone production to continue and potentially support a pregnancy if the egg is fertilized. If the egg is not fertilized, estrogen and progesterone production sharply decrease and FSH is then allowed to begin stimulation of another group of primordial follicles for the next cycle.

There are many factors that affect the recruitment of new follicles. Primarily, a woman must have an adequate reserve of competent eggs. As women age, the number of remaining ovarian follicles decline and becomes less sensitive to FSH. This results in decreased fertility with advancing age. Other hormones such as Inhibin B can have a profound effect on whether the eggs are healthy enough to be fertilized.[87] Figure 6-1 shows the various stages of the menstrual cycle graphically.

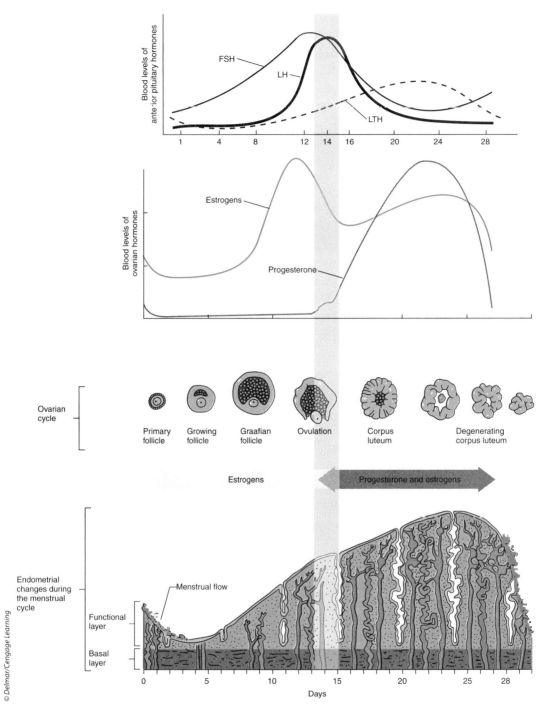

Figure 6-1 The menstrual cycle

Uterine Bleeding

As mentioned earlier, the follicular phase of the menstrual cycle begins with the onset of menstruation, or uterine bleeding. During the menstrual cycle, the endometrium, or lining of the uterus, undergoes several changes. These changes can be categorized into five phases:

1. menstrual endometrium
2. proliferative phase
3. secretory phase
4. preparation for implantation
5. endometrial breakdown.

The endometrium itself is divided into two layers: the functionalis (upper two-thirds *of the uterus*) and the basalis (lower third *of the uterus*). The functionalis is the layer that changes throughout the cycle and prepares for implantation to occur. This is also the layer that is sloughed, or shed, if implantation does not occur. The basalis layer is generally stable and provides support to regenerate the endometrium phase following menstrual sloughing of the functionalis (see Figure 6-1).

During the menstrual endometrium phase, which occurs during the follicular phase of the menstrual cycle, the endometrium is characterized by relatively thin but dense tissue that sheds due to the hormonal changes taking place, most notably the decrease in estrogen and progesterone and the increases in FSH and LH. Rapid loss of tissue during the first few days of menstruation generally indicates a shorter duration of flow. Delayed or incomplete shedding is associated with heavier flow and greater blood loss. Typically after five or six days of uterine bleeding, the entire cavity has sloughed and regenerated allowing for new endometrial growth.

The proliferative endometrium phase correlates with the follicular phase of the menstrual cycle and increasing estrogen levels. During proliferation, the endometrium grows from approximately 0.5 mm–5.0 mm in height. The maximum thickness of the lining occurs when the estrogen level is highest.

The secretory phase begins after ovulation. The endometrium is now under the influence of both estrogen and progesterone. During this phase, microscopic changes occur that will make the lining more hospitable for implantation of an embryo to occur.

Implantation usually occurs 7–10 days after ovulation (days 21–24 of the menstrual cycle). During this phase, there is an increase in the blood supply to the endometrium. If no implantation occurs during this time, estrogen and progesterone production begins to decrease and the endometrium begins to break down.

Endometrial breakdown begins about three days before menstruation (day 25 of the cycle) as the height and blood flow in the endometrium begins to decrease. Multiple proteins and enzymes are activated to facilitate the changes in preparation for menstruation. Normal clotting factors, for instance, are essential to ensure that menstrual flow eventually stops. Some women with abnormal clotting factors have extreme, and sometimes life threatening, menstruation. Menstrual flow ceases when the arteries in the endometrium constrict and estrogen begins to increase, causing a repair and regrowth of the lining.

The Normal Menstrual Cycle

Rate of blood flow, length of uterine bleeding, and overall length of the menstrual cycle are indicators of normal menses. Women with normal menstruation expel approximately 50% of the menstrual flow during the first 24 hours. The normal volume of menstrual blood loss is 30 ml, or about 1 ounce. More than 80 ml is considered abnormal. If the rate of flow is great, clotting and passing of large clots can occur. The usual duration of flow is 4–6 days, but many women routinely flow as little as two days and as long as eight days, and are still considered to have normal cycles.

In general, variations in menstrual cycle length reflect differences in the length of the follicular phase. Women who have a 25-day cycle ovulate on or about cycle day 10–12, and those with a 35-day cycle ovulate around day 21–22. (A simplified method to determine when a woman is ovulating is to subtract 14 days from the usual interval of the menstrual cycle; this is the ideal time for conception to occur.) Only 15% of cycles in reproductive women are actually 28 days in length.[55] Most women (80%) will have regular cycles that last between 24–35 days, but at least 20% of women will experience irregular cycles.[9]

Menstrual cycle length is also determined by the rate and quality of the growth of the oocytes and it is normal for the cycle to vary in individual women.[83] Cycle lengths are shortest with the least variability when a woman is in her late 30s.[45] The luteal phase is almost always 13–14 days, but the follicular phase begins to shorten when fewer follicles are growing which happens as women age. When the total number of follicles decreases to about 25,000 (usually around age 37–38),[31] a more rapid loss of oocytes begins and continues until the supply of follicles is depleted with the onset of menopause.[71] When this occurs the cycle length begins to shorten.

Variations in menstrual flow and cycle length are common at the extremes of reproductive age, during the early teenage years and the years preceding menopause. The onset of menses (called menarche) usually occurs around age 11–14. The first 5–6 years of menstruation usually consists of relatively long periods of bleeding which decrease naturally over time and become more regular. Around age 40, the cycle length decreases and is less variable. Over the next 8–10 years (before menopause), the cycle length and variability increase.

Average cycle length is also greater in women at the extremes of body mass and composition; both high and low body mass index are associated with an increased cycle length.

Abnormal Patterns of Menstruation

While the majority of women experience normal menses in terms of blood flow, duration, and cycle length, many women experience abnormal menstruation patterns. These include amenorrhea, oligomenorrhea, menorrhagia, and metrorrhagia.

Amenorrhea is the absence of menstruation for more than one year. This can be caused by failure to ovulate. Ovulation disorders are very common but can be present during times of great stress upon the body (such as anorexia and prolonged and unusually heavy exercise). Women who do not menstruate should always be evaluated by a physician to determine the cause as amenorrhea can be associated with a tumor of the pituitary gland.

Oligomenorrhea describes a menstrual cycle with intervals greater than 35 days. Women with unusually long cycles typically have a problem with regular ovulation. If the interval is prolonged greater than 3–4 months on a consistent basis, a woman should seek evaluation by her gynecologist for treatment options to better control the erratic bleeding.

Menorrhagia describes regular menstrual cycle intervals, but excessive flow or duration. This abnormality is very common but can be potentially harmful. Early identification and treatment is essential to ensure a woman does not become anemic as this can affect normal daily function. The vast majority of heavy menses in the reproductive age woman is from hormonal problems with ovulation. However menorrhagia can be due to endometrial hyperplasia (precancer) or cancer and should be evaluated with an ultrasound or office endometrial biopsy when it occurs in women over 35–40 years old. In younger women, especially those just starting menstruation, it is essential to rule out a bleeding disorder such as von Willebrands disease (although rare).[1,64] Other causes of heavy bleeding include conditions such as uterine fibroids (benign muscle tissue tumors) uterine polyps (benign growths in the uterus), endometritis (infection within the uterus) or adenomyosis (when the endometrium invades the muscle layer of the uterus).

Metrorrhagia describes a menstrual cycle of regular intervals with excessive flow or duration. These women often have problems with regular ovulation, but can also have similar abnormalities as those described in women with menorrhagia. These women bleed between normal cycles at unpredictable times. If this persists over a few months, the woman should be evaluated by a gynecologist to ensure that there is no underlying medical problem.

Treatments for Abnormal Menstruation

For many women, abnormal menstruation patterns can be improved with the use of oral contraceptives. This treatment supplies the hormones, estrogen and progesterone in the physiologic concentrations and at the proper time of the cycle. Other methods of controlling abnormal bleeding include progesterone injections, vaginal hormone contraception, or even transdermal hormone contraception (skin patches which deliver hormones similar to the birth control pill). Nonsteroidal anti-inflammatory drugs (NSAIDS) such as ibuprofen (Motrin) or naproxen are often used to reduce blood loss. In general, 400 mg–800 mg of Motrin taken 2–3 times a day can decrease blood loss by up to 40%.[38,78] Side effects are few because it is not necessary to treat for greater than a few days.

Although most patterns of abnormal menstruation can be easily treated, it is still essential for a thorough evaluation by a gynecologist to ensure more serious pathology is not present.

Hormones and Exercise

Exercise can induce changes in hormonal patterns without eliciting any changes in the menstrual cycle. For instance, Cumming et al.[17,18] and Loucks et al.[48] both found reduced LH pulse frequency in athletes who were normally menstruating, but found conflicting results with LH pulse amplitude. Cumming et al.[17,18] further stated that there appeared to be a central inhibition of the hypothalamic-pituitary-gonadal axis in eumenorrheic runners. This shows that there does not have to be disruptions in the menstrual cycle in order for changes to occur.

Other studies have shown short luteal phases in eumenorrheic athletes.[28,48,66] This short luteal phase translates into lower than normal progesterone levels and the interval between ovulation and menstruation onset is disrupted. De Souza et al.[20] conducted a comprehensive study looking at shortened luteal phases in athletes. They found that 43% of the cycles in the runners had luteal phase deficiencies and 12% of the cycles were anovulatory. They also found that the subjects with decreased luteal phases had lower FSH levels during the last five days of the previous cycle and lower mid-cycle LH levels. Beitins et al.[7] showed that initiation of strenuous endurance training in previously ovulating untrained women could induce menstrual changes. These changes lead to corpus luteum dysfunction, which was associated with insufficient free progesterone excretion. They also found short luteal phase cycles with decreased luteal phase length and a delay in the ovulatory LH peak.[7]

Oligomenorrhea and Hormones

With regards to the relationship between LH and oligomenorrhea, low, normal, and elevated LH levels have been reported in individuals who practice weight control.[6] It also appears that LH pulses are significantly affected with dietary restriction.[22] For instance, Dumoulin et al.[49] conducted a study showing the hormonal changes in relation to eating disorders. Their sample consisted of 74 oligomenorrheic individuals who were divided up into two groups. These two groups consisted of subjects who were classified as having an eating disorder (they scored above a 20 on the EAT and then had a follow-up psychological evaluation) and those who did not have an eating disorder. Their control group consisted of 18 normal cycling individuals. They showed that their eating disorder group had an increased variability in both LH and testosterone levels when compared to the controls. LH variability and lower testosterone levels were also found in individuals who had a low calorie intake but did not have an eating disorder.

Creatsas et al.[16] looked at the endocrinological profile of oligomenorrheic ballet dancers (ages 17–18) that were currently engaging in strenuous exercise. They found that LH serum baseline levels were significantly lower when compared to the control group. The control group in this study was matched for everything except that they were not strenuous exercisers. The strenuous exercisers were found to be anovulatory while the control group had ovulation cycles. The authors offered low LH basic serum levels as well as impaired FSH/LH ratio as the culprit. The authors also found that the subjects who started this type of exercise early had delayed menarche. The decreased LH secretion is in agreement with Schweiger et al.[76] Their study used 22 normal weight women with bulimia nervosa (BN), 16 of which had reported menstrual dysfunction and 6 had not had a menstrual cycle in three months. The authors found that individuals who fit the BN criteria and were of normal weight were associated with an increased rate of ovarian dysfunction, and the decreased pulsatile LH secretion appears to be an important factor along with increased cortisol levels, which might also play a role in the gonadal dysfunction in BN.[76]

Excessive Exercise and Hormones

With regards to hormonal changes and excessive exercise, females tend to have low levels of LH[81] that may be responsible for poor luteal function.[18,48,85] This is in contrast with other research that has shown conflicting results on changes in LH and FSH during exercise.[4,11] Boyden et al.[13] showed that the response of gonadotrophins to a gonadotrophin-releasing-hormone stimulation might be impaired in eumenorrheic endurance runners that were placed on a progressive running protocol for one year. The authors further concluded that endurance training of women is associated with frequent alterations in normal menstrual function and that the impaired gonadotropin response to releasing hormone stimulation is one important mechanism for these menstrual changes.[8]

The decrease in LH in female athletes that have engaged in daily physical exercise may be explained by inhibiting and facilitation neurotransmitters in the brain of ovariectomized rats.[10] For instance, this type of exercise increases the levels of cortisol and noradrenaline, which has been shown to alter the turnover of neurotransmitters in the brain, and ultimately inhibits pulsatile release of LH in rats.[10] This pulsatile release of LH may disappear completely in eumenorrheic women if extended bouts of intense exercise are continued.[44] Bonen[60] further stated that progressive loading of metabolic stressors (exercise, incorrect dieting, etc.) increases the extent of menstrual cycle changes. This may be done by stimulating the adrenal axis, which then stimulates the neurotransmitter corticotrophin-releasing hormone. This in turn suppresses gonadotropin releasing hormone (GnRH) release and results in suppressing LH pulse frequency. These factors may culminate in changes in the menstrual cycle that range from eumenorrhea to amenorrhea.[58]

Eating Disorders and the Menstrual Cycle

Anorexia nervosa has been linked to both amenorrhea and hypoestrogenism[12,66] whereas oligomenorrhea has been observed in bulimic individuals with normal body weight.[76] Furthermore, oligomenorrhea has also been reported in individuals that have participated in pathogenic weight control behaviors but do not have an eating disorder.[6,76] Physical training has also been associated with changes in a female's menstrual cycle.[41] Although the exact etiology of menstrual changes has not been elucidated, excessive body weight loss, low body fat, stress, and amount of training were all originally suggested as the cause.[5] In their research, Borrow and Saga[5] studied the results of 240 questionnaires regarding menstrual irregularity and stress fractures in collegiate female distance runners. The data that was received was divided into one of three groups, depending on the individual's menstrual history since menarche: very irregular (0–5 menses a year), irregular (6–9 menses a year), and regular (10–13 menses a year). Because this was a questionnaire, there were two limitations: there were sampling errors because the whole population was not included, and non-sampling errors that resulted from the individual's interpretation of the questions. They found that runners with irregular menstrual histories tended to weigh less and run more miles per week than both of the other groups. Runners with regular menstrual histories had a significantly younger age of menarche than either the irregular or very irregular group, but all three groups were significantly above the national average of 12.9 + 1.2 years.[35] In their study, they found that all three groups of runners averaged their onset of training before menarche, but the runners with very irregular menses started significantly earlier (16 months before menarche) than the runners with regular menses (6 months before menarche). It's interesting to note was that not all of the 120 runners with menstrual irregularities had athletically induced amenorrhea (lack of a menstrual cycle). Twenty-three had eating disorders (categorized by simply asking the question whether or not they thought they had an eating problem), but their menstrual irregularities were associated with low body weight and high running mileage. Menstrual dysfunction has also been reported to occur more in sports which emphasize leanness or a specific weight versus sports which focus less on such factors and controls.[81]

In two other studies, Carlberg et al.[15] and Lutter and Cushman[51] both found that low body weight and high mileage could have contributed to disrupted menstrual function in certain individuals with oligomenorrhea and amenorrhea. Nichols et al.[59] also studied the relationship between regional body composition to BMD in young females. They had two findings. First, they reported that the athletes in their study had significantly greater BMD than the non-athletes. Secondly, regional lean tissue mass (LTM) was more highly correlated with BMD than weight, total LTM, or fat mass and was the only significant predictor of BMD. Drinkwater et al.[23] showed that young female athletes who remain amenorrheic/oligomenorrheic for long periods of time could have severe residual effects on lumbar BMD, which may not be reversible. For these reasons, it is critical to be able to see the warning signs of the female athlete triad.

Amenorrhea

Amenorrhea, a known marker of anorexia nervosa,[2] can be divided into two categories; primary and secondary amenorrhea.[63] Primary amenorrhea is the delay of menarche past the age of 16,[86] while secondary amenorrhea is the cessation of periods for more than three consecutive months following menarche. Even more common is the occurrence of disrupted menstrual patterns, or oligomenorrhea.[19] These disruptions in the menstrual cycle can produce effects similar to those of menopause with a decreased ovarian hormone production. This decrease in hormone production has been shown to lead to decreased bone mineral density.[3,14,24]

Amenorrhea and Bone Density

Hetland et al.[39] found that the prevalence of amenorrhea increased from 1% in the normally active subjects to 11% in the elite runners, and the amenorrheic runners had a 10% reduction in lumbar bone density as compared with the normally menstruating runners. What was interesting was that the bone turnover between groups was similar. Snow-Harter[87] reported that amenorrheic endurance athletes have 15%-20% lower vertebral BMD than did their eumenorrheic teammates, and the amenorrheic endurance athletes showed hormonal patterns of a postmenopausal woman. Sanborn et al.[79] reported that female distance runners who increased their training mileage to more than 20 miles a week increased the risk for developing exercise associated amenorrhea. A study by Myburgh et al.[57] attempted to determine whether low BMD and other risk factors for osteoporosis were associated with stress fractures in athletes (mean age 32 ± 8 years). They examined 25 females with stress fractures and found three major findings. First and most importantly, they found that athletes with stress fractures had lower BMD (both in axial and appendicular skeleton) than did well-matched control athletes who had not previously had symptoms of either shin splints or a stress fracture. Secondly, injured subjects had a higher incidence of current menstrual irregularities and lower incidence of oral contraceptive use. Furthermore, menstrual status also was associated with low trabecular BMD of the spine and Ward's triangle. Lastly, they found that subjects with stress fractures had lower intakes of dietary calcium and histories of lower intakes of dairy products than did control subjects. There was also a positive correlation between calcium intake and BMD in the weight-bearing bones. Therefore, it not only appears that low BMD leads to stress fractures, but those individuals with stress fractures have lower intakes of calcium and oral contraceptive use.

Etiology of Amenorrhea

Frisch[34] originally theorized that body fat determined a minimum weight for the onset of a menstrual cycle. Further investigation then showed this to be inaccurate.[36,72,73,75,84] Other more recent theories exist. One more recent and accepted theory discussed by Loucks et al.[47] is the energy availability hypothesis. This hypothesis states that an individual exercises until in a negative caloric state and remains in this state for prolonged periods of time. This occurs when an individual does not ingest enough calories for the amount of exercise being performed. Loucks et al.[47] showed that dietary stress (low caloric intake) resulted in decreases in cyclical levels of luteinizing hormone (LH), and that LH was depressed in women with low dietary intakes. This is further supported by other research. For example, other researchers have shown that dietary restriction is the culprit for disruptions in the menstrual cycle, not the level of body fat.[49,56,66,89] Both Keizer and Rogol[43] and Prior et al.[69] stated that no one factor can be singled out as the primary cause of menstrual cycle dysfunction, since athletic amenorrhea results from a manifestation of nutritional deprivation, physical illness, stress, and excessive exercise.

So why is amenorrhea so important? Amenorrhea has not only been known as a marker for AN (DSM-IV), but other research has shown an important link between female athletes and disrupted menstrual cycles.[86] Low serum estrogen levels also appear to be associated with athletic amenorrhea and osteoporosis. This could be because one of the body's estrogen storage lies within adipose tissues, and low body fat compositions could lead to decreased estrogen stores. It is this body composition that many females and female athletes sometimes use as a gauge to assess their activity level. Eating disorders and the avoidance of dairy products could be a result of this behavior, which could lead to both amenorrhea and overall decreased bone health. Frisch[33] theorized that both high physical stress and psychological stress in athletes plays a vital role in weight loss and secondary amenorrhea. Epling et al.[29] further showed that food intake in athletes were reduced following high levels of exercise. West[88] also stated that patterns of eating disorders may lead to menstrual dysfunction and subsequent osteoporosis. Therefore, the availability of the body's energy stores appears to be crucial in the prevention of amenorrhea, a physical sign of an eating disorder.[27]

Even though menstrual irregularities have significant effects on the body, these effects can be reversible.[70,81] Diddle[21] showed that gaining weight, decreasing the intensity of training, or otherwise altering the physical and psychological stresses on the athlete usually restores normal menstrual cycling. More specifically, most athletes (secondary amenorrheic) will experience a return in their normal menstrual cycles within one year, even without an alteration in their training schedules.[37] Shangold[77] showed that future fertility was not interfered with in female marathon training. Drinkwater et al.[26] also showed that the resumption of menses increased the vertebral BMD of the former amenorrheic female athletes, but these increases in BMD did not return to normal levels. Other researchers have shown that premature osteoporosis in amenorrheic women is partially irreversible, even when normal menstruation is restored.[23,26] Therefore, it appears that menstrual irregularities do not have negative effects on future fertility, but increases in BMD associated with resumption of menses may not bring BMD back to normal levels.

Resumption of Menses

With regards to the resumption of menses and eating disorders, Golden et al.[36] showed that menses resumed at a mean (±SD) of 9.4 ± 8.2 months after patients were initially seen and required a weight of 2.05 kg more than the weight at which their menses were lost. Subjects who remained amenorrheic at one year had lower levels of LH and FSH at baseline and lower levels of LH and estradiol at follow-up. They also concluded that the resumption of menses required restoration of hypothalamic-piutitary-ovarian function, which was not dependent on the amount of body fat, but rather serum estradiol levels. In other studies, gains have been shown in lumbar-spine (6%-9% per year) have been evident in the first few years following the resumption of menses.[26,46,61] Though these gains were measured, they were not sufficient to restore bone-mineral density comparable to that versus controls or eumenorrheic athletes. Furthermore, there was also an absence of total lumbar-spine bone-mineral density back to normal after a longer recovery period and two other studies have shown that previously amenorrheic athletes continued to have low bone mineral density at the lumbar spine at a deficit of 15% compared with athletes who had always menstruated.[96, 97]

Infertility and Eating Disorders

Bates et al.[53] looked at infertility and eating disorders. Their subjects included 29 women with unexplained infertility and 18 with menstrual dysfunction. What was interesting was that 19 of the 26 infertile women (73%) conceived spontaneously when they increased their body weight to their ideal body weight when compared to the Metropolitan life Insurance Company tables for height and weight. Nine of the 10 women with secondary amenorrhea resumed menstruation. The authors then concluded that the practices of weight control might be a cause of unexplained infertility and menstrual disorders in otherwise healthy women. This issue will be discussed in greater detail in Chapter 14, Exercise and Fertility in the Female Athlete.

Other hormonal changes in individuals with eating disorders are as follows. Low estrogen levels and failure to ovulate during AN appears to be due primarily to gonadotropin deficiency.[77] Males with eating disorders, specifically those with AN appear to have the same deficiencies in gonadotropins as seen in females. This results in low testosterone levels.[79] There also appears to be a basal GH elevation in individuals with eating disorders.[80] IGF-1 levels are also low in individuals with both AN and BN.[81]

In summary, it appears that menstrual irregularities are more common in athletic populations when compared to the general population. Some examples of these menstrual irregularities are short luteal phases and a cessation of menstruation all together. This may put these individuals at a higher risk for more complicated medical conditions like premature osteoporosis and even sterility. Also, some inhibition of GnRH secretion does appear in individuals that engage in excessive exercise. This may then result in decreased secretions of hormones such as LH and FSH.

Summary

In recent years we have been able to study the menstrual cycle at depth and have a much better understanding of the physiology behind it. There are many different hormones that have a direct relationship with a normally functioning cycle. When a female's menstrual cycle does not occur on a regular basis, it could be a sign of a much greater problem, so it is imperative that a health care provider complete an evaluation right away.

It now appears that many different factors contribute to both normal and pathological menstrual cycles and the consequences can be major. For example, if an individual has not had a menstrual cycle in some time and has a history of skeletal injuries, a bone density scan may be warranted. Furthermore, even with the resumption of a normal menstrual cycle, one's bone density may not reach back to normal levels.

References

1. ACOG Committee Opinion, von Willeband's disease in gynecologic practice, *International Journal of Gynecology & Obstetrics.* 2002;76:336.

2. American Psychiatric Association. *Diagnostic and Statistical Manual of Mental Disorders (DSM-III-R).* 3rd ed., revised. Washington, DC: American Psychiatric Association; 1987.

3. Bachrach LK, Guido D, Katzman D, Litt IF and Marcus R. Decreased bone density in adolescent girls with anorexia nervosa. *Pediatrics.* 1990;86:440-447.

4. Baker ER, Mathur RS, Kirk RF, et al. Plasma gonadotrophins, prolactin and steroid hormone concentrations in female runners after along distance run. *Fertility and Sterility.* 1982;38:38-41.

5. Barrow GW and Saga S. Menstrual irregularity and stress fractures in collegiate female distance runners. *The American Journal of Sports Medicine.* 1988;16(3):209-215.

6. Bates GW, Bates SR, Whitworth NS. Reproductive failure in women who practice weight control. *Fertility and Sterility.* 1982;37:373-378.

7. Beitins IZ, McArthur JW, Trunbull BA, Skrinar GS, and Bullen BA. Exercise induces two types of human luteal dysfunction: confirmation by urinary free progesterone. *Journal of Clinical Endocrinology and Metabolism.* 1991;72:1350-1358.

8. Bergen H, Leung PCK. Norepinephrine inhibition of pulsatile LH release: receptor specificity. *American Journal of Physiology.* 1986;250.

9. Besley EM, Pinol APY, and Task Force on Long-Acting Systemic Agents for Fertility Regulation. Menstrual bleeding patterns in untreated women. *Contraception.* 1997;55:57.

10. Bonen A. Exercise-induced menstrual cycle changes: a function, temporary adaptation to metabolic stress. *Sports Medicine.* 1994;17:373-392.

11. Bonen A, Keizer HA. Pituitary, ovarian and adrenal hormone responses to marathon running. *International Journal of Sports Medicine.* 1987;8:161-167.

12. Boyar RM, Katz J, Finkelstein JW, et al. Anorexia nervosa: immaturity of the 24-hour luteinizing hormone secretory pattern. *New England Journal of Medicine.* 1974;291:861-865.

13. Boyden TW, Pamenter RW, Stanforth P, et al. Impaired gonadotropin response to gonadotropin releasing hormone stimulation in endurance-trained women. *Fertility and Sterility*. 1984;41:359-363.

14. Cann CE, Martin MC, Genant HK and Jaffe RB. Decreased spinal mineral content in amenorrheic women. *Journal of the American Medical Association*. 1984;251:626-629.

15. Carlberg K, Buckman MT, Peake GT et al. A survey of menstrual function in athletes. *European Journal of Applied Physiology*. 1983;51:211-222.

16. Creatsas G, Salakos N, Averkiou M, Miras K, and Aravantinos D. Endocrinological profile of oligomenorrheic strenuously exercising adolescents. *Journal of Obstetrics and Gynecology*. 1992;38:215-221.

17. Cumming DC, Vickovic MM, Wall SR, et al. Defects of pulsatile LH release in normally menstruating runners. *Journal of Clinical Endocrine Metabolism*. 1985;60:810-812.

18. Cumming DC, Vickovic MM, Wall SR, et al. The effect of acute exercise on pulsatile release of luteinizing hormone in women runners. *American Journal of Obstetrics and Gynecology*. 1985;153:482-485.

19. Dale E, Gerlach D and Wilhote A. Menstrual dysfunction in distance runners. *Journal of Obstetrics and Gynecology*. 1979;54:47.

20. De Souza MJ, Miller BE, Loucks AB, et al. High frequency of luteal phase deficiency and anovulation in recreational women runners: blunted elevation in follicle-stimulating hormone observed during luteal-follicular transition. *Journal of Clinical Endocrinol Metabolism*. 1988;83:4220-4232.

     a. *Disorders*, 38, 24–29.

21. Diddle A. Athletic activity and menstruation. *Sports Medicine*. 1984;76(5):619-624.

22. Dumoulin SC, de Glisezinski I, Saint-Martin F, et al. Hormonal changes related to eating behavior in oligomenorrheic women. *European Journal of Endocrinology*. 1996;135(3):328-34.

23. Drinkwater BL, Bruemner B, and Chestnut CH. Menstrual history as a determinant of current bond density in young athletes. *Journal of American Medical Association*. 1990;263(4):545-548.

24. Drinkwater B, Nilson, K, Ott S, and Chestnut CH III. Bone mineral density after resumption of menses in amenorrheic athletes. *Journal of American Medical Association*. 1986;256:380-382.

25. Drinkwater BL, Nilson K, Ott S, and Chestnut CH. Bone mineral density after resumption of menses in amenorrheic athletes. *Journal of American Medical Association*. 1986;256(3),380-382.

26. Drinkwater BL, Nilson K, Chesnut CH, Bremner WJ, Shainholtz S, and Southworth MB. Bone mineral content of amenorrheic and eumenorrheic athletes. *New England Journal of Medicine.* 1984;311:277-281.

27. Edwards JE, Lindeman AK, Nujesjtm AE, and Stager JM. Energy balance in highly trained female endurance athletes. *Medicine and Science in Sports and Exercise.* 1993;25:1398-1404.

28. Ellison PT and Lager C. Moderate recreational running is associated with lowered salivary progesterone profiles in women. *American Journal of Obstetrics and Gynecology.* 1986;154:1000-1003.

29. Epling W, Pierce W, Stefan L. A theory of activity-based anorexia. *International journal of eating disorders.* 1983;3:27-43.

30. Espey LL, Tanaka N, Adams RG, Okamura H, Ovarian hydroxyeicodatetraenoic acids compared with prostanoids and steroids during ovulation in rats. *American Journal of Physiology.* 1991;260:E163.

31. Faddy MJ, Gosden R, Gougeon A. Accelerated disappearance of ovarian follicles in mid-life: implications for forecasting menopause. *Human Reproduction.* 7: 1342, 1992.

32. Filicori M, Santoro N, Merriam GR, Crowley WF, JR. Characterization of the physiological pattern of episodic gonadotropin secretion throughout the human menstrual cycle. *Journal of Endocrinology & Metabolism.* 62: 1136, 1986.

33. Frisch R. Food intake, fatness, and reproductive ability. *Anorexia Nervosa.* New York, NY: Raven Press; 1977:149-160.

34. Frisch RE and McArthur JW. Menstrual cycles: fatness as a determinant of minimum weight for height necessary for their maintenance or onset. *Science.* 1974;185:949-951.

35. Frisch RE, and Revelle R. Height and weight at menarche and a hypothesis of menarche. *Archives of Disease in Childhood.* 1971;695-701.

36. Golden NH, Jacobson MS, Schebendach J, Solanto MV, Hartz SM, Shenker R. Resumption of Menses in Anorexia Nervosa. *Archives of Pediatrics & Adolescent Medicine.* 1997;151 (Jan):16-21.

37. Griffin, Letha Y. The Female Athlete. In: Delee JC. and Drez D, (Eds.), *Orthopedic Sports Medicine; Principles and Practice.* Philadelphia, Pennsylvania: W. B. Saunders Publisher; 1994:356-373.

38. Hall P, Maclachlan N, Thorn N, et al. Control of menorrhagia by the cyclo-oxygenase inhibitors naproxen sodium and mefenamic acid. *The British Journal of Obstetrics and Gynaecology.* 1987;94:554.

39.   Hetland ML, Haarbo J, Christiansen C, and Larsen T. Running induces menstrual disturbances but bone mass is unaffected, except in amenorrheic women. *The American Journal of Medicine*. 1993;95(1):53-60.

40.   Hoff JD, Quigley ME, Yen SSC Hormonal dynamics at midcycle; a reevaluation. *Journal of Clinical Endocrinology & Metabolism*. 1983;57:792.

41.   Jones KP, Ravnikar VA, Tulchinsky D and Schiff I. Comparison of bone density in amenorrheic women due to athletics, weight loss, and premature menopause. *Obstetrics & Gynecology*. 1985;66:5-8.

42.   Keen AD, Drinkwater BL. Irreversible bone loss in former amenorrheic athletes. *Osteoporosis International*. 1997;7:311-315.

43.   Keizer HA and Rogol AD. Physical exercise and menstrual cycle alterations: what are the mechanisms? *Sports Medicine*. 1990;10(4): 218-235.

44.   Keizer HA, Menheere P, Kuipers H. Changes in pulsatile LH secretion after exhaustive exercise and training. *Medicine & Science in Sports & Medicine*. 1987;19(supp):216.

45.   Lenton EA, Landgren B, Sexton L et al. Normal variation in the length of the follicular phase of the menstrual cycle: effect of chronological age, *The British Journal of Obstetrics and Gynaecology*. 1984:91:681.

46.   Lindberg JS, Fears WB, Hunt MM. Exercise-induced amenorrhea and bone density. *Annals of Internal Medicine*. 1984;101:647-648.

47.   Loucks AB, Verdun M, and Heath EM. Low energy availability, not stress of exercise, alters LH pulsatility in exercising women. *Journal of Applied Physiology*. 1998;84:37-46.

48.   Loucks AB, Mortola JF, Girton L, Yen SSC. Alterations in the hypothalamic-pituitary-ovarian and the hypothalamic-pituitary-adrenal axes in athletic women. *Journal of Clinical Endocrinology & Metabolism*. 1989;68:402-411.

49.   Loucks AB, Heath EM, Law T SR, Verdun M, Watts JR. Dietary restriction reduces luteinizing hormone (LH) pulse frequency during waking hours and increases LH pulse amplitude during sleep in young menstruating women. *Journal of Clinical Endocrinology & Metabolism*. 1994;78:910-915.

50.   Lumsden MA, Kelly RW, Templeton AA, Van Look PFA, Swantson IA, Baird DT. Changes in the concentrations of prostaglandins in preovulatory human follicles after administration of HCG. *Journal of Reproduction and Fertility*. 1986;77:119.

51. Lutter JM and Cushman S. Menstrual patterns in female runners. Physician in *Sportsmedicine.* 1982;10:60-72.

52. McNab D and Hawton K. Disturbances of sex hormones in anorexia nervosa in the male. *Postgraduate Medicine Journal.* 1981;57:254-256.

53. Micklesfield LK, Reyneke L, Fataar A, Myburgh KH. Long-term restoration of deficits in bone mineral density is inadequate in premenopausal women with prior menstrual irregularity. *Clinical Journal of Sports Medicine.* 1998;8:155-163.

54. Moore, J. Available at: http://www.uncharted-worlds.org/bodypolitics/meaningm.htm. 1996.

55. Munster K, Schmidt L, Helm P. Length and variation in the menstrual cycle – a cross sectional study from a Danish county. *The British Journal of Obstetrics and Gynaecology.* 1992;99:422.

56. Myerson M, Gutin B, Warren MP, et al. Resting metabolic rate and energy balance in amenorrheic and eumenorrheic runners. *Medicine & Science in Sports & Medicine.* 1991;23:15-22.

57. Myburgh KH, Hutchins J, Fataar AB, Hough SF, and Noakes TD. Low bone density is an etiologic factor for stress fractures in athletes. *Annals of Internal Medicine.* 1990;113(10):754-759.

58. Newman MM and Halmi KA. The endocrinology of anorexia nervosa and bulimia nervosa. *Endocrinology Metabolism Clinics of North America.* 1988;17:195-212.

59. Nichols DL, Sanborn CF, Bonnick SL, Gench B, and DiMarco N. Relationship of regional body composition to bone mineral density in college females. *Medicine and Science in Sports and Exercise,* 1995;27(2): 178-182.

60. Nillius SJ, Fries H, and Wide L. Successful induction of follicular maturation and ovulation by prolonged treatment with LH-releasing hormone in women with anorexia nervosa. *Fertility and Sterility.* 1975;25:453-458.

61. Otis CL. Exercise-associated amenorrhea. *Clinical sports medicine.* 1992;11:351-361.

62. Pall M, Friden BE, Brannstrom M. Induction of delayed follicular rupture in the human by the selective COX-2 inhibitor rofecosib: a randomized double blind study, *Human Reproduction.* 2001;16:1323.

63. Pauerstein CJ, Eddy CA, Croxatto HD, Hess R, Siler-Khodr TM, Croxatto HB, Temporal relationships of estrogen, progesterone, and

luteinizing hormone to ovulation in women and infrahuman primates, *American Journal of Obstetrics and Gynecology.* 1978;130:876.

64. Phillips MD, Santhouse A, von Willebrand disease: recent advances in pathophysiology and treatment, *American Journal of the Medical Sciences.* 1998;316:77.

65. Pirke KM, Fichter MM, Lund R, Doerr P. Twenty-four hour sleep-wake pattern of plasma LH in patients with anorexia nervosa. *Acta Endocrinology (Copenh).* 1979;92:193-204.

66. Pirke KM, Schweiger U, Broocks A, tuschl FJ, Laessle RG. Luteinizing hormone and follicle stimulating hormone secretion patterns in female athletes with and without menstrual disturbances. *Clinical Endocrinology,* 1989;33:345-353.

67. Pirke KM, Schweiger U, Broocks A, tuschl FJ, Laessle RG. Luteinizing hormone and follicle stimulating hormone secretion patterns in female athletes with and without menstrual disturbances. *Clinical Endocrinology.* 1990;33:345-353.

68. Priddy AR, Killick SR, Elstein M, et al. The effect of prostaglandin synthetase inhibitors on human preovulatory follicular fluid prostaglandin, thromboxane, and leukotriene concentrations *Journal of Clinical Endocrinology & Metabolism.* 1990;71:235.

69. Prior JC, Bigna YM, Schulzer M, et al. Determination of luteal phase length by quantitative basal temperature methods: validation against the mid-cycle LH peak. *Clinical and Investigative Medicine.* 1990;13:123-131.

70. Prior J, Yuen B, Clement P, Bowie L and Thomas J. Reversible luteal phase changes and infertility associated with marathon training. *Lancet.* 1982;2:269-270.

71. Richardson SJ, Senikas V, Nelson JF. Follicular depletion during the menopausal transition—evidence for accelerated loss and ultimate exhaustion, *Journal of Clinical Endocrinology & Metabolism.* 65: 1231, 1987.

72. Ridder CM, Thijssen JHH, Bruning PF, Van den Brande JL, Zonderland ML, and Erich WBM. Body fat mass, body fat distribution, and pubertal development: a longitudinal study of physical and hormonal sexual maturation of girls. *Journal of Clinical Endocrinology and Metabolism.* 1992;75:442-446.

73. Sanborn C, Albrecht BH and Wagner WW. Athletic amenorrhea: lack of association with body fat. *Medicine and Science in Sport and Exercise.* 1987;19:207-212.

74. Sanborn C, Martin BJ, and Wagner WW Jr. Is athletic amenorrhea specific to runners? *American Journal of Obstetrics and Gynecology*. 1982;143(8):859-861.

75. Schweiger U, Pirke KM, Laessle RG, and Fichter MM. Gonadotropin secretion in bulimia nervosa. Gonadotropin secretion in bulimia nervosa. *Journal of Clinical Endocrinology Metabolism*. 1992;74:1122-1127.

76. Schweiger U, Tuschl RJ, Platte P, Broocks A, Laessle RG, and Pirke KM. Everyday eating behavior and menstrual function in young women. *Fertility and Sterility*. 1992;57:771-775.

77. Shangold M, and Levine H. The effect of marathon training upon menstrual function. *American Journal of Obstetrics and Gynecology*. 1982;143:862.

78. Shaw RW, Assessment of medical treatments for menorrhagia, *British* **Journal of Obstetrics and Gynecology.** 1994;101(Suppl 11):15.

79. Snow-Harter CM. Bone health and prevention of osteoporosis in active and athletic women. *Clinics in Sports Medicine*. 1994;13:389-404.

80. Stager J, Ritchie-Flanagan G, and Robert-Shaw D. Reversibility of amenorrhea in athletes. *New England Journal of Medicine*. 1984;310:51-52.

81. Torstveit MK, and Sundgot-Borgen J. Participation in leanness sports but not training volume is associated with menstrual dysfunction: a national survey of 1276 elite athletes and controls. *British Journal of Sports Medicine*. March 2005;39(3):141-147.

82. Tracey R. Rich, Judaism 101. Available at: http://www.jewfaq.org/sex.htm#Niddah

83. Treloar AE, Boynton RE, Borghild GB et al. Variation of the human menstrual cycle through reproductive life, *International Journal of Fertility*. 1967;12:77.

84. Trussell J. Statistical flaws in evidence for the Frisch hypothesis that fatness triggers menarche. *Human Biology*. 1980;52:711-720.

85. Veldhuis JD, Evans WS, Demers LM et al. Altered neuroendocrine regulation of gonadotropin secretion in women distance runners. *Journal of Clinical Endocrinol Metabolism*. 1985;61:557-563.

86. Warren MP, and Stiehl AL. Exercise and female adolescents: effects on the reproductive and skeletal systems. *Journal of American Medical Women Association*. 1999;54:115-120.

87. Welt CK, Martin KM Taylor et al. Frequency modulation of follicle-stimulating hormone (FSH) during the luteal-follicular transition:

evidence for FSH control of inhibin B in normal women. *Journal of Clinical Endocrinology and Metabolism.* 1997;82:2645.

88.   West RV. The Female Athlete. *Sports Medicine.* 1998;26(2):63-71.

89.   Williams NI, Young JC, McArthur JW, Bullen B, Skrinar GS, and Trunbull B. Strenuous exercise with caloric restriction: effect on luteinizing hormone secretion. *Medicine and Science in Sport and Exercise.* 1995;27:1390-1398.

90.   World Health Organization Task Force Investigators, Temporal relationships between ovulation and defined changes in the concentration of plasma estradiol-17B, luteinizing hormone, follicle stimulating hormone and progesterone, *American Journal of Obstetrics and Gynecology.* 1980;138:383.

CHAPTER 7

Osteoporosis in the Female Athlete

David Kahler, MD and Margaret Kuhn, MD

Introduction

It has become well recognized that decreased bone density may be a consequence of over-training and participation in certain sports, particularly in the presence of nutritional deficiencies.[30] Abnormally low bone density results in an increased susceptibility to stress fractures during participation, but may also be completely asymptomatic. If this problem is unrecognized and left untreated, the young female athlete may never attain a normal peak bone density. The normal gradual loss of bone mass during aging may then predispose the former athlete to develop typical osteoporotic fractures at a relatively young age. In this era of outcome-driven health care, fracture management alone is not enough; prevention of osteoporosis-related fractures has assumed an equally important role.[44] It is not possible to properly care for the female athlete without knowledge of the profound skeletal effects of overtraining, eating disorders, and prolonged amenorrhea as they relate to the potential for significant lifelong problems.

Historical Perspective

In the late 1950s, it was noted that female athletes in endurance sports sometimes reported menstrual disturbances that were apparently associated with training. By the 1980s, amenorrhea (defined as absence of a normal menstrual period for three consecutive months) was recognized as a common occurrence in female endurance athletes. In the past decade, the potentially severe problems associated with athletic amenorrhea and osteoporosis have received considerable attention in the medical literature. Unfortunately, there is a popular misconception among coaches, athletes, and some physicians and trainers that athletic amenorrhea is not a significant health problem. Indeed, some athletes consider amenorrhea to be a convenient side effect of overtraining. Although it has been shown that amenorrheic athletes are no more competitive than their eumenorrheic counterparts, the perception persists that amenorrhea and extremely low body fat percentage offer some advantage in endurance sports.[48]

The increased participation of women in sports over the past two to three decades produced a rash of overuse injuries and stress fractures. This type of injury accounts for the fact that girls cross-country has the highest injury rate of any organized high-school sport, surpassing football and wrestling (Table 7-1).[41] Initially, the increased incidence of stress fracture in female athletes was attributed to lack of conditioning and increased body fat percentage compared to male athletes. It later became evident, however, that even with improved conditioning, women continued to have a greater risk of stress fracture than men participating in similar sports.[3] These injuries were concentrated in sports that favored a small body habitus with low body fat percentage, such as cross-country running, ballet, and figure skating. These findings have led to to the recognition of the "Female Athlete Triad," which consists of disordered eating, amenorrhea, and

TABLE 7-1   •   Injury Rates for Specific High School Sports - Seattle, 1979–1992

RANK	SPORT	TOTAL ATHLETES	INJURIES PER 100 ATHLETES	PERCENTAGE OF ATHLETES INJURED
1	Girls cross country	1,299	61.4	33.1
2	Football	8,560	58.8	36.7
3	Wrestling	3,624	49.7	32.1
4	Girls soccer	3,186	43.7	31.6
5	Boys cross country	2,481	38.7	24.6

Adapted from Rice, SG. University of Washington. Data Presented at American College of Sports Medicine Annual Meeting, Seattle, 1993.

osteoporosis.[31, 30] These three conditions are interrelated; eating disorders increase the susceptibility to amenorrhea, and either condition may result in premature osteoporosis and susceptibility to stress fractures. The reader is referred to the Chapter 4 and 5 on this topic for further information. The following case report will serve to illustrate the significance of this triad.

The Natural Course of Bone Mass in a Healthy Athlete

The skeleton of the normal male or female athlete rapidly accumulates mineral content during skeletal growth, and this increase will gradually continue for several years following skeletal maturity. Peak bone density is usually reached between the ages of 20–30 for both males and females, and gradually decreases naturally after this peak. Estrogen is the key hormone for maintaining bone mass and estrogen deficiency, the hallmark of menopause, is the major cause of age-related bone loss. At a cellular level, estrogen mediates a balance between bone resorption and formation by regulating the activity of osteoclasts and osteoblasts respectively.[36] Estrogen also effects bone metabolism indirectly through cytokines, growth hormones and through systemic hormones that regulate calcium balance, such as calcitonin and parathyroid hormone.[2] In addition to these known actions, recent evidence suggests that estrogen also plays a critical role in mediating the skeletal response to biomechanical strain,[36] a finding that may ultimately shed additional light on the association between exercise and bone density.

In the first seven years following menopause, bone loss accelerates at a rate of two to three percent per year. This rapid decrease in bone loss is entirely due to decreased estrogen production by the ovaries. A normal woman may lose up to 0.5% of her bone mass each year until menopause. Although intermittent strenuous physical activity generally helps to maintain bone mass during this period, exercise cannot completely eliminate this natural process of bone loss.

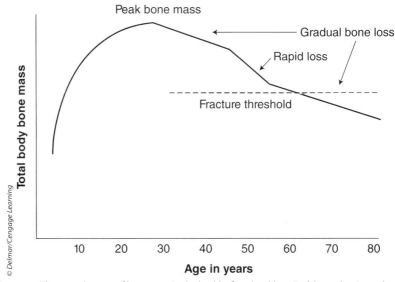

Figure 7-1 The natural course of bone mass in the healthy female athlete. Peak bone density and mass is reached during the third decade of life. Bone mass then steadily declines, with accelerated bone loss in the seven years following menopause. An increase in the risk of osteoporotic fractures occurs when the "fracture threshold" is crossed. This may occur at a relatively young age in the athlete who never reaches a normal peak bone mass by around age 30.

The same rapid bone loss is seen in women whose, ovaries have been surgically removed prior to menopause. It has been shown in controlled studies that this bone loss can be prevented, though not reversed, simply by taking oral estrogen supplements to counteract the loss of natural estrogen production.[23] If bone mineral density falls below a certain critical level, the so-called "fracture threshold" is crossed and the athlete is at risk for the typical fractures associated with osteoporosis (Figure 7-1).

The Significance of Decreased Peak Bone Mass

When natural bone loss with aging is taken into account, it is easy to see that the untreated amenorrheic female athlete that never attains a normal peak bone density will be at a disadvantage for the remainder of her life. Natural history dictates that she will gradually lose bone mass, and that her bone density may pass below the fracture threshold.

The classic fractures associated with osteoporosis involve the hip, the wrist (distal radius), the proximal humerus, and the spine and pelvis. These are all areas of the skeleton that rely on normal cancellous bone density for their strength. One out of every three American women will suffer a hip fracture after the age of 55.[35] Furthermore, Osteoporosis disproportionately affects women, who account for 71% of fractures and 75% of costs;[5] even though the majority of women aged 45 and older have at least two risk factors for osteoporosis, only 15% of those women not diagnosed by a doctor believe they are at risk for the disease.[29] In general, the patients that sustain these osteoporotic fractures have much lower bone densities than normal for their age. Recent reports have confirmed that patients over age 50 suffering a hip fracture usually have mean femoral neck bone densities, approximately two standard deviations below those of age matched controls.[10] Low bone mineral density is unquestionably a significant risk factor for fracture.

In 1991, the treatment of osteoporotic fractures accounted for $10 billion in health care costs. A more recent statistic revealed nearly a 50% rise in incidence and economic burden of osteoporotic fractures is projected by the year 2025 (total osteoporotic fractures will increase from greater than 2 million/year to greater than 3 million/year; direct health care costs increase from over $19 billion a year to nearly $29 billion a year).[5] In the year 2020, with the inevitable aging of the population, it is estimated that the annual cost will spiral to $60 billion for the care of fractures related to osteoporosis.[8] These numbers could be even greater if we persist in ignoring the problem of athletic amenorrhea and the female athlete triad, and allow a population of young athletes to mature without ever reaching a normal peak bone density.

The Effects of Training on the Skeleton

Regular physical exercise is important for development and maintenance of normal bone density. Numerous studies have shown a clear association between activity level and overall skeletal health. Weight bearing exercise (defined as impact loading of the legs, as in running, jumping, and brisk walking) has a clearly beneficial effect on bone density. It has been demonstrated that postmenopausal women with osteoporosis may be able to increase their bone mineral density by simply increasing their level of activity, especially if weight-bearing activity is added.[15,32] Women who have been active throughout their lives tend to have better skeletal health than more sedentary women.[21]

In general, increasing levels of physical activity leads to increased bone mineral density, even in well-trained female athletes.[42] At the start of a competitive collegiate season, healthy eumenorrheic (normally menstruating) gymnasts will have a lower body fat percentage and higher average bone mineral density than eumenorrheic non-athletic controls. During the course of training and competition, the gymnasts will increase their lean tissue mass, and will have significant increases in their lumbar bone density over a relatively short period of time.[33] Gymnasts have a relatively low incidence of athletic amenorrhea, and their increased weight bearing activity leads, as expected, to increased bone mass.

The beneficial effects of exercise on the skeleton are dependent on normal circulating levels of sex hormones. Both male and female athletes involved in strength training tend to have higher sex hormone levels than endurance athletes. The highest levels of bone mineral density (BMD) are also seen in strength and power training athletes. Eumenorrheic endurance athletes tend to have higher BMD than sedentary control subjects as a result of their increased activity level. Sport-specific increases in BMD are seen in runners, dancers, and skaters, all of whom have increased BMD in their legs. Rowers have higher lumbar spine BMD than distance runners. Female volleyball players have significantly higher bone mineral content in the humerus and radius of their hitting arm, while this effect is absent in non-active females.[1]

The paradox of athletic amenorrhea is that, in the highly trained female athlete, increasing levels of activity may lead to a decrease in bone mineral density.[45,30] This over-training effect is seen most commonly in endurance athletes. In the absence of other disorders, this decrease in BMD is almost never seen in normally menstruating athletes with normal estrogen levels. Amenorrheic endurance athletes have 15%–20% lower vertebral bone mineral density than their eumenorrheic teammates.[40] As a distance runner increases her training mileage to greater than 20 miles per week, her risk for developing exercise associated amenorrhea increases in a linear fashion.[39] This "dose-related" effect is not confined to women; male runners training 15–20 miles per week have increased bone density in their lower legs, while those who train by running 60–75 miles per week have decreased testosterone levels and decreased BMD.[26] The reported prevalence of athletic amenorrhea is up to 66% in endurance sports and in those sports emphasizing a thin appearance, compared with 2%–5% in the general population.

This effect is most profoundly noted in athlete runners and ballet professionals.[6,46] However, athletes participating in other endurance sports, such as swimmers and cyclists, have a baseline 10% incidence of athletic amenorrhea. That increasing training miles or hours does not appear to increase the risk of decreased BMD in these athletes, even at seemingly excessive levels of training,[32] suggests that exercise alone may not be the primary cause of reproductive abnormalities seen in female athletes. Research to explain such trends may help to further elucidate the relationship between exercise and amenorrhea.

The Cause of Athletic Amenorrhea and Osteoporosis

While there may be many underlying causes of amenorrhea, athletes often share the same hypothalamic-amenorrhea profile.[13] Hypothalamic dysfunction is characterized by a decrease in the pulsatile secretion of gonadotropin-releasing hormone which governs pituitary function. Pituitary dysfunction, then, results in decreased secretion of lutenizing hormone (LH) and follicle-stimulating hormone (FSH), both of which are responsible for stimulating the ovary to produce estrogen.[43] Both athletic amenorrhea and the associated decrease in bone mineral seen among this population have historically been attributed to this resulting hypoestrogenic state.

While the etiology of this hypothalamic dysfunction in the amenorrheic athlete remains to be definitively proven, the current consensus is that it is directly related to a relative energy deficiency. In patients with the Female Athlete Triad, disordered eating most often results in inadequate caloric intake for high exercise energy expenditures. The result is that the athlete, like her anorexic counterpart, has a relative energy deficiency. Net caloric deficits in both populations, in turn, stimulate compensatory mechanisms, such as weight loss or energy conservation. It is thought that central suppression of reproductive function results as metabolic fuels are shunted away from the costly processes of reproduction and towards the more essential, life-sustaining metabolic functions. The result is concomitant hypoestrogenism.[9] The precise mechanisms whereby this hypometabolic state is communicated to the hypothalamus and whereby metabolic fuels are shunted away from it remains to be determined. The relatively recent emergence and acceptance of this "energy availability" hypothesis for athletic amenorrhea has minimized the historic emphasis on body weight and/or body fat per se as the critical link between athletics and reproductive function.

That estrogen replacement therapy in women with hypothalamic amenorrhea only minimally increases bone density[16,17,7,34,11,14,50] suggests that a mechanism other than hypoestrogenism may also be involved with the osteopenia associated with athletic amenorrhea.[47] Hypothesized mechanisms include the impact of nutritional factors, such as micronutrient deficits, caloric restriction, and chronic under nutrition deficiencies or reductions in bone trophic factors such as Insulin-Like Growth Factor I (IGF-I) and possibly leptin.[9] If an estrogen-independent mechanism for decreased BMD in athletic amenorrhea exists, it remains to be identified.

High serum cortisol levels have also been found in amenorrheic athletes, and have historically been implicated in the development of osteoporosis. A relative catabolic state may be the result of the high levels of endogenous opiates (endorphins) seen in distance runners.[38] The "runners high" resulting from distance training has been linked to endorphin production, and may explain the prevalence of osteoporosis in distance runners.

Although the causes of hypoestrogenic amenorrhea in the athlete are multifactorial, there appear to be decreased circulating levels of all cyclical sex hormones in the amenorrheic athlete. Low levels of androgens (the male equivalent of estrogen) are also seen in male endurance athletes, and these levels increase when their level of activity is decreased.[25] Recent research has determined a possible link between low levels of circulating sex hormones and osteoporosis. Bone remodeling in response to stress occurs primarily in areas of cancellous bone where fatty marrow is in contact with bone trabeculae, or the inner surface of cortical bone. Cellular messengers, or cytokines, have been implicated in promoting the activity of osteoclasts, the cells that absorb bone during the normal remodeling process. Production of the interleukin-6 cytokine is suppressed by sex hormones such as estrogen and testosterone. It has been hypothesized that normal circulating levels of sex hormones are necessary to prevent overactivity of the osteoclasts and the resulting osteoporosis.[12]

It should be noted that exercise-induced amenorrhea is a diagnosis of exclusion. Any athlete with unexplained primary amenorrhea (absence of menarche by age 16) or secondary amenorrhea (lack of a normal menstrual period for three consecutive months) should undergo a thorough diagnostic evaluation to rule out other causes of amenorrhea. A pregnancy test is the first step, as pregnancy is the most common cause of amenorrhea. Polycystic ovaries are a common cause of both primary and secondary amenorrhea. Failure of a progesterone challenge test to induce vaginal bleeding can lend support to a tentative diagnosis of hypoestrogenic amenorrhea.

The presence of these risk factors should be explored in all female athletes that present with a stress fracture. The following risk factors have been associated with development of amenorrhea and decreased bone mass in the athlete and should be screened for in the female athletic population:

- athletes who began competitive distance running prior to menarche
- late onset of menses (age 14 or older)
- low body fat percentage
- running more than 20 miles per week.

The Significance of Athletic Amenorrhea

Studies have shown that the amenorrheic athlete has about 15% lower total body bone mass than normally menstruating control athletes.[18] There is some controversy regarding the site specificity of bone loss. When ovarian function suddenly ceases, the rate of bone loss from the spine is initially five times greater than that from the legs. In amenorrheic endurance athletes, it appears that the weight bearing bones of the lower extremity are spared somewhat, and the bone loss is most prominent in the spine, or axial skeleton.[37] Other studies, though, suggest that the bone loss may be more generalized.[27] Although, one would expect the portions of the skeleton exposed to repetitive impact loading to be somewhat protected from the effects of athletic amenorrhea, this has not been conclusively shown.

There is little question that decreased bone mass can affect athletic participation. The risk of stress fracture is higher in the athlete with decreased bone mineral density, as the bone is less able to withstand the cyclical loading associated with sports in general and running in particular. In athletes with similar training habits, those with stress fractures are more likely to have lower bone density, lower dietary calcium intake, and menstrual irregularity.[28] Normal menstrual cycling has proven to be a good indicator of skeletal health. The risk of stress fracture in an amenorrheic distance runner is approximately twice as high as that of a normally menstruating control athlete.[3]

The diagnosis of a stress fracture in an athlete at risk should raise a red flag in the mind of the clinician. Identification of any single component of the female athlete triad (amenorrhea, eating disorders, and osteoporosis) should prompt evaluation for the other two components.

Treatment of Athletic Amenorrhea and Osteoporosis

Multiple factors must be considered in treatment of exercise-induced menstrual irregularities, including the type of athletic activity, duration and intensity of training, age of the athlete, the diet and caloric balance, the duration of menstrual problems, and the estrogen status. As the loss of BMD is directly related to the duration of amenorrhea, both prevention and treatment of osteoporosis in the female athlete are dependent on the restoration of menses.[13] Historically, estrogen replacement in the form of oral contraceptive pills (OCPs) has been the mainstay of treatment. The effectiveness of this treatment, however, remains controversial. Though the pharmacological effects of both estrogen and progesterone on bone metabolism are well established in the literature,[22] the clinical effects of OCP use on BMD remain unclear. Conflicting views over effectiveness of this treatment, especially with respect to the female athlete, likely stems from the many confounding variables that affect BMD, particularly weight, exercise, diet, and estrogen status. Though there is good evidence for a positive effect of oral contraceptives on bone density in perimenopausal women, evidence is only fair for a positive effect in hypothalamic oligo/amenorrheic premenopausal women and only limited for a positive effect in healthy and anorexic premenopausal women. However, current literature does not show any evidence of a negative effect of OCP use on BMD in women.[24] Hence, in oligo/amenorrheic athletes, the best therapeutic option to support BMD remains to reestablish menses with estrogen treatment in the form of OCPs. Although the optimal estrogen dosage for this condition has not been established, it is assumed that resumption of normal menstrual cycling indicates sufficient dosage. It must be remembered that, though estrogen replacement may help prevent further loss of bone mass in an amenorrheic athlete, it will not reverse the bone loss that has already occurred, which may be significant.

Estrogen supplementation is rarely contraindicated in the young athlete, but may be inadvisable in the older athlete with a history of hypertension, stroke, deep venous thrombosis, or malignancy. Estrogen replacement therapy in amenorrheic athletes has also been associated with significant, predominantly beneficial, changes in body composition, including increases in weight and fat mass. Despite these changes, little impact on physical performance has been observed. However, it cannot be excluded that a marked increase in fat mass might have unfavorable effects for athletic performance in individual women.[34]

Given the absence of conclusive evidence of OCPs to prevent and treat exercise and diet associated bone loss, it is important that caretakers also address other potential avenues whereby BMD may be decreasing. Individuals with energy restricting behaviors must be provided with clear information regarding the potential consequences of their actions on skeletal health and should be advised on proper nutritional practices for their activity levels.[49] As the energy availability theory of athletic amenorrhea is widely supported in the literature, and as evidence to support a non-estrogen dependent pathway of athletic amenorrhea, the importance of caloric balance must be addressed.

As athletic amenorrhea most often occurs within the context of the Athletic Triad, disordered eating habits must be addressed and adequate dietary intake of vitamin D, calcium, and phosphorus ensured. The most rational approach to this affect is to attempt to restore menses by decreasing the intensity of exercise and/or increasing nutritional intake. This treatment is easy to suggest to a patient, but many female athletes are unwilling to decrease their exercise load and are scared of gaining weight. Once decrease of exercise intensity and increase of caloric intake are rejected, or if they fail to restore menses, pharmacological restoration of menses should be pursued.[13]

Ultimately, the decision to prescribe OCs to support BMD in the female athlete should be made on an individual basis, taking into account lifestyle and hormonal factors.[24] All three components of the female athlete triad must be addressed. If a bone density study has not been performed during the diagnostic workup, it is important to obtain a baseline study. The effectiveness of treatment may then be established with a follow-up study in six to twelve months. The most difficult aspect of treatment is convincing the athlete that the problem is severe enough to warrant a significant change in lifestyle. The athlete may be unwilling to start using OCPs for fear of weight gain. The distance runner will be extremely resistant to suggestions that she decrease her training miles by 10%–20% and attempt to increase her body fat percentage. The elite athlete may refuse to consider any of these interventions until she has been sufficiently disabled by a series of stress fractures. The importance of treatment of athletic amenorrhea must be emphasized to both athletes and their coaches.

Athletes with persistent bone pain, despite adequate treatment are sometimes treated with a trial of Calcitonin administered via injection or nasal spray. The postmenopausal athlete with established osteoporosis may also benefit from treatment with one of the newer biphosphonates, such as alendronate. However, no rule exists for use of potential antiresorptives such as bisphosphonates, as they have not been studied in young women and have potential for effects during pregnancy because of their long half-life in bone.[13] Although both of these interventions have been shown to increase bone density in some studies, their optimal use in the treatment of exercise-induced osteoporosis has yet to be established.

The down side of treatment for this condition is that the results are somewhat discouraging. Failure to reestablish normal menstrual cycling with treatment results in continued accelerated bone loss. Even if normal menstrual cycling returns following treatment, the female athlete's bone mass will probably not return to normal for her age. The best that can be hoped for is maintenance of current bone density, or perhaps a modest increase in lumbar spinal bone density.[20] As medical treatment of the female athlete triad may be ineffective, special emphasis should be placed on education for prevention of this disorder.

Prevention of the Problem: Awareness and Surveillance

Early identification of the female athlete triad in athletes at risk may help to decrease the morbidity associated with this condition.[30] If any single limb of the triad is suspected, the following questions should be asked at the preparticipation physical:[30]

Eating Disorders:

- Have you ever used laxatives, diuretics, or diet pills?
- Do you sometimes skip meals?
- Have you ever made yourself vomit to get rid of a big meal?
- What have you eaten in the last 24 hours?
- Compared to your current weight, what is your ideal weight?

Menstrual History:

- When did you start having your period?
- How regular has it been?
- Have you ever missed a period? How many months in a row? How many cycles do you have in a usual year?
- Have you ever used birth control pills?

Stress Fractures (osteoporosis):

- Have you ever had a stress fracture or other broken bone?
- How many hours (or miles) per day and per week do you train? Any sudden changes?
- Have you ever had to stop training because of an overuse injury?
- Have you ever taken thyroid supplements or corticosteroids (prednisone)?

The problem of athletic amenorrhea and osteoporosis will persist until the attitudes concerning this disorder are changed. Skin fold calipers should not be used by trainers or coaches to assess the adequacy of training. Young athletic women must not treat acquired amenorrhea as a natural consequence of their sport. The high prevalence of eating disorders in endurance and appearance sports must be addressed. Finally, athletes and caregivers must be made aware of the potential consequences of decreasing bone density at the stage of life when bone mass should naturally be increasing.

PERSONAL ENCOUNTER:

A 20-year-old highly-recruited Caucasian female distance runner was referred for evaluation of persistent left-sided low back pain. This pain had been treated unsuccessfully with sacroiliac joint manipulation, and had prevented competition and training runs longer than about a mile. The pain was always well localized and associated with activity.

The patient had been a distance runner since age 13, and had her first menstrual period at the age of 15. Her cycles had been irregular since then, and she had not had a normal menstrual period in the two years prior to evaluation. Although she had not been diagnosed as having an eating disorder, she admitted to frequently skipping meals and avoiding dairy products in attempt to keep her body fat percentage below 10%.

Physical examination revealed localized tenderness, and the FABER test localized pain to the region of the left sacroiliac joint. Serum calcium, phosphorus, and alkaline phosphatase levels were within normal limits. Radiographs of the lumbar spine and pelvis appeared to show decreased bone density with an irregularity in the left sacrum. A bone scan showing increased uptake in this region was consistent with the radiographic diagnosis of a sacral insufficiency fracture. This type of stress fracture is most commonly seen in severely osteoporotic women over 80 years of age, and is extremely rare in the active young athlete. A bone density determination revealed lumbar bone density to be severely decreased to more than two standard deviations below normal for her age, or approximately normal mean density for an 80-year-old woman (Figure 7-2A and 7-2B). Further endocrine evaluation revealed that the most likely explanation for this athlete's severe osteoporosis was secondary amenorrhea, with a low estrogen level and a possible eating disorder.

The athlete was treated with oral contraceptives and dietary counseling to achieve adequate estrogen levels and a body fat percentage

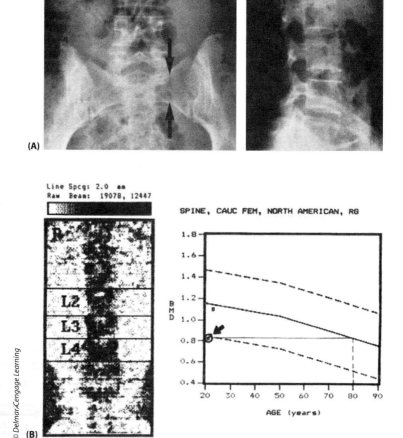

Figure 7-2 Pelvis and lateral lumbar spine radiographs demonstrate osteopenia and suggest a sacral insufficiency fracture in this 20 year old collegiate distance runner. This type of stress fracture is most commonly seen in severely osteoporotic elderly women. The bone density study in Figure I(b) shows that the patient's vertebral bone density at the start of treatment (bold arrow) would be normal only in an 80 year old woman.

of approximately 20%. She resumed normal menstrual cycling and her lumbar spine bone mineral density increased by 15%. Although her sacral insufficiency fracture eventually healed, she was bothered by persistent low back pain at the site of her stress fracture and was treated with a course of injectable Calcitonin. Although she graduated from college and went on to Veterinary graduate school, she was never able to run competitively again. After four years of treatment, the exercise prescription for this former elite cross-country runner now reads: "Low impact aerobic exercise and 2–3 brisk 30-minute walks per week." At the age of 24, she remains at increased risk of osteoporotic fractures, and will probably always have decreased bone density for her age.

It is not unusual to have persistent pain at the site of a stress fracture, despite radiographic evidence of fracture healing. Stress fracture of the femoral neck is frequently a career ending injury in the elite runner, even if diagnosed early and not allowed to progress to a complete fracture.[19] It is clear that prevention of the problem is better than treatment.

Summary

Though osteoporosis is normally accounted for in the elderly, it can and does occur in the young. Physical activity is also normally associated with increases in bone density, but when taken to extremes it can have a reverse effect. Therefore it is imperative to understand the limitations of the skeletal system and the impact that exercise can have on it. Exercise, when performed in the correct dosages can be beneficial but can be just as devastating when taken out of context. Therefore, recognizing the early signs of poor menstrual function can help an athlete combat early bone loss. This bone loss may not pose an acute risk but does set the stage for osteoporosis later in life.

References

1. Alfredson H, Nordstrom P, Pietila T, and Lorentzon R. Long-term loading and regional bone mass of the arm in female volleyball players. *Calcified Tissue International*. 1998;62:303-8.

2. Balasch J. Sex steroids and bone: current perspectives. *Human Reproduction Update*. 2003;9:207-22.

3. Barrow GW, and Saha S. Menstrual irregularity and stress fractures in collegiate female distance runners. *American Journal of Sports Medicine*. 1988;16(3):209-216.

4. Bonci CM, Bonci LK, Granger LR et al. National Athletic Trainer's Association position statement: preventing, detecting and managing disordered eating in athletics. *Journal of Athletic Training*. 2008;3(1): 80-108.

5. Burge R, Dawson-Hughes B, Solomon D et al. Incidence and economic burden of osteoporosis-related fractures in the United States, 2005-2025. *Journal of Bone and Mineral Research*. 2007;22:465-475.

6. Calabrese LH, and Kirkendall DT. Nutritional and medical considerations in dancers. *Clinics in Sports Medicine*. 1983;2(3):539-48.

7. Cumming DC. Exercise associated amenorrhea, low bone density, and estrogen replacement therapy. *Archives of Internal Medicine* 1996;156:2193-5.

8. Cummings SR, Rubin SM, and Black D. The future of hip fractures in the United States: numbers, costs, and potential effects of postmenopausal estrogen. *Clinical Orthopaedics*. 1990;252:163-166.

9. De Souza MJ, and William NI. Physiological aspects and clinical sequalae of energy deficiency and hypoestrogenism in exercising women. *Human Reproduction Update*. 2004;10(5):433-448.

10. Dirschl DR, Henderson RC, and Oakley WS. Correlates of bone mineral density in elderly patients with hip fractures. *Journal of Orthopaedic Trauma*. 1995;9(6):470-475.

11. Gibson JH. Treatment of reduced bone mineral density in athletic amenorrhea: a pilot study. *Osteoporosis International*. 1999;10:284-9.

12. Girasole G, Jilka RI, Passeri G et al. 17-B estradiol inhibits interleukin-6 production by bone marrow-derived stromal cells and osteoblasts in vitro: A potential mechanism for the antiosteoporotic effect of estrogens. *Journal of Clinical Investigation* 1992;89:883-891.

13. Goodman LR, and Warren MP. The female athlete and menstrual function. *Current Opinion in Obstetrics and Gynecology*. 2005;17:466-470.

14. Gremion G, Rizzoli R, Slasman D et al. Oligo-amenorrheic long-distance runners may lose more bone in spine than in femur. *Medicine and Science in Sport and Exercise*. 2001;3:15-21.

15.   Grove KA, and Londeree BR. Bone density in postmenopausal women: high inpact vs. low impact exercise. *Medicine and Science in Sport and Exercise.* 1992;24:1190-4.

16.   Gulekli B, Davies MC, and Jacobs HS. Effect of treatment on established osteoporosis in young women with amenorrhea. *Clinical Endocrinology (Oxford)* 1994;41:275-81.

17.   Haenggi W, Casez JP, Birkhaeuser MD et al. Bone mineral density in young women with long-standing amenorrhea: limited effect of hormone replacement therapy with ethinylestradiol and desogestrel. *Osteoporosis International.* 1994;4:99-103.

18.   Heinrich C, Going S, Pamenter R, Perry C, Boyden T, and Lohman T. Bone mineral content of cyclically menstruating female resistance and endurance trained athletes. *Medicine and Science in Sport and Exercise.* 1990;22:558-563.

19.   Johansson C, Ekenman I, Tornkvist H, and Eriksson E. Stress fractures of the femoral neck in athletes. The consequence of a delay in diagnosis. *American Journal of Sports Medicine.* 1990;18(5):524-8.

20.   Jonnavithula S, Warren MP, Fox RP, and Lazaro MI. Bone density is compromised in amenorrheic women despite return of menses: a 2-year study. *Obstetrics and Gynecology.* 1993;81(5):669-74.

21.   Krall EA, and Dawson-Hughes B. Walking is related to bone mineral density and rates of bone loss. *American Journal of Medicine.* 1994;96:20-26.

22.   Kuohung W, Borgatta L, and Stubblefield P. Low-dose oral contraceptives and bone mineral density: an evidence based analysis. *Contraception.* 2000;61:77-82.

23.   Lindsay R, Hart DM, and Clark DM. The minimum effective dose of estrogen for prevention of postmenopausal bone loss. *Obstetrics and Gynecology.* 1984;63(6): 759-63.

24.   Liu SL, and Lebrun CM. Effect of oral contraceptives and hormone replacement therapy on bone mineral density in premenopausal and perimenopausal women: a systematic review. *British Journal of Sports Medicine.* 2006;40:11-24.

25.   MacConnie SE, Barkan A, Lampman RM, Schork MA, and Beitens IZ. Decreased hypothalamic gonadotropin-releasing hormone secretion in male marathon runners. *New England Journal of Medicine* 1986;315:411-417.

26.   MacDougall JD, Webber CE, Martin J et al. Relationship among running mileage, bone density, and serum testosterone in male runners. *Journal of Applied Physiology.* 1992;73:1165-70.

27.   Myburgh KH, Bachrach LK, Lewis B, Kent K, and Marcus R. Low bone density at axial and appendicular sites in amenorrheic athletes. *Medicine and Science in Sports and Exercise.* 1993;25:1197-202.

28.   Myburgh KH, Hutchins J, Fataar AB, Hough SF, and Noakes TD. Low bone density is an etiologic factor for stress fractures in athletes. *Annals of Internal Medicine.* 1990;113:754-9.

29. National Osteoporosis Foundation Survey, April 2004.

30. Nattiv A, Loucks AB, Manore MM et al. The American College of Sports Medicine. Position Statement on the Female Athlete Triad. *Medicine and Science in Sports and Exercise.* October 2007;39(10):1867-1882.

31. Nattiv A, and Lynch L. The female athlete triad: Managing an acute risk to long term health. *The Physician and Sportsmedicine.* 1994;22(1):60-68.

32. Nelson ME, Fiatarone MA, Morganti CM, Trice I, Greenberg RA, and Evans WJ. Effects of high-intensity strength training on multiple risk factors for osteoporotic fractures. A randomized controlled trial. *Journal of the American Medical Association.* 1994;272(24):1909-14.

33. Nichols DL, Sanborn CF, Bonnick SL, Ben-Ezra V, Gench B, and DiMarco NM. The effects of gymnastics training on bone mineral density. *Medicine and Science in Sports and Exercise.* 1994;26(10): 1220-1225.

34. Rickenlund A, Carlstrom K, Ekblom B et al. Effects of oral contraceptives on body composition and physical performance in female athletes. *Journal of Clinical Endocrinology and Metabolism.* 2004;89:4364-70.

35. Riggs BL. Pathogenesis of osteoporosis. *American Journal of Obstetrics and Gynecology.* 1987;156(5):1342-1446.

36. Riggs BL, Khosla S, and Melton LJ III. Sex steroids and the construction and conservation of the adult skeleton. *Endocrine Reviews.* 2002;23:279-302.

37. Risser W, Lee E, Leblanc A, Poindexter H, Risser J, and Schneider V. Bone density in eumenorrheic female college athletes. *Medicine and Science in Sport and Exercise.* 1990;22:570-74.

38. Samuels MH, Sanborn CF, Hofeldt F, and Robbins R. The role of endogenous opiates in athletic amenorrhea. *Fertility and Sterility.* 1991;55(3):507-12.

39. Sanborn CF, Martin BJ, and Wagner WW Jr. Is athletic amenorrhea specific to runners? *American Journal of Obstetrics and Gynecology.* 1982;143(8):859-61.

40. Snow-Harter CM. Bone health and prevention of osteoporosis in active and athletic women. *Clinics in Sports Medicine.* 1994;13:389-404.

41. Stephen GR. Presented at American College of Sports Medicine Annual Meeting, University of Washington, June 1993.

42. Taafe DR, Robinson TL, Snow CM, and Marcus R. High-impact exercise promotes bone gain in well-trained female athletes. *Journal of Bone and Mineral Research.* 1997;12:255-60.

43. The Practice Committee of the American Society for Reproductive Medicine. Current evaluation of amenorrhea. *Fertility and Sterility.* 2004;82(Suppl 1): S33-S39.

44. Tosi LL, and Lane JM. Editorial: Osteoporosis prevention and the orthopaedic surgeon: when fracture care is not enough. *Journal of Bone and Joint Surgery.* 1998;80A:1567-1569.

45. Voss LA, Fadale PD, and Hulstyn MJ. Exercise-induced loss of bone density in athletes. *Journal of the American Academy of Orthopaedic Surgeons.* 1998;6: 349-357.

46. Wakat DK, Sweeney KA, and Rogol AD. Reproductive system function in women cross-country runners. *Medicine and Science in Sport and Exercise.* 1982;14(4):263-9.

47. Warren MP, Brooks-Gun J, Fox RP et al. Persistent osteopenia in ballet dancers with amenorrhea and delayed menarche despite hormone therapy: a longitudinal study. *Fertility and Sterility.* 2003;80(2):398-404.

48. Wilmore JH, Wambsgans KC, Brenner M et al. Is there energy conservation in amenorrheic compared to eumenorrheic distance runners? *Journal of Applied Physiology.* 1992;72(1):15-22.

49. Zanker CL, and Cooke CB. Energy balance, bone turnover, and skeletal health in physically active individuals. *Medicine and Science in Sport and Exercise.* 2004;36(8):1372-1381.

50. Zanker CL, Cooke CB, Truscott JG et al. Annual changes of bone density over 12 years in an amenorrheic athlete. *Medicine and Science in Sport and Exercise.* 2004;36:137-42.

SECTION 3

Managing the Athlete with an Eating Disorder

CHAPTER 8

Components of an Eating Disorder Program

Shari Bartz, PhD, ATC

Introduction

There are several components to preventing eating disorders that should be addressed when developing a health care intervention policy. While the institutional policy should be overly comprehensive covering as much as possible, it should also include how to prevent a disorder or how to prevent further development of a disorder that has already manifested itself. Prevention starts with the ability to identify an individual with a disorder, knowing how and when to intervene, and finally how to manage a disorder after recognition and intervention have taken place. This chapter focuses on these components, while the details on how to develop a policy are covered in Chapter 9.

Prevention

Prevention should be addressed through all stages of an eating disorder program (i.e. recognition, intervention, and management) and can be broken down into primary, secondary, and tertiary components. In its 2007 Position Stand, the American College of Sports Medicine stresses the importance of having a good prevention program. It also stresses the need for early diagnosis and treatment to deter the possible irreversible consequences that often manifest as a result of the inter-related components of the female athlete triad, including low energy availability, amenorrhea, and osteoporosis.[17]

The goal of primary prevention is to prevent the onset of an eating disorder. Primary prevention programs should be directed mainly at the elementary, middle, and high school levels, where eating disorders often begin, but should be a focus of all eating disorder policies.

The goal of secondary prevention is to intervene early in the development of a health problem or eating disorder. This portion of the policy would target the population that has already had some experience with an eating disorder or has already begun to exhibit characteristics associated with an eating disorder, such as weight obsession or performing excessive exercise techniques as a form of purging. The objective of secondary prevention is to limit the extent of abuse and, if possible, to reduce it.[13] Overall, this group tends to be older than those persons targeted in primary prevention.

The goal of tertiary prevention is treatment and/or rehabilitation, as well as the prevention of relapse. Having policies and procedures for treatment and/or rehabilitation will ensure that the target population of the policy receives information regarding stance and/or protocol for helping an athlete who is in any stage of an eating disorder. It is important to remember that eating disorders can develop at any age; therefore, policy should target all aspects of prevention, including primary, secondary, and tertiary.

Identification

A primary area of importance in planning prevention interventions is having knowledge of or being able to recognize the risk factors involved.[27,29, 24] There are several methods that can be used to identify an athlete who is suspected of having an eating disorder, including the use of surveys and questionnaires, observing the population, talking with the athletes either individually or in a group setting, or combining any of the above mentioned methods.[20]

Part of understanding the problem is understanding the nature of the problem in different settings (i.e. whether the setting involves a physical education teacher working with students at the middle school level or a collegiate coach working with an athlete). Barriers to identification of eating disorders include avoidance of the topic by coaches because of the complicated nature of the subject and/or because of the fear that they may have contributed to the development of the problem. The athlete's teammates may be uncertain about how to help or may fear that the behaviors seen in their teammate may also be seen in themselves. It is important to realize that there is no quick fix to this problem and that a multifaceted approach is necessary to address all associated issues. Recognizing potential barriers and educating individuals about the contributing factors are often the first step in understanding and identifying eating disorders.

There are many methods that can be used to identify an individual with an eating disorder. One method is the use of a survey or questionnaire, which can be given at a preparticipation physical examination or at a separate team meeting to discuss nutrition and performance. Other methods include observing the population for signs and symptoms of eating disorders, and talking with the athletes. Talking with athletes can be done in several ways, including one-on-one interviews with the individual, a group interview, a written interview, or anonymous response process. The important thing to remember is that there is not one single method of identifying the problem and that often a combination of methods is the best approach.

Prevention efforts aim to reduce the incidence of eating disorders.[27,28] Primary prevention of eating disorders refers to programs that are designed to prevent the occurrence of the target disorder before it begins as a means of promoting and sustaining healthy development. Rosen and Neumark-Sztainer[19] introduced a comprehensive approach to primary prevention by addressing at all levels, which eating disturbances may occur, from individual counseling to efforts for changing societal norms, and suggested that primary prevention programs coexist with secondary and tertiary prevention efforts and remain a high priority because of the prevalence of the conditions and the large amounts of suffering that these conditions impose.

Education

Secondary prevention is designed to facilitate identification and correction of a disorder in its early stages, when the disorder is less likely to be a "lifestyle" and more likely to be associated with other significant problems. Secondary prevention involves education about signs and symptoms, effective ways to reach out to people in distress, and referral to appropriate sources of treatment. According to Rosen and Neumark-Sztainer,[19] in choosing the factors to be addressed in prevention programs, it is essential to consider the intervention setting. Prevention strategies need to involve the education of coaches, athletic trainers, parents, athletes, and anyone else working closely with the athletes.[29, 19, 12]

Not educating individuals about their role in preventing or identifying a potential eating disorder only contributes to the problem. According to Williamson et al.,[30] social pressure for thinness from coaches and peers, as well as anxiety about athletic performance and negative self-appraisal of athletic achievement, were associated with increased concern about body size and shape. Institutional rules enforced by coaching and support staff can also contribute to the development of an eating disorder. Standards that require a minimum number of individuals to compete in a minimum number of contests, such as the standards of the NCAA,[5] place pressures on coaches that could lead to poor health care decisions regarding their athletes. Such standards place a coach in the contradictory position of knowing that an athlete should not compete because of health status, but also of knowing that, if the athlete does not compete, the university would be in jeopardy of being placed in a probationary status. This situation, in effect, could place the coach in a position in which his or her job may be held in jeopardy. Certainly, coaches generally hold the health care of the athlete in high priority; however, the pressure to produce winning teams and high-level, competitive athletes is also of paramount concern at some institutions.

Coaches and athletes alike are concerned with performance outcome and with being the best they can be. It is a common misperception, often on the part of coaches, that talking about eating disorders will encourage their manifestation. This is a myth that must be overcome. It should be emphasized that the disorders do not develop from talking about them or from educating oneself about the risks.[20] Coaches, according to Ryan, must learn to distinguish the variables that affect body weight as a performance factor, and must also learn to identify those athletes who may be likely to develop an eating disorder. By identifying characteristics early, coaches and athletic trainers may be able to reach these athletes before they display all of the characteristics of a clinically diagnosed eating disorder.

Classifying an individual as being at risk begins with knowledge of the contributing factors of eating disorders. Contributing factors in the athletic setting have a tendency to stem from environmental, social, and psychological factors.[20] Environmental factors may include being vulnerable to the media and advertising, which emphasize sexual stereotypes. Social factors may include family histories such as having someone in the family who has a history of alcoholism or having an individual in the family who has a history of sexual abuse. Psychological risk factors include sensitivity to criticism, perfectionism, or a need for approval.

Although coaches may not have all of this information available to them, parents, friends, or the athletes themselves may have such information.

By educating as many individuals as possible, including coaches, administrators, the athletes themselves, support staff, parents, and others, to recognize the contributing factors and the early signs and symptoms of eating disorders, the risk of development of an eating disorder can be minimized. Typically, athletes do not set out to manifest an eating disorder; however, one may develop if any or all of these contributing factors are present. There is no set number of risk factors that an athlete must have to develop a disorder; one can be the key number. If educated about the predisposing factors, athletes can minimize their risk themselves. These athletes want to reach peak performance in the best way possible. It is the job of the coaches, administrators, and support staff to educate them about what the best way is.

Coaches and athletic trainers must not become so focused on one component of a disorder, for example the psychological component, that the interrelationship among the components is lost. It is known that there is a large psychological component to athletic participation, but it is also known that proper nutrition is also a key contributor to optimal performance. Both psychological stress and improper nutrition have effects on the health and well-being of the body, which also demonstrates the link to the general health status of an athlete.

Athletes are typically highly-trained, competitive, achievement oriented, disciplined, often perfectionist individuals who have goals to perform to the best of their abilities. These characteristics are also commonly seen in women with eating disorders.[9] For example, they tend to possess poor coping skills when dealing with issues, such as: academic demand, injury, perceived poor sports performance, social relationships, financial concerns, or family issues. Instead of managing these problems in a healthy way, athletes often try to manage their weight, thus providing a sense of control.[11] Coaches and support staff must understand these interrelationships because what they say to an athlete may have implications far beyond the intended behavior change. The institution must make the roles of the coaching and support staff clear. Just as the athletes are expected to attend informational meetings regarding health, nutrition, and performance, so should the coaching and support staff be expected to attend educational meetings regarding institutional policies, including those related to eating disorders, on an annual basis.

Assessment Tools

Educational Benchmarks

Over the years, there have been several attempts to create materials to assist athletic personnel in educating their athletes regarding eating disorders. In 1989, Randa Ryan[20] published the first policy on eating disorders in collegiate athletics. This policy helped to educate athletic administrators, coaches, athletic trainers, medical personnel, and student athletes about the potential risks and associated health hazards of disordered eating. Other available materials include videotapes and written supplements that were sent to each NCAA member institution in 1998 to be reviewed as part of the NCAA project, "Nutrition and Eating Disorders in College Athletes."[15] In 1992, the ACSM began developing material specific to the female athlete triad and three national organizations published position statements related directly to the triad and the timeline is as follows. In 2005 the International Olympic Committee published thiers while in 2007 the Americian College of Sports Medicine revised thier original position stand and most recently in 2008, the National Athletic Trainer's Association came out with theirs entitled Preventing, Detecting, and Managing Disordered Eating in Athletes.[2]

The Process

As discussed in greater detail earlier in the text, there are several well-known assessment tools in existence, including the EDI,[7] the Diagnostic Survey for Eating Disorders, Revised,[10] the EAT,[6] and the National Eating Disorder Screening Program.[16] These assessment tools collect data on areas, such as weight history, body image, dieting behaviors, binge-eating and purging behavior, menstruation, and medical and psychiatric history. Once again, the earlier these disorders can be identified, the greater the chance of minimizing the harmful effects on the health and sport performance of the athletes.

The assessment and diagnoses of athletes should begin at the pre-participation physical examination. The primary purpose of this examination is to identify athletes who may be at risk before they participate in a specific sport.[8] Information that is gathered in the examination establishes baseline data that can be used for comparison in the future. For athletes who may develop an eating disorder during their college careers, these data will allow the medical personnel to look back at baseline height, weight, body composition, heart rate, blood pressure, and numerous other pieces of valuable information. The college or university team physician, rather than the athlete's personal physician, is the best individual to perform the examination. This allows team physicians to get to know athletes who will be under their care. Because of the broad population that family physicians treat, they often do not have an extensive background in sports-related injuries or disorders unless they had specific training in their schooling.

Having solid knowledge of the factors that can lead to eating disorders and having knowledge about performance factors can help coaches in preventing a disorder from happening. Often, by using qualitative analysis, a coach determines that an athlete is overweight and needs to lose a few pounds to help improve performance. If a proper assessment to determine whether losing weight is what the athlete really needs is not done, further decrease in performance is often seen. What coaches must realize is that there is a difference between losing fat and losing lean body weight. Coaches, along with the general population, often assume that, if an athlete loses body weight when already overweight, the effects will be positive. Losing nonlean or fat weight is good; however, losing lean weight, or muscle weight, is not good. This is where proper education of coaches; placing an emphasis away from body weight and composition and instead focusing more on athlete performance can be an invaluable tool in the prevention of an eating disorder.

Knowing that coaches can be a precipitating factor in the development of a disorder, it is important to stress that discussions with athletes should be well thought out before any consultation occurs. This could mean that the focus of the conversation be on performance factors and not directly on how much the athlete weighs or specific numbers on the scale as this can lead to additional complications. Coaches may want to either hire a nutritionist or have one speak to student athletes on topics to take the pressure off of them to discuss how proper nutrition impacts their performance. Example topics to be discussed could be performance enhancing foods, how to shop for success on a college student budget, or what to eat when time is at a premium. By shifting discussions away from the negative and ambiguous task of losing weight and focusing more on the positive aspect of improving performance, we can once again work to prevent eating disorders from manifesting themselves.

Both body weight and body composition have received much attention as possible causes of athletic amenorrhea, which shows increased prevalence rates among runners and ballet dancers.[22] Physicians typically obtain information on height and weight during a pre-participation physical examination.

But, what is done with this information? Is it beneficial to use an accepted range of values to help identify those individuals at greater risk for development of the Female Athlete Triad? Other questions arise as to who will collect the information. If the information is being collected to evaluate the health care of the athlete, it would be appropriate to have the data collected by a health care professional and not a coach. By placing this task in the hands of the health care provider, the coach is removed from the controversial position of pressuring an athlete to "lose weight," which is discussed as a possible precipitating factor in the development of eating disorders in athletes.

Arguments exist about whether to focus on body weight or on body fat when evaluating sport performance. According to Smith,[25] tables of weight for height, sex, and frame size are of little relevance to the serious athlete. Thompson and Trattner-Sherman[29] believe that "the individual with an eating problem is usually someone who is pursuing the ideal body, shape or weight" (p. 32–33). This implies that the individual has not yet achieved "ideal" weight and body composition, but is striving to reach these goals. Distance runners tend to be below the weight standards for the general population, but this tendency does not mean that all distance runners who fall below standards have an eating disorder.

Height and Weight

The most common method used to determine appropriate body has been to compare individual height and weight values with growth grids or tables.

According to Peterson,[18] the first height-to-weight values used were published by the Metropolitan Life Insurance Company, but the accuracy of these documents was highly questioned. The tables were developed in 1959, and weight ranges were specific to individuals who were insured and of the lowest mortality rates. However, these values are not reflective of the athletic population. Today, the most common assessment tool used by health care professionals to determine appropriate height-to-weight values are the body mass index (BMI) tables that were created in 1977[4] and then adopted for international use in 1978 and updated in May 2000.

The BMI is a single number that evaluates an individual's weight in relation to the individual's height. BMI, along with skinfold (SF), is one of the first indicators used in assessing body fat and is one of the most common methods of tracking weight problems and obesity among adults.[4] BMI is also the tool most widely used by health practitioners to track growth and development in children and to assist in identifying signs of potential developmental problems. This index divides weight in kilograms, by height in meters squared, and has a high correlation with SF measurement.[18]

In addition to height and weight, some tables also take into consideration the frame size of the individual. According to Peterson,[18] after the 1971–1974 U.S. Health and Nutrition Survey (HANES) was completed a classification system of body-frame size was developed that used elbow breadth, which is reported to be a reliable indicator of frame size independent of obesity and age.

In addition to body weight, which is largely determined by genetics and depends on an athlete's body size and body type, body composition can also be explored. The most common methods of predicting body composition are bioelectrical impedance anthropometry (BIA), skeletal anthropometric width (SAW), near infrared (NIR), computed tomography-magnetic resonance imaging (CT-MRI), hydrostatic weighing (HW), and SF. Choosing the appropriate method must take into consideration cost, availability, time constraints, validity, and reliability. One of the most economical and widely used assessment tools is the SF.

The SF is used widely among the athletic population. The two most standard SF calipers used are the Lange and Harpenden brands. There are standard SF sites, depending on whether the subject is male or female. The sites are marked, identified, and then gently palpated. The SF and underlying fat are then elevated by using the thumb and index finger of the left hand to pinch the skin. The calipers are held in the right hand and perpendicular to the site, and measurements are taken.[23]

In 1974, Frisch and McArthur proposed the "critical-fat" theory. This theory suggested that a critical level of 17% body fat was necessary for menarche to take place and that 22% body fat was needed for regular menstrual cycles to be maintained. This theory has since been refuted through a critical review of the methods and statistical analysis.[24] In addition, the critical-fat theory has been refuted further in more recent studies. No significant differences in the percentage of body fat of amenorrheic and regularly menstruating subjects were found within a group of athletes.[3,21,22] Despite the refutable nature of this topic, it is still widely discussed today. The question that coaches and health care providers must continue to ask themselves is how they plan to use information regarding body fat and body composition.

Only after proper education occurs regarding the factors that contribute to the development of an eating disorder, along with knowledge on how to identify an individual with a disorder, can the true focus be on preventing a disorder from occurring. It is important to know that this is not the job nor the responsibility of one individual; coaches and health care providers must work together to ensure the health and well-being of their athletes.

Intervention

As discussed previously, the goal of secondary prevention is to intervene early in the development of a health problem or eating disorder. Those involved in this type of prevention should ask themselves a series of questions before moving forward. For example, "What do I say to the person?" "How should I say it?" "What if she gets angry with me?" The person intervening should also have the appropriate referral resources in place before approaching the subject. This should be defined in the eating disorder policy. Because every situation is unique, and every individual responds different in various situations, the health care practitioner should have multiple resources for referral. The referral process is discussed in detail in a later chapter.

Non-Threatening Atmosphere

After having appropriate resources are in place, the health care practitioner should decide on a location in which to speak with the athlete. This should be in a public, but private area, such as an office. This allows the conversation with the athlete to stay confidential. Next, decide what to say to the athlete. One recommended approach is to use open-ended questions to allow the athlete an opportunity to open up. Ask the athlete how she is doing and give her an opportunity to respond. The coach or athletic trainer may find that she is very busy; overwhelmed with school, working, studying, trying to fit in at college and is having trouble balancing it all. She may also respond that she is "fine" with no elaboration. Any answer that the athlete gives, either verbally or non-verbally can lead additional questions. A statement such as; "You seem a little tired in practice lately" can lead to further discussion. The athlete may open up further that she just doesn't have time to eat with how busy her schedule is.

The intervener, then has an opportunity to discuss healthy alternatives to not eating or to suggest that the athlete sit down with the team nutritionist to come up with a customized plan for that athlete. Although some cases may appear to be obvious, an intervener should not assume that an individual has an eating disorder until they have an opportunity to sit down and speak with the athlete. The coach and athletic trainer may find that due to all of the stress in the athlete's life that she is having stomach pains and therefore doesn't eat because the food won't stay down. Clinically, according to DSM-IV criteria the athlete may meet the criteria for anorexia, falling below required weight for height; remembering that this is very different from an individual with anorexia nervosa who has an obsession with the characteristics of their body. Treatment and referral for this individual may be very different from the individual with suspected anorexia nervosa.

Management

Management of the program begins after the athlete has been referred to the appropriate individual(s) for treatment. Because of the nature of eating disorders, a multifaceted approach is usually best and should include a medical examination by a physician; a counseling session with a psychiatrist, psychologist, or licensed counselor; and nutritional counseling by a registered dietician or nutritionist who specializes in eating disorders.[14,1,29,2,17] Development of intervention goals should be addressed, as well as the development of long-term strategies to alleviate the factors. Eating disorders have medical, nutritional, and psychological associations. Striegel-Moore[27] wrote about the tremendous gains made by women as a result of the women's liberation movement and about how women still struggle with the age-old gender-role expectation of beauty as the "quintessential female achievement." Women are now confronted with the "superwoman" ideal, which describes ideal femininity as encompassing beauty, motherhood, and career success. By combining these society stresses placed on women with the added pressures and desires to optimize performance in the female athlete, the risk factors for developing inappropriate nutritional habits are greatly increased in the female athlete.

Should management of an individual with an eating disorder include the coach? This is a controversial issue, to say the least. Institutional rules and regulations often require athletes to maintain a certain weight or body-fat percentage to make a team. Once the athlete has made a team, this process often continues, with maintenance checks once a week or once every two weeks. If the athlete does not maintain the desired weight, a financial scholarship or position on the team may be jeopardized. Two sports in which this commonly occurs are cheerleading and dance teams.

Policies may require that a certain number of individuals in a team participate in a set number of events. An example of this is evident in NCAA Policy 20.9.3.3, which requires Division I track and field teams to enter a minimum of 14 contestants in a minimum of six contests over the duration of one season.[5] According to Policy 20.3.5.1.2, failure to meet the minimum sports sponsorship requirements can result in a one-year probation for the college. If the college fails to meet the sports sponsorship criteria at the end of the probationary period, the institution will be placed in a restricted-membership category, making the college ineligible for NCAA championship competition in all sports, for both men and women.[5] Although coaches generally hold the health care of the athlete in high priority, pressures of policy can often place coaches in a conflicted role concerning the health of the athlete. These pressures can encourage coaches to enter an athlete into competition who may not be medically fit because of injury or an eating disorder. This practice may be seen in teams that are struggling to meet the minimum number of contestants required.

Having information available for athletes, coaches, and support staff regarding the prevention, intervention, and management of eating disorders is a start toward reducing prevalence rates in athletics but is not enough. Training all involved individuals about how to prevent, treat, and manage an individual suspected of having an eating disorder also needs to take place. Before training can occur, the institution should have a written policy regarding its stand on the issues involved. It could be argued that the importance of having a written eating-disorder policy in the athletic setting parallels other more traditional policies such as those concerning sexual harassment and drug testing.

Summary

It should be clear how important it is to have an eating disorder program in place. Although identification of eating disorders remains extremely important and many different programs exist, if your institution does not have policy, or, dire consequences may occur. Therefore, it is imperative that your institution has a program in place.

References

1. Baer J, Walker W, and Grossman J. A disordered eating response team's effect on nutrition practices in college athletes. *Journal of Athletic Training.* 1995;30(4):315-317.

2. Bonci C, Bonci L, Granger L et al. National Athletic Trainers' Association Position Statement: Preventing, Detecting, and Managing Disordered Eating in Athletes. *Journal of Athletic Training.* 2008;43(1):80-108.

3. Carlberg K, Buckman M, Peake G, and Riedesel M. Body composition of oligo/amenorrhoeic athletes. *Medicine and Science in Sport and Exercise.* 1983;15:215-217.

4.   Centers for Disease Control (CDC). *BMI Tables*. Available at: http://www.cdc.gov. Accessed June 8, 2001.

5.   Earle M. *2002-03 NCAA Division I Manual*. Indianapolis: National Collegiate Athletic Association; 2002.

6.   Garner D, and Garfinkel P. The eating attitudes test: an index of the symptoms of anorexia nervosa. *Psychological Medicine*. 1979;9:273-279.

7.   Garner D, Olmsted M, and Polivy J. *Eating Disorders Inventory*. Odessa, FL: Psychological Assessment Resources; 1983.

8.   Herbert D. Professional considerations related to conduct of pre-participation exams. *Sports Med Stand Malpractice Report*. 1994;6(4):49.

9.   Jackson S, and Marsh H. Athletic or antisocial? The female sport experience. *Journal of Sport Psychology*. 1986;8:198-211.

10. Johnson C, and Pure D. Assessment of bulimia: a multidimensional model. In: Brownell KD and Foreyt JP eds, *Handbook of Eating Disorders: Physiology, Psychology, and Treatment*. New York: Basic Books; 1986.

11. Johnson M. Disordered eating in active and athletic women. *Clinics in Sports Medicine*. 1994;13(2):355-369.

12. Joy E, Clark N, Lloyd-Ireland M, Martire J, Nattiv A, and Varechok S. Team management of the female athlete triad: part 2: optimal treatment and prevention tactics. *The Physician and Sportsmedicine*. 1997;25(4):12.

13. Levinthal C. *Drugs, Behavior, and Modern Society*. 3rd ed. Boston, MA: Allyn and Bacon; 2002:346-347.

14. Linnell S, Stager J, Blue P, Oyster N, and Robertshaw D. Bone mineral content and menstrual regularity in female runners. *Medicine and Science in Sport and Exercise*. 1984;16:343-348.

15. National Collegiate Athletic Association (NCAA). Eating disorders. In: Earle M. ed. *NCAA Sports Medicine Handbook* 11th ed., Overland Park: NCAA; 1998:24-26.

16. National Eating Disorder Screening Program (NEDSP). *National Eating Disorder Screening Program*. Screening for Mental Health, Inc. June 8, 2001.

17. Nattiv A, Loucks A, Manore M, Sandborn C, Sundgot-Borgen J, and Warren M. Position Stand: The Female Athlete Triad. *Medicine and Science in Sport and Exercise*. 2007;39(10):1-9.

18. Peterson M. *Eat to compete* 2nd ed., St. Louis: Mosby; 1996.

19. Rosen D, and Neumark-Sztainer, D. Review of options for primary prevention of eating disturbances among adolescents. *Journal of Adolescent Health*. 1998;23(6):354-363.

20. Ryan R. Management of eating problems in athletic settings. In: Brownell KD, Rodin J, and Wilmore JH eds, *Eating, Body Weight and Performance in Athletes; Disorders of Modern Society.* Malvern, PA: Lea and Febiger; 1992:334-361.

21. Sanborn C, Albrecht B, and Wagner W. Athletic amenorrhoea: lack of association with body fat. *Medicine and Science in Sport and Exercise.* 1987;19:207-212.

22. Sanborn C, Martin B, and Wagner W. (1982). Is athletic amenorrhoea specific to runners?

23. Scott J. (2001, February 21). *Body composition.* Paper presented at the Student Athletic Training Inservice, Grand Valley State University.

24. Sinning W, and Little D. Body composition and menstrual function in athletes. *Sports Medicine.* 1987;5:34-45.

25. Smith N. Weight control in the athlete. *Clinics in Sports Medicine.* 1984;3:693-704; *American Journal of Obstetrics Gynecology.* 1984;143: 859-61.

26. Spear B, and Stellefson-Meyers E. Position of the American Dietetic Association: nutrition intervention in the treatment of anorexia nervosa, bulimia nervosa, and eating disorders not otherwise specified (EDNOS). *Journal of The American Dietetic Association.* 2001;101(7):810-9.

27. Striegel-Moore R. Risk factors for eating disorders. *Annals of Sports Medicine.* 1997.

28. Sundgot-Borgen J. Eating disorders in female athletes [Review]. *Sports Medicine.* 1994;17(3):176-188.

29. Thompson R, and Trattner-Sherman R. *Helping Athletes with Eating Disorders.* Champaign: Human Kinetics; 1993.

30. Williamson D, Netemeyer R, Jackman L, Anderson D, Funsch C, and Rabalais J. Structural equation modeling of risk factors for the development of eating disorder symptoms in female athletes. *International Journal of Eating Disorders.* 1995;17(4):387-393.

CHAPTER 9

Development of the Eating Disorder Policy

Shari Bartz, PhD, ATC

Introduction

Although it is important that policies and procedures exist to guide the course of actions to be taken in particular circumstances, it is also important that policy development does not become lost in current "hot" issues and theories.[9] From policies regarding gender equity to drug testing, controversy exists about their effectiveness and constitutionality. Eating disorders, although a hot topic, are something health care professionals and coaches can help to minimize by simply recognizing the signs and symptoms and knowing how to act. The problem is that many coaches and athletic trainers don't know how to recognize these conditions or what to do if they suspect that an athlete is afflicted. The purpose of this chapter is to provide a framework to development of a policy that will address all aspects of eating disorders from prevention, to intervention, to management of eating disorders.

The Significance of an Eating Disorder Policy

With the high rate of eating disorders in collegiate athletics, creating an eating-disorder policy is a proactive approach toward helping to ensure the health and welfare of student athletes, as well as reducing the chance of litigation against the university. Eating disorders have been recorded to occur at a ratio of 10:1 women to men. It could be argued that, without an eating-disorder policy, women athletes are not receiving the standard of care owed to them under the law, specifically, Title IX of the Education Amendment of 1972.

Although mortality is by far the most significant problem and morbidity the most prevalent problem associated with eating disorders, the concern of litigation at any institution is an area of importance. From a risk-management perspective, Bickford[3] investigated the legal duty of college athletic departments to athletes with eating disorders. More important, the focus of her study was to address the issue of the role of the athletic department in the well-being of the student athlete. Bickford points out that it is established and accepted that athletes at the collegiate level are owed a duty of care under reasonable and ordinary circumstances.

Just as a coach would not allow an athlete who is injured or sick to compete if additional harm could come to the athlete, a coach or athletic trainer must not allow an athlete with an eating disorder to continue to compete. Depending on the stage of the eating disorder, an athlete who continues to participate in sports, risks decreases in health and performance. More specifically, there is a risk of osteoporosis; stress fractures; and, although rare, death from cardiac arrhythmias.[19] Failing to act in a reasonable and prudent manner, (i.e. allowing an athlete to continue to compete without evaluation by a physician) could lead to a coach or athletic trainer being found negligent in a court of law; all the more reason to employ a policy that delineates prevention, intervention, and management procedures.

Another reason for a formal policy is illustrated in Macrina et al.,[16] which examines the use of the Glasgow Coma Scale (GCS) by emergency-department personnel. The GCS is a valid and reliable tool used to assess neurological status in patients and its effectiveness has been well documented in the literature. Analysis revealed that when the results of the GCS were present in a medical chart, the patient was more likely to be referred for formal rehabilitation. The study also found that injury severity, as measured by the GCS score, predicted referral to rehabilitation and that the greater the severity of the injury was determined to be, as indicated by the GCS, the greater the level of rehabilitative care. The problem was that, although the personnel understood the importance of the tool, they continued either to not use it or to use it very inconsistently. They found that simply conveying the benefits of a particular protocol or practice was insufficient to bring about change in patient-care practice and also found that the most significant changes in usage occurred in emergency departments that required or encouraged the use of the GCS through formal policy. In addition, they also found that an on-site advocate of change was a significant factor that influenced the potential for behavior change.

There are various reasons why institutions may not have policies regarding eating disorders, such as ???? a lack of resources, funding, or in extreme cases even knowledge. The GCS example demonstrated that when policies and procedures were followed, the staff was better able to recognize the problem and more likely to refer. A formal eating disorder policy can improve patient care could also create better recognition and treatment for individuals with eating disorders. Some individuals may feel that eating disorders are not a problem at their institution, but one could that is the result of not having a staff trained on how to recognize the problem.

The GCS example also demonstrated that having an on-site advocate for policy implementation, such as an athletic director who requires mandatory training sessions regarding eating disorder policies and procedures, resulted in better recognition and treatment of athletes with this condition.

Current Organizations with Eating-Disorder Policies and Position Statements

In a study conducted in 2000,[2] it was discovered that 19% of NCAA Division I athletic programs stated that they had an eating-disorder policy and an additional 28% reported that they had one in progress. These findings indicate that approximately 50% of responding institutions felt that the issue of eating disorders was important enough to warrant policy development. The first published eating disorder policy at the collegiate level was created at the University of Texas at Austin (UTA). This is a comprehensive policy that has been in publication for over 10 years.[23] It addresses the areas of recognition, prevention, treatment, and management of eating disorders in the collegiate population.

Several professional organizations have also written statements and policies regarding eating disorders. In 1992, the American College of Sports Medicine (ACSM) introduced the term *female athlete triad*.[1] The term *triad* was created as physicians began to see correlations among individuals with amenorrhea, osteoporosis, and disordered eating. In 1997, the ACSM issued a position statement on the female athlete triad, stating that it is a serious syndrome that needs further research. In addition, this organization strongly advised that specific strategies be developed to prevent, recognize, and treat this problem.[18] In 2007, the ACSM issued a position statement which replaced the one created in 1997. This statement focused on three inter-related spectrums; low energy availability (with or without eating disorders), amenorrhea, and osteoporosis and stressed the importance of developing a prevention program, early diagnosis, and treatment due to the possible irreversible consequences of these conditions.[17]

Other organizations, including the Society for Adolescent Medicine and the American Dietetic Association[24] have policies relating to eating disorders. In 2001, the Committee on Sports Medicine and Fitness of the American Academy of Pediatrics issued a position statement on medical concerns of the female athlete.[20] In 2003, the American Academy of Pediatrics issued a policy statement for pediatricians on identifying and treating eating disorders.[13] In 2008, the National Athletic Trainers' Association created a position statement with the purpose of providing recommendations to athletic healthcare personnel, coaches, and support personnel working with athletes who may present or be at risk for disordered eating.[4]

The Policy Development Process

When the decision is made by an organization to create a policy, the next question becomes, "How are policies created?" Is there a sharing of information among universities and professionals in the field? Yes, of course there is. Although, it is positive to think that a profession is open to the sharing of information, from where is the initial information coming? Consider this scenario: Did Professional 1 research how to properly write a policy or work with a university board to create this policy? Alternatively, did Professional 1 simply brainstorm a list of ideas that this person felt should go into a so-called policy, put the ideas down on paper, label them as a policy, and share them with Professional 2, who modified the ideas to meet their needs and decide to call those ideas their policy?

Administratively, the individuals that are involved with policy development must understand what constitutes a policy. One study demonstrated that when collecting eating disorder policies from NCAA Division I institutions there were five separate interpretations of what constituted a policy.[2] Programs submitted policies, protocols, procedures, guidelines and some not labeled at all. It is difficult to stress the need for or the importance of a policy for athletes suspected of having an eating disorder until we know what a policy is. By providing a framework for policy development it is our hope that programs will have an educated starting position for the development of an eating disorder policy. According to Karger,[14] a policy framework is a systematic means for examining a specific policy or series of policies and can be used to evaluate the congruence of a policy with the missions and goals of the department or university.

Some may argue that what a document is called is simply an issue of semantics, whereas others may cite the difference between a standard and a guideline. The Commission on Accreditation of Allied Health Education Programs states that standards are the minimum requirement to which an accredited program is held accountable, whereas guidelines are intended to assist in interpreting standards. If athletic program administrators do not convey to their staff that standards are required and not optional, then the staff may not be very inclined to enforce the policy.

When the policy is being created, it is important to first conceptualize and to be sure that the following three content areas are addressed:

- prevention, including identification and education
- intervention
- management of individuals who are either identified as having an eating disorder or suspected of having one

Each of these areas is well supported in the literature as an important factor in the holistic treatment of an individual with an eating disorder. The framework will assist in the development of a comprehensive eating disorder policy.

Developing the Framework or Purpose

Once the conceptualization of the policy is completed and it is time to put pen to paper, there are four sections that should be included in a strategic planning process that will guide the development of the policy:[14]

- Historical background.
- Description of the problem(s) that necessitate the policy.
- Description of the policy which includes the three areas previously mentioned above.
- Policy analysis; including policy goals, political feasibility, economic feasibility, and administrative feasibility.

After the strategic planning has been completed, the next step is to make the plan operational through the development of the policies, processes, and procedures. The following section provides the framework to guide individuals through this process. The first place to start is with a description explaining the purpose of the eating disorder policy; acknowledged by Karger[14] to be a main component of policy development. As part of the purpose the population for whom the policy is intended and who your "at-risk" population is needs to be defined.

Developing the Policy

A policy, as defined by Ray[21] and Castetter,[7] is a plan for expressing the organization's intended behavior. Policies are broad statements of intended action created and do not answer detailed questions about operation. Policies should be created by a board of individuals; in this case the athletic trainer, coach, nutritionist, team physician, and mental health professional. After the board creates the policy it should then be endorsed by an administrator, in this case the athletic director. According to Ray,[21] the policy should be consistent with the vision and mission of the program, department, and/or university to help ensure its effectiveness. For example, a sample policy statement may read as follows:
The Smith University Athletic Department is committed to

- preventing athletes from developing disordered eating patterns or clinically diagnosed eating disorders
- establishing a protocol to be followed by all athletic department personnel and athletes, should an athlete be diagnosed with disordered eating or clinically diagnosed with a specific eating disorder.

A second example of a policy statement may read:
The Smith University Athletic Department will

- provide guidelines to all athletic department personnel for the recognition of individuals with an eating disorder or those who are suspected of having disordered eating and/or unhealthy exercise habits
- provide procedures for all athletic department personnel on intervention of these individuals
- provide a referral system for all athletic department personnel in the event that an athlete is diagnosed with having an eating disorder.

Developing the Processes

Once the policy is formed, the processes and procedures should follow. Processes are the next step down from a policy, and are the incremental and mutually dependent steps that direct the most important tasks.[21] Examples of process may include prevention of eating disorders, intervention of individuals suspected of having an eating disorder, management of eating disorders, organization and administration, and education and counseling. An example of a process for the prevention of eating disorders may read:

> The eating disorder management team, including the physician, athletic trainer, nutritionist, and psychologist, shall work together to provide student athletes, coaches, and support staff with a prevention program appropriate to the collegiate athletic setting. Considerations will be given to the specific dynamics of each athletic team.

Developing the Procedures

Procedures provide specific interpretations of processes, and are often referred to as protocols. Procedures tend to be fairly detailed and do not leave the employee much discretion on how to carry out the processes. The procedures should provide step-by-step instructions as to how the processes should be carried out. While developing procedures it is important for XXX to go back to the purpose of the policy and review for whom is the policy intended (i.e. athletes, coaches, or support staff). Procedures need to address all parties for whom the policy is intended.

If administration and/or the health care team evaluates the process of prevention, will coaches and support staff be required to go through training to recognize individuals with eating disorders or disordered eating behaviors? If deemed *Again, by whom?* important to educate athletic department personnel on how to recognize the signs and symptoms of eating disorders and/or disordered eating in their athletes, then a procedure explaining this would be required. To address the issue of communication between the eating-disorder-management personnel and the initial intervener, a procedure needs to be developed explaining who the intervener should refer to. Procedures provide structure and guidance to assist individuals with understanding their roles in the processes.

Training an athletic department can be done through several different modes, such as mandatory educational seminars, optional educational seminars, one-on-one meetings, etc. If performance outcome, proper nutrition, and mental status are all related, stress the importance that each of these areas in the processes and procedures.

Prevalence rates of eating disorders in college athletics have been reported to be as high as 73%,[12] with rates in the general population at approximately 3%-5%[15]. With such high rates, institutions may want to think hard whether training will be mandatory or optional. A problem with an optional approach to training is that a coach, athletic trainer, or support staff may not think training is necessary and many athletes with disordered eating do not realize that they have a problem. Admitting to a problem is the first step in an athlete's recovery process.

A myriad of methods of identification, including scrutinizing the pre-participation physical examination, observing the athletes, and talking with the athletes can be used. Additionally, other methods can be used to screen athletes like standardized health questionnaires designed to identify eating disorders, determining whether or not an athlete had been previously diagnosed as having an eating disorder or menstrual dysfunction, as well as examining BMI ratings as they can serve as useful tools in identification of a potential problem when used correctly. Talking with athletes as a group may prove to be one of the more controversial methods. A one-on-one meeting with an athlete should not be an issue, but discussing concern about an athlete with other athletes is cause for alarm because of the issue of confidentiality.

Questions to consider when writing procedures include

- Is the role of the support staff addressed?
- Is the role of the coach addressed?
- When will training take place?
- Will follow-up training be required?
- How will training be delivered?
- Will a procedure for referral be addressed?

Summary

Administratively, institutions need to address the issue of what constitutes a policy versus a guideline, protocol, or procedure. Prevalence rates of disordered eating in the athletic population have been shown to be significantly higher than in the general population.[5,6,12,22] The health and well-being of the athlete are often compromised, not only in the short term, but also in the long term. Health issues such as dehydration, malnutrition, amenorrhea, and osteoporosis have been associated with individuals with eating disorders.[8,10,11,22] In the short term, these health issues can lead to decreases in performance because of the lack of proper nutrients in the body.

Over time, problems such as fractures, caused by repeated stresses being placed on a body may develop, leading to increased time away from competition. The severe consequences of eating disorders, should lead an institution to provide a standard of care to its athletes as it is their legal duty to do so. This stresses the importance for the development of an eating disorder policy. To create a comprehensive policy, one must have knowledge of the basic components of policy development (i.e. the purpose, policy, processes, and procedures). When each of these areas is addressed an institution can be assured that they are meeting the needs of their athletes, coaches, and support staff in dealing with a serious condition. The framework for policy development included in this chapter is designed to assist institutions with this process.

References

1. American College of Sports Medicine. The female athlete triad: disordered eating, amenorrhea, osteoporosis: call to action. *Sports Med Bull.* 1992;27, 4.

2. Bartz S. *An exploration of eating disorder policies at NCAA division I institutions.* A dissertation. 2003; Birmingham.

3. Bickford BJ. The legal duty of a college athletics department to athletes with eating disorders: a risk management perspective. *Marquette Sports Law Journal.* 1999;10(1), 87-116.

4. Bonci C, Bonci L, Granger L, et al. National Athletic Trainers' Association Position Statement: Preventing, Detecting, and Managing Disordered Eating in Athletes. *Journal of Athletic Training.* 2008;43(1): 80-108.

5. Brooks-Gunn J, Warren M, and Hamilton L. The relationship of eating disorder to amenorrhea in ballet dancers. *Medicine and Science of Sports Exercise.* 1987;19, 41-44.

6. Burckes-Miller M, and Black D. Eating disorders: a problem in athletics. *Health Education.* 1988b;19, 22-25.

7. Castetter W. *The personnel function in educational administration* (4th ed.). New York: Macmillan; 1986.

8. Constantini N, and Warren M. Special problems of the female athlete. *Bailliere's Clinical Rheumatology.* 1994;8(1), 199-219.

9. Desai U, Holden M, and Shelley M. The politics of policy: prospects and realities. *Policy Studies Journal.* 1998;26(3), 423.

10. Drinkwater B, Nilson K, Chesnut III C, Bremner W, Shainholtz S, and Southworth M. Bone mineral content of amenorrheic and eumenorrheic athletes. *New England Journal of Medicine.* 1984;311(5), 277-281.

11. Frisch R, Gotz-Welbergen A, McArthur J, et al. Delayed menarche and amenorrhea of college athletes in relation to age of onset of training. *Journal of American Medical Association.* 1981;246(14), 1559-1563.

12. Guthrie S. Prevalence of eating disorders among intercollegiate athletes: contributing factors and preventative measures. In: Black (Ed.), *Eating Disorders Among Athletes*; 1991;43-66.

13. Kaplan D, Blythe M, Diaz A, Feinstein R, et al. Identifying and treating eating disorders. *Pediatrics.* 2003;111(1), 204.

14. Karger H. Social welfare policy research: a framework for policy analysis. In: P Quinlin (Ed.), *American social welfare policy: a pluralist approach* (4th ed.). Boston: Allyn and Bacon; 2002.

15. Leon G. Eating disorders in female athletes. *Sports Medicine*. 1991;12(4), 219-227.

16. Macrina D, Macrina N, Horvath C, Gallaspy J, and Fine P. An educational intervention to increase use of the glasgow coma scale by emergency department personnel. *International Journal of Trauma Nursing*. 1996;2(1), 7-12.

17. Nattiv A, Loucks A, Monroe M, Sandborn C, Sundgot-Borgen J, Warren M. Position Stand: The Female Athlete Triad. *Medicine and Science of Sports Exercise*. 2007;39(10), 1-9.

18. Otis C, Drinkwater B, Johnson M, Loucks A, and Wilmore J. American College of Sports Medicine Position stand: the female athlete triad. *Medicine and Science in Sport and Exercise*. 1997;29(5), i-ix.

19. Powers P, Tyson I, Stevens B, and Heal A. Total body potassium and scrum potassium among eating disorder patients. *International Journal of Eating Disorders*. 1995;18, 269-276.

20. Preboth M. Medical concerns of the young female athlete. *American Family Physician*. 2001;63(6), 1239.

21. Ray R. *Management strategies in athletic training* (2nd ed.). Champaign: Human Kinetics; 2000.

22. Rosen L, McKeag D, Hough D, and Curley V. Pathogenic weight-control behaviors in female athletes. *Physician Sportsmedicine*. 1986;14, 79-86.

23. Ryan R. Management of eating problems in athletic settings. In: Brownell KD, Rodin J, and Wilmore JH, (Eds.). *Eating, Body Weight and Performance in Athletes; Disorders of Modern Society*. Malvern, PA: Lea and Febiger; 1992:334-361.

24. Spear B, and Stellefson-Meyers E. Position of the American Dietetic Association: nutrition intervention in the treatment of anorexia nervosa, bulimia nervosa, and eating disorders not otherwise specified (EDNOS). *Journal of The American Dietetic Association*. 2001;101(7), 810-819.

CHAPTER 10

Development of the Eating Disorder Referral Program

Shari Bartz, PhD, ATC

Introduction

Eating disorders are a complex condition and therefore require a versatile approach to referral and treatment. As discussed in the previous chapter, what works for one athlete may not work or be appropriate for the next. Therefore, athletic department personnel, and health care personnel should be prepared to identify multiple resources as referrals.

The Referral Process

Coaches and support staff should be informed as to whom they should refer an athlete who is suspected of having an eating disorder. The referral is often the certified athletic trainer or another designated health care provider. The next step is to establish who the certified athletic trainer (ATCs) or designated health care provider will refer the athlete to for additional follow-up. For some athletes it is more appropriate to see a licensed counselor, for others a medical doctor, and yet others, a registered dietician. The health care provider or ATC must remember the uniqueness of each situation and that its management is equally as important.

Activation of the Referral Process

Once the athlete is in the system and accepts that she needs further treatment, a multifaceted approach to caring for the athlete is usually recommended, including a medical examination by a physician, a counseling session with a psychiatrist, psychologist, or licensed counselor; and nutritional counseling by a registered dietitian or nutritionist who specializes in eating disorders.[6,7,2]

The referral process and procedures of the institution's eating disorder policy should be defined to avoid any confusion. Furthermore, when determining a contact person for referral, the institution should also be sensitive to the fact that the coach might be part of the problem. Note also that contacting the parents may be a violation of the Health Insurance Portability and Accountability Act (HIPAA) of 1996 relating to confidentiality, especially if the athlete is considered to be a legal adult within the state. Confidentiality is a universal principal of health care ethics.

Because coaches are not considered health care providers, they should be counseled on the importance of this issue. Athletic trainers responsible for the electronic filing of insurance claims must follow the appropriate confidentiality rules set forth by HIPAA. HIPAA regulations only affect "covered entities," including all health care entities that utilize patients' medical records, such as certified athletic trainers in all employment settings.

HIPAA's privacy rule, which took effect on April 14, 2001, created national standards to protect individuals' personal health information and gave patients increased access to their medical records. This rule states that health care providers cannot disclose the personal health care information of a patient to a third party, unless authorized to do so by the patient; and the third party must be specified by the patient. This also means that the medical staff and the coaching staff must be told that authorization by a student athlete is required before the health care provider can discuss the condition of the athlete with the coaching staff, administration, support staff, or any other individuals, including the athlete's teammates. It is also important to note that an authorization is more specific and more detailed than consent. An authorization covers only the uses and disclosures of stipulated information, contains an expiration date, and can state the purpose for which the information may be used or disclosed. State law governs disclosure to parents if the individual is a minor. This situation develops less frequently at the collegiate level but still occurs.

Support for Multi-Faceted Referral

There are true health consequences related to eating disorders, including physiological changes in the body that may lead to dry skin, brittle hair and nails, cold intolerance, amenorrhea, delayed menarche, lightheadedness, and constipation. Physical signs for which the physician may also look include decreased subcutaneous fat and muscle, bradycardia, lanugo, changes in orthostatic blood pressure, and discolored hands and feet. All of these characteristics are superficial indications of more serious conditions, including stress fractures, premature osteoporosis, disturbances in reproductive function, psychological issues, and cardiovascular and gastrointestinal problems. This stresses the importance of having a physician available who is trained to recognize the signs and symptoms associated with eating disorders.

Medical problems are not independent of psychological problems, and both have ties to eating disorders. Individuals diagnosed with anorexia nervosa or bulimia nervosa often display perfectionism, obsessional symptoms, anxiety, and rigid cognitive styles, which are also traits common in a majority of athletes.[8] Physicians now commonly treat anxiety with prescription drugs and do not refer the patient for psychological intervention. The psychological stress associated with competitive athletics has also been found to be associated with decreased levels of hypothalamic GnRH, which is a key component associated with normal menstrual functioning. This is a fundamental example of the interrelationship between the health care disciplines and provides support for multiple resources for referral. Creating a system of communication among the following identified resources is equally important:

- Physician
- Nutritionist or dietitian
- Psychologist

- Psychiatrist
- Licensed Counselor
- Certified Athletic trainer

Communication Between Health Care Providers

If the decision is made to hold an athlete out of competition, the athlete's return to competition will most likely be determined by the individual with the power to keep the athlete out of competition; that individual may be the physician or mental health provider. Rarely does the nutritionist or dietitian make this decision without consulting with a physician or mental health provider; in this case, the physician or mental health provider would be deemed more appropriate to make this decision on the basis of the overall health status of the individual. Once again, communication between all members of the health care team will be of great importance.

To assist with communication, and to ensure that everyone knows exactly what it will take for the athlete to return to competition if held out, a written medical clearance or a written contract signed by the student athlete, stating the terms regarding return to play would be options. Requiring the signature of the athlete on such a contract may increase the sense of control that the athlete has in the recovery process. This requirement would allow athletes to have ownership in the decision to get well, and would increase the sense of control in their own rehabilitation process. Having the athlete participate in the writing of the contract can also potentially increase the sense of control of the athlete in the process. As stated earlier, one factor that may contribute to the development of eating disorders is the sense of a lack of control that the athlete may be experiencing.

Treatment

The interrelationship among the subcomponents of nutrition, mental health, and physical health cannot be stressed enough when exploring treatment options. The first step toward any type of treatment is to understand that eating disorders can and do pose a serious problem to the health status of the athlete. Thompson and Trattner-Sherman[7] define treatment as "the application of therapeutic techniques in an attempt to modify the behavioral, cognitive, and affective components of the athlete's eating disorder."

Treatment Approaches

There are several types of treatment that exist for individuals suspected of having an eating disorder including: individual, group, or family therapy. Treatment may be provided on either an inpatient or an outpatient basis. Decisions must be made on how, when, and to whom to refer an athlete. In other words, at what point and to whom, is a suspected athlete referred? These are common questions that coaches, support staff, athletic trainers, and even the athletes themselves often face.

Because of the nature of eating disorders, a multifaceted treatment approach is usually recommended, including a medical examination by a physician; a counseling session with a psychiatrist, psychologist, or licensed counselor; and nutritional counseling by a registered dietician or nutritionist who specializes in eating disorders.[6,7] Several existing programs have taken on this team approach, including the University of Tennessee Knoxville[3] and the University of Oregon.[2] Regardless of the type of treatment received, the primary focuses are to normalize weight and eating behaviors, modify unhelpful thought processes that maintain the disorder, and deal with the emotional issues of the individual that create the need for the disorder.[4]

According to the APA,[1] there are numerous steps of treatment for individuals with anorexia nervosa. The first step is to restore patients to a healthy weight. At a normal healthy weight, menses and normal ovulation occur in females, normal sexual drive and hormone levels occur in males, and normal physical and sexual growth and development occur in children and adolescents.

The second step is to treat physical complications. Next is enhancing patient motivations to cooperate in the restoration of healthy eating patterns and to participate in treatment. After the patient has been convinced to cooperate, education regarding healthy nutrition and eating patterns should be provided.

The next step in the process is to correct core maladaptive thoughts, attitudes, and feelings related to the eating disorder. At this point, clinicians should begin to treat associated psychiatric conditions, including defects in mood regulation, self-esteem, and behavior. Enlisting family support, as well as providing family counseling and therapy if needed, should also be considered. The last goal is to prevent relapse.

Role of the Certified Athletic Trainer

The certified athletic trainer can be essential in the prevention of eating disorders in the collegiate athlete. Athletic Trainers have been acknowledged by the American Medical Association as an allied health profession. In 1999, the Board of Certification (BOC) redefined the profession of athletic training and what certified athletic trainers were required to know in the role delineation study.[4] Individuals striving to pursue a career in athletic training are required to pass a national certification examination covering several domains established by BOC which are listed below;

- Prevention
- Clinical evaluation and diagnosis
- Immediate care

- Treatment, rehabilitation, and reconditioning
- Organization and administration
- Professional responsibility

Each of these domains focuses on increasing health and wellness in athletes and those engaging in physical activity.

Most collegiate athletic programs have at least one certified athletic trainer on staff. The certified athletic trainer is often the first individual on the sports medicine team to intervene on behalf of the athlete in the event of injury. Certified athletic trainers are educated in the prevention, recognition, evaluation, and assessment of athletic injuries and illnesses, including eating disorders.

The certified athletic trainer works under the supervision of a team physician, who is responsible for the direction of the total health care of the athlete. At the collegiate level, the team physician is responsible for conducting pre-participation examinations of all athletes. This is usually done in conjunction with the certified athletic trainer to help identify any information that may prove to be a threat to the health of the athlete. Early recognition of eating disorders begins with the pre-participation exam. The physician determines when a recommendation should be made that an athlete be disqualified from practice or competition on medical grounds and must have the final say about when an injured athlete may return to activity. The physician's decision should be based on recommendations made by the certified athletic trainer, who sees the athlete on a daily basis and may be able to provide valuable insight into the daily activities of the athlete, the physical demands currently in the sport or coming up in the sport, and whether the athlete has been receiving treatments. Because of their role as health care providers, certified athletic trainers play an important role in the development of programs to promote the health and well-being of the athlete, including the development of eating-disorder programs.

Summary

Developing the following referral system checklist and having resources identified prior to an athlete being diagnosed with an eating disorder is essential to proper intervention and management:

- Have resources for treatment and referral been identified?
- Has a process for referral been identified?
- Has confidentiality been addressed?
- Have criteria for return to participation been considered if athlete participation is discontinued?
- Has the role of the coach been defined in the management process?
- Have consequences of not following the policy been created?

TABLE 10-1   ·   **Overview of the Development of an Eating Disorder Referral Program**

Have resources for treatment and referral been identified?
Has a process for referral been identified?
Has confidentiality been addressed?
Have criteria for return to participation been considered if athlete participation is discontinued?
Has the role of the coach been defined in the management process?
Have consequences of not following the policy been created?

The roles of all individuals involved in the referral and treatment process, including coaches, support staff, administrators, and health care personnel, must be made clear to ensure the best care possible for the athlete. Having a written policy and clarifying the roles of all individuals involved in the process will help to ensure that the athlete's right to privacy is protected. If this privacy is threatened, there is a risk that an athlete may choose to not come forward for treatment. A choice to not come forward may be detrimental to health, wellness, and performance.

References

1.   American Psychiatric Association. *Diagnostic and Statistical Manual Of Mental Disorders* (4th, text revision ed.). Washington DC: American Psychiatric Association; 2000b.

2.   Bonci C, Bonci L, Granger L, et al. National athletic trainers' association position statement: Preventing, detecting, and managing disordered eating in athletes. *Journal of Athletic Training*. 2008;43(1):80–108.

3.   Knoxville, University of Tennessee. *Enhancing nutrition health athletic performance networking community and education* (Brochure). Knoxville: University of Tennessee; 2000.

4.   National Athletic Trainers Association Board of Certification (NATABOC). National athletic trainers' association board of certification: role delineation study. Raleigh, NC: Columbia Assessment Services; 1995.

5.   Oregon, University of Oregon. *Eating Disorder Program Description* (Program). Eugene: University of Oregon; 2000.

6. Spear B, and Stellefson-Meyers E. Position of the American Dietetic Association: nutrition intervention in the treatment of anorexia nervosa, bulimia nervosa, and eating disorders not otherwise specified (EDNOS). *Journal of the American Dietetic Association*. 2001;101(7):810–819.

7. Thompson R, and Trattner-Sherman R. *Helping athletes with eating disorders*. Champaign: Human Kinetics; 1993.

8. Zerbe K. The emerging sexual self of the patient with an eating disorder: implication for treatment. *Eating Disorders: Journal of Treatment and Prevention*. 1995;3:197–215.

CHAPTER 11

Screening Tools for Eating Disorders

Mike Brunet, PhD, ATC, CPT, STS

Introduction

Despite the amount of literature that exists regarding disordered eating and eating disorders, managing these pathologies remains a challenge due to the secretive nature of them. Not everyone is willing to come forward stating that they have a problem and they want some help. Furthermore, there may be consequences that follow these actions, such as the health care practitioner temporarily removing the individual from sport. Secrecy, lying, and covering up their problem(s) are all reasons why it is important for the Certified Athletic Trainer to be sensitive to the signs of eating disorders and disordered eating behaviors. Fortunately, four new tools have been developed to identify those who may need help. This chapter shows that when used correctly, the tools are an effective way to reveal those who need help.

Eating Disorder Assessment

According to Allison,[1] the most common and widely used assessment tools are the Eating Disorder Inventory (EDI) questionnaire,[11] the Eating Attitudes Test (EAT) questionnaire,[9] and the Eating Disorder Examination (EDE.)[4] The Michigan State University Weight Control Survey (MSUWCS)[21] questionnaire takes a comprehensive look at the type, and the frequency of different pathogenic weight control measures. All four assessment tools have clinical utility in the diagnosis of patterns of eating disorders and pathogenic weight control measures.

Eating Disorder Inventory

The EDI questionnaire was designed to assess psychological characteristics and symptoms common to anorexia nervosa and bulimia nervosa (BN). It contains 64 items that form eight sub-scales:

- drive for thinness
- bulimia, body dissatisfaction
- ineffectiveness
- perfection
- interpersonal distrust
- interoceptive awareness
- maturity fears

A later revised version of the EDI, the EDI-2 included just three original sub-scales: drive for thinness, bulimia, and body dissatisfaction. Both versions of the questionnaire are reliable and internally consistent.[11] Though it has been used diagnostically, it was originally designed for profiling purposes to track changes that occur with treatment. Recently, the EDI-2 was enhanced and the EDI-3 was created. EDI-3 is a more user-friendly version that takes around 20 minutes to complete and yields information that was not possible using the EDI-2. It also has computer compatible software that makes user interface easier for the clinician. For more information, please visit Psychological Assessment Resources, INC. Table 11-1 lists the differences between the EDI-2 and the EDI-3.

Eating Attitudes Test

The EAT questionnaire was originally designed to assess anorexia nervosa, but now is being used as a tool to screen for eating disorders. The EAT is a 40-item self-report measure, with each item being answered on a 6-point Likert scale (1 = never, 6 = always), where extreme anorexic values receive 3 points, the next to anorexic value receives 2 points, and the next adjacent receives just 1 point. The remaining three questions all receive 0 points. A year later, a revised version of the EAT was created: the EAT-26. It contains 26 of the original 40 questions, disregarding 14 redundant questions. Both are highly correlated and have high test and re-test reliability and internal consistency.[12]

Michigan State University Weight Control Survey

Many different instruments have been designed to detect pathologic dieting behaviors. What makes the MSUWCS different is that it was designed to assess the pathological weight control behaviors (PWCB)s of athletes and does not attempt to classify individuals with eating disorders. Though it is different in that aspect, the framework is similar to other questionnaires. It is divided into sections with a number of subscales. Some questions throughout the survey involve questions that include teammates rather than just opinions of other people. This makes the MSUWCS more specific to athletes versus the widely used Eating Attitudes Test (EAT) that was designed to detect eating disorders in clinical populations.[10] Many people have used the EAT in athletic populations, but given the fact that the test was originally formulated from clinically diagnosed anorexics and bulimics, there is a level of difficulty that exists to be able to use the EAT in athletic settings.

Eating Disorder Examination

The EDE is a semi-structured interview for the assessment of general eating disorders and is considered a criterion measure for the assessment of eating disorder psychopathology.[23] It is designed to assess a broad range of specific psychopathology of anorexia nervosa and bulimia nervosa along with their variants.[8] The EDE contains 62 questions that are divided into 4 sub-scales: dietary restraint, eating concern, weight concern, and shape concern. All questions refer to functioning over the previous four weeks, and each question

TABLE 11-1 • Comparison of EDI-2 and EDI-3

EDI-2	EDI-3	CHANGES TO EDI-3
Eating Disorder Risk Scales	**Eating Disorder Risk Scales**	**Item changes from the EDI-2 Scales**
Drive for thinness (DT)	Drive for thinness (DT)	No change
Bulimia (B)	Bulimia (B)	1 item from IA
Body dissatisfaction (BD)	Body dissatisfaction (BD)	1 item from IA
Psychological scales	**Psychological Scales**	**Psychological Scales**
Ineffectiveness (I)	Low self-esteem (LSE)	5 items from I
	Personal alienation (PA)	4 items from I; 3 from SI
Social insecurity (SI)[1]	Interpersonal insecurity (II)	4 items from ID; 3 from SI
Interpersonal distrust (ID)	Interpersonal alienation (IA)	3 items from ID; 3 from IR; 1 from SI
Interoceptive awareness (IA)	Interoceptive deficits (ID)	8 items from IA; 1 from IR
Impulse regulation (IR)[1]	Emotional dysregulation (ED)	8 items from IR
Perfectionism (P)	Perfectionism (P)	No change
Asceticism (A)[1]	Asceticism (A)	7 items from A
Maturity fears (MF)	Maturity fears (MF)	No change
	Composite Scales[2]	**EDI-3 Composite: T-score**
	Eating disorder risk composite (EDRC)	T-score for DT + B + BD
	Ineffectiveness composite (IC)	T-score for LSE + PA
	Interpersonal problems composite (IPC)	T-score for LSE + PA
	Affective problems composite (APC)	T-score for ID + ED
	Overcontrol composite (OC)	T-score for P + A
	General psycological maladjustment (GPMC)	T-score for all psychological scales
	Response Style Indicators[2]	
	Inconsistency (IN)	
	Infrequency (IF)	
	Negative impression (NI)	

[1]These scales were not on the original EDI.
[2]Composite scales and response style indicators are completely new to the EDI-3.
Note: Item 71 from the EDI-2 is included on the EDI-3 item sheet, but is not scored on the EDI-3
Source: Eating Disorder Inventory TM-3 by David M. Garner. Psychological Assessment Resources Inc.

is scored on a 6-point rating scale with regards to severity and frequency of a particular feature. It is scored from 0 (absence of feature) to 6 (feature present to an extreme degree).[8]

The original items in the EDE were selected by using three different methods. First, the authors completed a literature review on anorexia nervosa and bulimia nervosa to obtain a comprehensive description of the specific psychopathology of the two disorders.[4] Next, the psychopathology was broken down into its key elements. The elements distinguished between behavioral and attitudinal features. From that list, the authors were able to complete a list of items that included a broad range of specific psychopathologies.[4] Lastly, a series of lengthy unstructured interviews were conducted with clinically diagnosed anorectics and bulimics for purposes of eliciting detailed descriptions of various aspects of their specific behavior and attitudes.[4] This helped the authors formulate further items. Now on its 12th edition, four subscales remain. These four subscales identify two key behavioral aspects of overeating and using extreme measures of weight control.[4,8] Weight control measures included self-induced vomiting, laxative misuse, diuretic misuse, and intense exercising.

With regard to the validation of the EDE and why it has been called a criterion measure, Cooper et al.[5] administered the interview to a group of 100 patients with either anorexia nervosa or bulimia nervosa and to 42 controls. They had two major findings. First, the EDE discriminated well between patients with eating disorders and controls.[5] Secondly, they found that the EDE was able to distinguish between groups of AN and BN.[5] Wilson and Smith[24] further showed that the EDE was able to distinguish between groups of bulimics and other weight preoccupied women.

Though the EDE is relatively new in the literature, many studies have established the inter-rater (between those who are using the tool) reliability and validity[14,5,22,8,13] along with the test re-test reliability.[20] More recently, a questionnaire version of the EDE was made, the EDE-Q[7] and validated.[7,16,2] The EDE's four subscales and question descriptions are as follows:

1. Restraint
   - Restraint over eating
   - Avoidance of eating
   - Food avoidance
   - Dietary rules
   - Empty stomach

2. Eating Concern
   - Preoccupation with food, eating, or calories
   - Fear of losing control over eating
   - Social eating
   - Eating in secret
   - Guilt about eating

3. Shape concern
   - Flat stomach
   - Importance of shape
   - Preoccupation with shape or weight
   - Dissatisfaction with shape
   - Fear of weight gain
   - Discomfort seeing body
   - Avoidance of exposures
   - Feelings of fatness

4. Weight Concern
   - Importance of weight
   - Reaction to prescribed weighing
   - Preoccupation with shape or weight
   - Dissatisfaction with weight
   - Desire to lose weight

Athlete Specific Assessment Tools

Although the assessment tools just discussed are the ones most frequently used, they were originally developed for the general population, not athletes. This led researchers to construct other questionnaires that are more athlete-specific. The National Collegiate Athletic Association (NCAA) Eating Disorder Project[15] used parts of different questionnaires to make one big assessment tool that included questions from the Eating Disorder Inventory-2 (EDI-2), the Rosenberg Self-Esteem Scale, and the Body Cathexis Scale for a total of 133 items. The questions from the EDI-2 included three scales; body dissatisfaction, drive for thinness, and the bulimia scale. Other items that were designed to assess demographics, athletic involvement, eating behaviors, alcohol and drug behaviors, and body image questions were also included in the questionnaire. Other questionnaires include the Female Athlete Screening Tool (FAST),[17] the Athletic Milieu Direct Questionnaire (AMDQ),[18] the Physiological Screening Test (PST),[3] and the Survey of Eating Disorders among Athletes (SEDA).[14]

The Questionnaire versus the Interview

Now that two types of assessment tools have been discussed (the questionnaire and the interview), which one is best to use? Black and Wilson[2] discussed the advantages of using both the interview and the questionnaire. In their study they compared the results of the EDE and the EDE-Questionnaire, or simply stated the questionnaire form of the EDE which is meant to be conducted in an interview format. They found that the EDE-Questionnaire identified eating disorders symptoms and purging techniques, but difficulties existed with multidimensional topics. These findings should not be surprising. The face-to-face interview was able to assess the individual more thoroughly versus just answering specific questions on the questionnaire.

Generally speaking, the possibility of the athlete lying on questionnaires will always remain. One way to combat this limitation is to make sure that confidentiality is upheld. Another factor to consider is the time of year when administering these tools. For instance, if the questionnaires are given to an athlete in the off-season, she might answer differently when compared to an in-season athlete.

Another strategy may be to incorporate these assessment tools into the pre-participation physical exam. This way the health care provider does not single out one individual, but rather asks everyone the same questions. This approach may provide a less intrusive means of evaluating a large number of athletes at one time. Ideally, a combination of both a questionnaire and an interview would probably serve as the best means to evaluate.

Be sure that the tool used as a health care provider has been sufficiently evaluated for reliability and validity.

Other Screening Methods

While the scientific literature does show the clinical utility of using surveys and interviews to help identify those who need help, other techniques can be used. For instance, different physiological measurements can be taken to risk stratify someone that may have an eating disorder or may be engaging in pathological eating behaviors. The first method is simply acquiring the individual's body mass index (BMI) which is a measurement of the relationship between height and weight. It is calculated by using the following formula: weight (kg)/height (cm).[11] It is commonly known that one's BMI is associated with percentage person's health, but this formula has only shown clinical utility at the extremes. This method is not able to distinguish fat mass from fat-free mass when calculating weight, which means that it cannot differentiate the individual who weighs 150 pounds and has 10% body fat versus someone who weighs the same but has 35% body fat. Therefore, this method has definite limitations.

Another physiological measurement that can be used is calculating body fat. This method can be both helpful as well as dangerous. It can be helpful when an individual is evaluated that has a low body fat percentage coupled with other physiological pathologies (low bone density, amenorrhea, etc), but it can be detrimental when used incorrectly. For instance, it has been documented that body composition assessment does have the potential to act as a trigger to engage in pathological eating behaviors.[18] Another challenge to the acquisition of someone's body composition is the technique used. It is commonly known that the use of calipers can be unreliable, (either through faulty equipment or tester error), but not everyone may have use of criterion measures, such as a dual energy x-ray absorptiometry (DEXA) machine, an air displacement plethysmography machine (BODPOD), or an underwater weighing tank. Therefore, the use of assessing body composition needs to be conducted with much consideration when using it for means of eating disorder and disordered eating pathology screening or identification. It can cause more harm than good.

Summary

While many different tools exist regarding the examination of eating disorders and disordered eating, it is imperative that the health care practitioner be aware of what each tool is designed to do and use the information gathered correctly. There many assessment tools available, but not all of them have been examined for their validity and usefulness. Therefore it is the responsibility of the clinician to know exactly what the chosen tool is designed to do, and to verify that the tool has been validated against another like criterion measure. Lastly, clinicians need to know how to properly deliver the information gathered, because the tools used incorrectly, can inflict more harm than good.

References

1. Allison (Ed.). *Handbook of Assessment Methods for Eating Behaviors and Weight Related Problems; Measures, Theory, and Research.* Thousand Oaks, Ca: Sage; 1995.

2. Black CM, and Wilson CT. Assessment of Eating Disorders: Interview versus Questionnaire. *International Journal of Eating Disorders.* 1996; 20(1):43–50.

3. Black Dr, Larkin LJ, Coster DC, Leverenz LJ, and Abood DA. Physiologic screening test for eating disorders / disordered eating among female collegiate athletes. *Journal of Athletic Training.* 2003;38:286–297.

4. Cooper Z, and Fairburn C. The eating disorder examination: A semi-structured interview for the assessment of the specific psychopathology of eating disorders. *International Journal of Eating Disorders.* 1987;6:1–8.

5. Cooper A, Cooper PJ, and Fairburn CG. The validity of the Eating Disorder Examination and its subscales. *British Journal of Psychiatry.* 1989;154:807–812.

6. Cooper PJ, Taylor MJ, Cooper Z, and Fairburn CG. The development and validation of the body shape questionnaire. *International Journal of Eating Disorders*. 1987;6(4): 485–494.

7. Fairburn, and Beglin. Studies of the epidemiology of bulimia nervosa. *American Journal of Psychiatry*. 1990;147(4):401–408.

8. Fairburn CG, and Cooper Z. The eating disorder examination (12th ed.). In Fairburn CG, and Wilson GT (Eds). *Binge Eating: Nature, Assessment, and Treatment*. New York: Guilford Press;1993:317–360.

9. Garner DM, and Garfikel PE. The Eating Attitudes Test: An index of the symptoms of anorexia nervosa. *Psychological Medicine*. 1979;9:273–279.

10. Garner DM, and Garfinkel PE. *Handbook of Treatment for Eating Disorders*. NY: Guilford Press; 1997.

11. Garner DM, Olmsted MP, and Plivy. Development and validation of a multi-dimensional Eating Disorder Inventory for anorexia nervosa and bulimia. *International Journal of Eating Disorders*. 1983;2:15–34.

12. Garner DM, Olmsted MP, Bohr Y, and Garfinkel PE. The eating attitudes test: psychometric features and clinical correlates. *Psychological Medicine*. 1982;12:871–878.

13. Guest T. Using the Eating Disorder Examination in the assessment of builimia and anorexia: issues of reliability and validity. *Social Work in Health Care*. 2000;31(4):71–83.

14. Guthrie SR. Prevalence of eating disorders among intercollegiate athletes: contributing factors and preventive measures. In: Black DR, ed. Eating Disorders Among Athletes: Theory, Issues, and Research. Reston, VA: Association for Girls and Women in Sport, Associations for Health, Physical Education, Recreation, and Dance; 1991:43–66.

15. Johnson C, Powers PS, and Dick R. Athletes and eating disorders: The National Collegiate Athletic Association study. *International Journal of Eating Disorders*. 1999;26:179–188.

16. Luce KH, and Crowther JH. The reliability of the Eating Disorder Examination-self report questionnaire version (EDE-Q). *International Journal of Eating Disorders*. 1990;25:349–351.

17. McNulty KY, Adams CH, Anderson JM, and Affenito SG. The development and validation of a screening tool to identify eating disorders in female athletes. *Journal of the American Diet Association*. 2001;101:886–892.

18. Nagel DL, black DR, Leverenz LJ, and Coster DC. Evaluation of a screening test for female college athletes with eating disorders and disordered eating. *Journal of Athletic Training*. 2000;35(4):431–440.

19. Otis C, Drinkwater B, Johnson M, Loucks A, and Wilmore J. Position stand on the female athlete triad. *Medicine and Science in Sports and Exercise.* 1997;29:i–ix.

20. Rizvi SL, Peterson CB, Crow SJ, and Agras S. Test-retest reliability of the Eating Disorder Examination. *International Journal of Eating Disorders.* 2000;28:311–316.

21. Rosen LW, McKeag DB, and Hough DO. Pathogenic weight-control behavior in female athletes. *Physician Sportsmedicine.* 1986;14(1): 79–86.

22. Rosen JC, Vara L, Wendt S, and Leitenberg H. Validity studies of the Eating Disorder Examination. *International Journal of Eating Disorders.* 1990;9:519–528.

23. Wilson GT. Assessment of binge eating. In Fairburn CG, and Wilson GT (Eds.). *Binge Eating: Nature, Assessment, and Treatment.* New York: Guilford Press; 1993:227–249.

24. Wilson GT, and Smith D. Assessment of bulimia nervosa: An evaluation of the Eating Disorder Examination. *International Journal of Eating Disorders.* 1989;8:173–179.

CHAPTER 12

The Role of the Certified Athletic Trainer in Managing Athletes with Disordered Eating and Eating Disorders

Ron A. Thompson and Roberta Trattner Sherman

Introduction

In general, disordered eating and eating disorders are difficult problems to manage and treat. However, when these problems occur in the female sport world, a unique set of issues and circumstances can further complicate the identification, the management, and the treatment of the affected athletes.[25] As a result, athletes and treatment providers require specialized approaches in treating such problems.[20]

A recent survey of athletic trainers regarding managing female athletes with eating disorders suggests that certified athletic trainers[26] often do not feel they have what they need to address the complex problems of eating disorders. Ninety-one percent of those surveyed indicated they had worked with such athletes, but only 27% felt confident in identifying them and only 38% felt confident asking the athlete if she had a disorder. At the same time, the certified athletic trainer is probably the person in the athletic environment who is most often given the responsibility for managing such athletes.

Evidence for this is provided by a recent study of how collegiate coaches manage female athletes with disordered eating.[18] The study recommends that certified athletic trainers should receive special training in that regard. Our extensive experience in working with collegiate athletes suggests that certified athletic trainers are in an ideal position to effectively handle the identification and management of this special subpopulation. Thus, the purpose of this chapter is to provide specific information and recommendations designed to enhance the certified athletic trainer's effectiveness in identifying, managing, and preventing disordered eating and eating disorders in the sport environment.

This chapter focuses primarily on the role of the certified athletic trainer in the management process. It should be noted that we make a distinction between the terms "management" and "treatment." Management is a much broader term than treatment. A discussion of the treatment process is well beyond the scope of this chapter. (For such a discussion, the reader is directed to Petri and Sherman [2000]). However, the treatment primarily involves nutritional counseling to normalize eating and weight, and psychotherapy to assist the patient in making the cognitive, affective, and behavioral changes necessary for recovery. Even though the certified athletic trainer is not usually directly involved in either of these specific treatment processes, the ATC certified athletic trainer can play a significant role in helping manage them.

Rationale for Involving the Certified Athletic Trainer

The certified athletic trainer is in a unique and very important position. The "worlds" of sport and health care are usually quite different. Psychologists, like most other health care professionals, are not usually a part of the sport world. Sport personnel, other than the certified athletic trainer, are not part of the health care world. The certified athletic trainer can act as a bridge between the two worlds.

Focus on Health

In order for an individual with disordered eating or an eating disorder to recover, the patient must take a "health" focus as opposed to a weight focus. To facilitate recovery, health care professionals must also have a primary health focus. The focus on health is even more important in an athletic environment driven by athletic performance; therefore the focus on health is even more important and must be communicated to the athlete.

For several years, a prevailing notion in the sport world has suggested that thinner or leaner athletes perform better. Because of this belief, it is easy for some athletes to rationalize their disordered eating/eating disorder by saying that they must keep their weight down in order to perform better. Therefore, the certified athletic trainer must be the person in the athletic environment that puts the athlete's health before her performance.

Ideal Vantage Point

Certified athletic trainers spend a significant amount of time with their athletes and thus have a special vantage point from which they observe and manage an athlete. They are usually at practices, competitions, road trips, and team meetings, in addition to seeing the athletes during treatment and rehabilitation sessions. Thus, the certified athletic trainer has numerous opportunities to observe the athlete in a variety of situations. In addition to the medical information they have based on their treatment, they are usually privy to the athlete's medical history. Given the observational data and medical information certified athletic trainers have about the athlete, they are apt to be the first persons to notice an actual or potential problem with an athlete.

Liaison Between the Athlete and Coach

The athletic trainer bridges the gap between the health care and sport worlds. Coaches have considerable power with their athletes.[7,27] Sometimes the athlete has difficulty talking to a coach, particularly about an issue or problem which she may have, such as an eating disorder. Non-athletes with eating disorders are often concerned about pleasing (or at least not displeasing) others, especially significant others. Athletes with eating disorders or disordered eating are no different; they don't want to displease the coach. The athlete may feel more comfortable talking with the certified athletic trainer, who may serve as a "go between" with the coach.

Liaison Between the Athlete and Health Care Providers

Another rationale for involving certified athletic trainers is that they can also be the bridge between the athlete and other health care providers that she may need regarding the treatment of her disordered eating. The athletic trainer can also be a helpful part of the health care team in a variety ways (i.e. observation, monitoring, and reporting of symptoms), which will be discussed later.

Identification of At-Risk and Symptomatic Athletes

Certain aspects of the sport environment can complicate the identification of disordered eating in athletes; for example, sport body stereotypes, the belief that thinness/leanness enhances performance, the misperception of eating disorder symptoms as being "normal" or even desired athlete traits, and the presumption of health with good performance. These identification issues were discussed in earlier chapters and will not be recounted here. Suffice it to say that these stereotypes, beliefs, misperceptions, and false assumptions serve to complicate identification for certified athletic trainers, as well as for other sport personnel, thereby delaying treatment.

Signs and Symptoms

Despite identification difficulties with athletes, research suggests that it is still possible to identify athletes with eating problems using common signs and symptoms.[18] Although, signs and symptoms do not necessarily indicate a problem, they do suggest a risk and that risk increases as the number of signs and symptoms increase. The following sections discuss the common signs and symptoms of disordered eating, which fall into two major categories: Physical/medical and psychological/behavioral.

Physical/Medical Signs and Symptoms

Common physical/medical signs and symptoms of disordered eating and eating disorders include, but are not limited to, amenorrhea, dehydration, gastrointestinal problems (constipation and/or diarrhea), hypothermia, stress fractures/overuse injuries, significant weight loss, muscle weakness/cramps/fatigue, and dental/gum problems. For a more complete list of physical/medical signs and symptoms of disordered eating and eating disorders, the reader is directed to Thompson and Sherman.[20]

Psychological/Behavioral Signs and Symptoms

Common psychological/behavioral signs and symptoms of disordered eating and eating disorders include but are not limited to anxiety, depression, claims of feeling "fat" despite being thin, excessive exercise, excessive use of the restroom (especially after eating), decreased concentration, preoccupation with eating/food/weight, avoidance of eating and eating situations, and misuse of diet pills and purgatives (laxative, diuretics, enemas, and emetics). Again, for a more complete list of psychological/behavioral signs and symptoms of disordered eating and eating disorders, the reader is directed to Thompson and Sherman.[20]

Management of the Symptomatic Athlete

The management process should begin once an athlete has been identified as having an eating disorder or engaging in disordered eating. The first step in this process involves approaching the athlete regarding treatment.

Approaching the Athlete

Perhaps the most important step in the management process is approaching the athlete because this can determine if she accepts or rejects treatment. It is not uncommon for individuals with eating problems (regardless of whether they are athletes or not) to be unreceptive to offers of assistance. For a variety reasons, these individuals have difficulty in this regard. Those whose symptoms are more characteristic of anorexia nervosa (i.e. weight loss, severe dietary restriction, excessive exercise, etc.) often do not believe that they have a problem. They believe that they know what they are doing, that they are in control, and that they are simply doing what many other young women are doing—dieting/attempting to lose weight. Those whose symptoms are more characteristic of bulimia nervosa (i.e. self-induced vomiting, laxative/diuretic abuse, etc.) are often so embarrassed or ashamed of their symptoms that they feel they must deny them. Add this to the fact that many athletes fear losing playing time or status by admitting to a disorder, it becomes even more difficult to approach the athlete.

Clearly, the person approaching a symptomatic athlete must be a person who can do so with considerable care and sensitivity. It has been suggested that this individual should be a person of some authority who has a good relationship with the athlete or at least has a comfortable manner of relating.[9] The certified athletic trainer fits this description because he/she already knows how to talk with the athlete about her body and how it functions. Additionally, because these are health issues and the certified athletic trainer is the health care professional most often involved with the athlete's health, the certified athletic trainer is an ideal choice for approaching the athlete.

More important than *who* approaches the female athlete is *how* she is approached. The athlete should be approached privately. In order to minimize her discomfort, the communication needs to be made non-critically. The athlete should be told by the person approaching her that individuals within her sport are concerned about her health. Focusing on health rather than an eating problem per se is less emotional for the athlete. Also, a direct confrontation about her eating can be too easily rejected by the athlete by simply denying that she has a problem.

Making a Referral

An athlete with disordered eating or an eating disorder ideally should be treated by health care professionals who have experience and expertise in working with eating disorders, preferably with athletes.[10,20] The certified athletic trainer assigned to manage the athlete's treatment should be aware of treatment providers and programs in his or her geographic area. Having a specific person to refer the athlete to will greatly facilitate her getting into the treatment she needs.

For a variety of reasons, eating disorders frequently occur on college campuses. As a result, there is often a staff member at the counseling center on campus who has experience treating eating disorders. There are also several resources for finding qualified treatment providers and programs, such as the Academy for Eating Disorders, the National Eating Disorders Association, and Anorexia Nervosa and Associated Disorders (contact information for these sources is provided at the end of this chapter). A more in-depth discussion on how to develop and facilitate an Eating Disorder Referral Team can be found in Chapters 8–10 in this book.

The athlete should be told that an evaluation will be arranged out of concern for her welfare. Hopefully, she agrees to the referral. If the athlete refuses the referral, she should be considered *injured* until an evaluation proves otherwise. In such a case, it is recommended that the athlete be withheld from training and competition until an evaluation clears her.[6,9,17] In such a situation, the certified athletic trainer needs to reassure the athlete that she is not being punished, but rather that the medical staff is following protocol for injured athletes. It is very important to communicate to the athlete that the primary concern is for her physical and emotional well-being rather than her sport performance.

Contact Outside of Treatment

The seriousness of the eating problem determines the frequency with which the athlete is seen in treatment. In the majority of cases, she will be seen on an outpatient basis by the treatment staff (mental health professionals, physician, and dietitian). This may involve only a few hours per week. The certified athletic trainer can be very helpful to the athlete and to the treatment staff by talking with the athlete on a frequent basis. This allows the athlete to have a contact outside of treatment and the treatment team; someone with whom she can be accountable to regarding her therapy homework, compliance with her treatment plan and health maintenance criteria, symptom management, and any immediate or emergency issues that might need attention when treatment staff professionals are not available.

Liaison Between Athlete and Treatment Team

As mentioned previously, the certified athletic trainer can be a liaison between the athlete and the treatment team. The information obtained from being with the athlete frequently can be quite helpful to the treatment staff. Depending on the arrangement with the athlete, the treatment team may or may not be able to provide the certified athletic trainer with information. Confidentiality dictates that the treatment providers can release information only to individuals for whom the patient has designated with written consent to release information.

In the event that the athlete does not give this consent, treatment providers can still receive information from the certified athletic trainer.

Monitoring Symptoms

The certified athletic trainer can play a significant role in monitoring symptoms. One of the more important symptoms involves hydration, which is concern for athletes without eating problems, as well. For eating disorder patients, fluid intake can vary from too much (to water load to appear heavier, to feel full, to suppress appetite, to facilitate vomiting) to conscious and unconscious attempts to under- or dehydrate.[5] Intuitively, the idea of an athlete dehydrating herself seems unreasonable, given the probable negative effect on performance. It should be remembered that disordered eating, especially at the level of a clinical eating disorder, is not reasonable, rational, or logical. Thus, the certified athletic trainer who assumes that a symptomatic athlete would not dehydrate herself because of the negative effect on performance, especially if she is an endurance athlete, is probably making a mistake.

Liaison Between Athlete and Coach

Serving as the liaison between the coach and athlete (and perhaps as a liaison between the treatment team and the coach) can be a difficult. Coaches have reported that one of the biggest difficulties or frustrations with their athletes being in treatment is that they often cannot get information from treatment providers regarding the athlete's progress. As one coach said, "It's like they go into a black hole when they go into treatment." As a consequence, it is not surprising that many coaches report that they refer within their athletic department (i.e. athletic trainers), rather than to health care professionals outside the department.[18]

In essence, coaches sometimes have difficulty with the constraints of confidentiality with which health care professionals must ethically and legally comply. The certified athletic trainer can again play an instrumental role by not only reiterating the necessity for privacy and confidentiality to the coach, but by assisting the coach in obtaining the information he/she needs. With a good relationship and frequent contact with the athlete, the certified athletic trainer will most likely know how she is doing and how treatment is progressing.

Bridge Between Sport and Treatment Worlds

Many health care professionals who work with eating disorders believe that coaches often play a significant role in an athlete developing an eating disorder. To some degree, this belief has probably been based on their experience, and based on accounts in the popular press[16] and the professional literature.[15,21] As mentioned previously, there is a considerable gap between the "worlds" of sport and health care as they relate to disordered eating and eating disorders—a gap that has only recently begun to be addressed.[22]

There is considerable responsibility on both parts to better understand and appreciate the other. Many eating disorder treatment specialists have had little exposure, and thus have little information regarding the training, special skills, and responsibilities of the certified athletic trainer. As the certified athletic trainer plays a more integral role in the identification and management of athletes with disordered eating and eating disorders, it behooves those in the eating disorder treatment world to learn more about certified athletic trainers, and it behooves certified athletic trainers to provide that information.

Making Decisions Related to Training and Competition

One of the more difficult roles for the certified athletic trainer with symptomatic athletes involves having to make decisions about training and competition. Recent research suggests that the certified athletic trainer is often the person in the sport world who must make these difficult decisions,[18] especially when the symptomatic athlete is not in treatment. It is believed that these athletes should not be training or competing unless they are in treatment and meet specific criteria while symptomatic, a belief that has recently been endorsed by some sport governing bodies.[6,9,17] Certified athletic trainers can provide an invaluable service to symptomatic athletes in the following ways:

- by recommending that they not be considered for sport participation without being in treatment
- by becoming informed as to the specific diagnostic and health maintenance criteria necessary for an athlete to be considered for training and/or competition
- by providing consultation to treatment providers regarding the type, intensity, and duration of physical activity that would be appropriate for the athlete at various stages of treatment and recovery

Contact and Support When not Training or Competing

Opposing sport participation without treatment protects the athlete and sends a very important message that the athlete's health is not to be subordinated to her sport. Individuals with eating disorders often believe that they are valued primarily because of what they are able to do (rather than for who they are). One of our the author's goals in treatment is to help the patient begin to value herself for whom she is, rather than for what she does or how she looks. A decision to allow a symptomatic athlete to train and compete without being in treatment will likely confirm her unhealthy belief that she is primarily valued because of her sport performance. The Team Physician and the Certified Athletic Trainer obviously need to take part in this decision.

The decision to withhold treatment is an important one that can be difficult for the athlete, the athlete's family of origin, and the athlete's "sport family" (coaches, teammates, etc.) The certified athletic trainer can provide an invaluable service to the athlete in two ways. First, the certified athletic trainer can again be the link between groups and individuals by talking with the "families" involved as desired and permitted by the athlete. Second, even though the athlete cannot train or compete, the certified athletic trainer can assist the athlete in continuing to feel a part of the team through regular contact and by arranging for the athlete to participate in all sport and team activities (i.e. team meetings) other than training and competition.[10] From a treatment standpoint, feeling a part of a team—a sense of attachment—can facilitate treatment. Also, having the athlete still involved with the team allows for closer and better monitoring of her symptoms and ongoing condition.

Monitoring Treatment Compliance

The following recommendations should be considered for adoption of specific diagnostic and health maintenance criteria necessary for an athlete to train and compete:

- Athletes who meet diagnostic criteria for anorexia nervosa (weight less than 85% of expected based on height, irrational fear of being/becoming fat, body image disturbance, and amenorrhea) should not be permitted to train or compete.

- Athletes who do not meet criteria for anorexia nervosa may be permitted to train and compete if medically and psychologically cleared, if their disordered eating is not directly related to their sport, or if they are in treatment and progressing, and comply with all treatment recommendations and health maintenance criteria. Note that health maintenance criteria will differ depending on the needs of the individual, but generally at a minimum they include maintenance of at least 90% of expected body weight and ingestion of sufficient calories to comply with all treatment goals and recommendations.

These criteria should be monitored by the treatment staff and by the certified athletic trainer. If the athlete fails to comply, sport participation should be withdrawn. As mentioned previously, the certified athletic trainer working with the athlete may be consulted regarding the type, intensity, frequency, and duration of activity that is safe and appropriate for the athlete to engage in at various stages of treatment and recovery.

Being the Middleperson

In many of the roles discussed, the certified athletic trainer has been cast as a liaison between individuals or groups. In essence, the certified athletic trainer often seems to be in the "middle," which sometimes can be the worst place to be. The certified athletic trainer may experience pressure to make decisions based on what the athlete, families, coaches, and health care providers want. The best way to resolve this potential dilemma is to remember with whom the certified athletic trainer's responsibility rests; the patient.

Finally, if certified athletic trainers are going to be asked to take such responsibilities (and they are), then they should be granted the power and control commensurate with those responsibilities. Again, this shows the importance of having an institutional eating disorder referral program in place within the athletic department.

Prevention

In a recent survey, 93% of certified athletic trainers indicated that attention should be paid to the prevention of eating disorders among female athletes.[26] Unfortunately, very little has been reported in the literature on prevention program outcomes in the general population, and even less regarding the special subpopulation of athletes. This section focuses on primary prevention, which involves strategies and programs that are designed to lower the incidence of eating disorders by reducing the risk and enhancing protective factors.[12] However, before providing recommendations regarding primary prevention, a brief discussion on secondary prevention is presented.

Previous discussions involving identification have focused on secondary prevention, which involves early identification and intervention.[12] The focus provided information on aspects of the sport environment that complicate or interfere with the identification process,[20,23] with the goal of improving identification to expedite treatment.

Secondary prevention efforts often involve screening procedures. Most of the available screening instruments are paper and pencil, self-report inventories. However, a new and promising approach involves a physiologic screening test recently proposed for the purpose of detecting eating and disordered eating among female collegiate athletes.[1] An in-depth discussion on eating disorder assessment tools are found in Chapter 11 of this book.

A recent review of prevention studies suggested that targeted or selective primary prevention interventions may reduce potential risk factors in older adolescents and college-age women.[19] In this regard, most of the prevention literature on athletes has stressed reducing the risk through a de-emphasis of weight and dieting, in addition to providing education to athletes and sport personnel (see NCAA, 2005; Powers & Johnson, 1996; Thompson & Sherman, 1993b; Thompson & Sherman, 1999b). Dieting and a desire to be thin are related to the development of eating disorders,[4,13] and a decrease in pressure to diet reduces the risk. Thus, a de-emphasis on weight is essential for the prevention of eating disorders and disordered eating.

De-emphasize Weight

Because dieting (dietary restriction) is related to the development of eating disorders, any situation or issue that encourages the loss of weight or body fat constitutes a risk. A de-emphasis on weight will reduce the risk. Obviously, the notion that a decrease in weight or body fat can enhance performance not only emphasizes weight; worse yet, it emphasizes weight loss.

There are several issues that are apt to arise with regard to de-emphasizing weight. The first involves the inevitable issue of weight and performance. If an athlete is not performing well, a coach or athlete may view (excess) weight as the problem, and weight loss as the solution. Using performance as the rationale for weight loss does not diminish the potential risk of disordered eating to the athlete if she attempts to lose weight. This is a complicated issue that has been discussed elsewhere (IOCMC, 2005; NCAA, 2005; Sherman & Thompson, in press), and are not be recounted here. Suffice it to say that weight issues regarding are health issues and should be managed by health care professionals, and there are numerous non-weight-focused strategies for enhancing performance that should be tried before the athlete is asked to lose weight.[9]

Decrease Competitive Thinness

Many girls and young women engage in "competitive thinness,"[23] a term used to define the enormous emphasis on thinness in our society in which many girls and young women feel competitive about being thinner than others. This is manifested in their being tempted to lose weight when encountering others who they believe to be thinner. This competitiveness is often accomplished through body comparisons. For athletes, this competitiveness can relate to thinness as the athletes can begin to compare their thinness to each other just as it occurs in non-athletes, but it can also be related to sport performance. For example, if an athlete notices that a competitor or a teammate who has outperformed her looks thinner or leaner, she may use the rationale of enhanced performance as her reason for dieting.

Competitive thinness can create a weight (loss) focus. Thus, this focus needs to be discouraged and decreased. The certified athletic trainer can again play an integral role. By assisting in de-emphasizing weight, the certified athletic trainer is also decreasing part of the impetus for competitive thinness. Additionally, some athletes tell us the authors of this chapter that difficulties for them sometimes occur when a coach compares their body and performance to that of their teammates. (This is actually encouraging competitive thinness.) Depending on the relationship the certified athletic trainer has with the coach, it may be difficult to discuss the need for eliminating this kind of comparison. Nonetheless, it needs to be done.

Many girls and young women are uncomfortable with their bodies. Another risk for competitive thinness is related to revealing uniforms. Revealing uniforms cannot only exacerbate feelings of body dissatisfaction; they can facilitate unhealthy body comparisons. Even if the certified athletic trainer has little or no input into the type of uniform worn, he or she can watch and listen for signs of the athlete being uncomfortable or self-conscious about how she looks (and feels) in her uniform.

As an example, one observant coach indicated that through the years she had noticed that athletes in her sport with eating problems often chose to cover their "bunnies" (bunhuggers) with shorts. An athlete who is constantly tugging on her shorts may be trying to "cover up." For these athletes, it is recommended to approach her privately and inquire as to her (dis)comfort with her uniform.

Education of Athletes and Sport Personnel

Education can be a primary contributor to prevention. There are several areas in which education is needed for athletes, coaches, and other sport personnel. One of the greatest needs in this regard involves nutrition, eating, weight, and weight loss. It is believed that the sport world is a microcosm of the world at large. In the larger world, there is no greater area so driven by myth, misconception, and misinformation than topics surrounding nutrition, eating, weight, and weight loss. Often athletes with disordered eating and eating disorders, incorrectly believe that they are knowledgeable about nutrition and weight. It is highly recommended that athletes, coaches, and other sports personnel take a basic course in nutrition.

Athletes, coaches, and other sports personnel should be given access to factual sources, such as *Nancy Clark's Sports Nutrition Guidebook* (3rd ed.)[2] and the NCAA Web site on nutrition and performance (www.ncaa.org). The certified athletic trainer could play an integral role in arranging for this information and encouraging its use. It is also recommended that a dietitian be added to the sport management staff, if not full-time at least on a part-time or consulting basis. Specialists are needed to deal with the very special problems of disordered eating and eating disorders. Dietitians are the nutrition and eating health care specialists.

is an additional area of education that is needed by athletes and sport personnel involves. Because the Female Athlete Triad involves three health issues (disordered eating, amenorrhea, and osteoporosis), this is an area in which the certified athletic trainer can play a significant role. As important as it is to monitor athletes for disordered eating, it is equally important to monitor the menstrual status of athletes. In a survey of collegiate team physicians and certified athletic trainers, only 35% of the respondents saw their screening programs for menstrual dysfunction as successful.

In a survey of collegiate coaches regarding how they manage athletes with disordered eating, only 48% viewed amenorrhea as abnormal and in need of intervention, and only 35% had ever referred an amenorrheic athlete for a medical evaluation.[18] This could mean that there is no one checking on the female athletes' menstrual status which has shown to be a reliable health predictor. Therefore, someone in the athletic department needs to know, or inquire about, the menstrual status of its athletes. This should be the role of the Certified Athletic Trainer as this is a health issue. Again, the certified athletic trainer could again play a significant role in identifying these potentially devastating pathologies. There are sources available with information on how to identify, manage, treat, and prevent the Female Athlete Triad via websites (IOCMC, 2005; Female Athlete Triad Coalition, 2005) and printed materials (ACSM, 2007; NCAA, 2005). Again, the certified athletic trainer can play a significant role by making these sources and materials available and encouraging their use by athletes, coaches, and other sport personnel.

PERSONAL ENCOUNTER:

An interesting aspect of treating individuals with disordered eating or an eating disorder is that many people are coming for an evaluation at the request of someone who is concerned about them—a concern they do not often share. I always greet them on the first visit by asking "How are you?" Their response is almost always "Fine." I usually say to them that their coach and athletic trainer are concerned about them, and I ask if they themselves are concerned. The response is usually, "No, I think they are overreacting." When asked if they have any medical problems, they almost always reply they are fine and do not have any problems. I have learned to be more specific in my questions and ask if they have a regular menstrual cycle (the answer is usually "No"), if they feel "lightheaded" when standing up quickly (the answer is often "Sometimes"), or if they experience diarrhea or constipation (the answer is often "Sometimes"). Some of their responding may be the denial that often accompanies eating difficulties, but it often relates as well to their mental toughness, or to the fact that they accommodate or habituate to their symptoms and do not notice them. Athletes may also not report fully for fear that identification of an eating problem will negatively affect their playing status or even result in being withdrawn from sport participation.

- Is it better to ask open ended questions or specific questions regarding their health?

PERSONAL ENCOUNTER:

Most individuals with an eating disorder tend not only to believe that they can get over their difficulties without assistance but also believe that they *should*. They seem almost afraid that I am going to change them. Perhaps this is a part of the control issues that are often a part of an eating disorder. I suggest to them, "I am not going to change you. I don't think I could change you if I wanted to. If you change, it will be because you changed you. My role is to help you change—or, more accurately help you change you." This often seems to reassure them. I suggest that they think of me as a consultant or advisor. If the individual is an athlete, I suggest that he/she think of me as a coach. I remind athletes that their coach does not compete for them. Rather, he/she assists them with their training and performance. One athlete responded to this by saying, "Oh, you're like my mental coach." I responded, "Yes, and you can think of your treatment with me as your *training*." Putting treatment in a sport or training context, seems to be helpful to many of them.

- How can putting the treatment in a sport training context be helpful?

Summary

This chapter discussed the many ways the certified athletic trainer is the appropriate person to take on the multiple and varied tasks, roles, and responsibilities of the athlete with disordered eating or an eating disorder. Though it is well within the Certified Athletic Trainer's scope of practice, screening and maintaining treatments in athletes with disordered eating may be a challenging and formidable job. Research and literature clearly identify a need for the identification, management, and prevention of disordered eating and eating disorders in athletes. The certified athletic trainer may be the person best equipped to identify, address, and manage this aspect of the athlete's care.

Resources

Academy for Eating Disorders (AED): www.aedweb.org

National Association of Anorexia and Associated Disorders (ANAD): www.anad.org

National Eating Disorders Association (NEDA): www.nationaleatingdisorders.org

Female Athlete Triad Coalition: www.femaleathletetriad.org

References

1. American College of Sports Medicine. (2007). Position stand: The female athlete triad. *Medicine & Science in Sports & Exercise, 39,* 1867–1882.

2. Black DR, Larkin LJS, Coster DC, Levernz LJ, and Abood DA. Physiologic screening test for eating disorders/disordered eating among female collegiate athletes. *Journal of Athletic Training,* 2003;38:286–297.

3. Clark N. *Nancy Clark's sport nutrition guidebook* (3rd. ed.). Champaign, IL: Human Kinetics; 2003.

4. Female Athlete Triad Coalition. The female triad website. 2005. Available www.femaleathletetriad.org.

5. Garfinkel PE, and Garner DM. *Anorexia nervosa: A multidimensional perspective.* New York: Brunner/Mazel; 1982.

6. Hart S, Abraham S, Luscombe G, and Russell J. Fluid intake in patients with eating disorders. *International Journal of Eating Disorders.* 2005;38:55–59.

7. International Olympic Committee Medical Commission. Position stand on the female athlete triad. 2005. Available at: http://multimedia.olympic.org/pdf/en_report_917.pdf .

8. LeUnes AD, and Nation JR. *Sports psychology: An introduction.* Chicago: Nelson Hall; 1989.

9. National Collegiate Athletic Association. The NCAA nutrition and performance website. 2003. Available at: www.ncaa.org/nutritionandperformance.

10. National Collegiate Athletic Association. *Managing the female athlete triad: NCAA coaches handbook.* Indianapolis: The National Collegiate Athletic Association; 2005.

11. Petrie TA, and Sherman RT. Recognizing and assisting athletes with eating disorders. In: Ray R, and Wiese-Bjornstal DM (Eds.). *Counseling in Sports Medicine.* Champaign, IL: Human Kinetics; 1999: 205–226.

12. Petrie TA, and Sherman RT. Counseling athletes with eating disorders. In: Andersen MB (Ed.), *Doing Sport Psychology.* Champaign, IL: Human Kinetics; 2000:121–137.

13. Piran N. Prevention of eating disorders. In Fairburn CG, and Brownell KD (Eds.), *Eating Disorders and Obesity: A Comprehensive Handbook* (2nd ed.). New York: The Guilford Press; 2002:367–371.

14. Polivy J, and Herman CP. Diagnosis and treatment of normal eating. *Journal of Consulting and Clinical Psychology.* 1987;55:635–644.

15. Powers PS, and Johnson C. Small victories: Prevention of eating disorders among athletes. *Eating Disorders: The Journal of Treatment and Prevention.* 1996;4:364–377.

16. Rosen LW, and Hough DO. Pathogenic weight control behaviors of female college gymnasts. *Physician and Sportsmedicine.* 1988;16:141–144.

17. Ryan J. *Little Girls in Pretty Boxes: The Making and Breaking of Elite Gymnasts and Figure Skaters.* New York: Warner Books; 2000.

18. Sherman RT, and Thompson RA. (2006). Practical use of the international Olympic committee medical commission position stand on the female athlete triad: A case example. *International Journal of Eating Disorders; 39,* 193–201.

19. Sherman RT, DeHaas D, Thompson RA, and Wilfert M. (2005). NCAA coaches survey: The role of the coach in identifying and managing athletes with disordered eating. *Eating Disorders: The Journal of Treatment and Prevention, 13,* 447–466.

20. Taylor CB. Update on the prevention of eating disorders. In Wonderlich S, Mitchell J, de Zwaan M, and Steiger H (Eds.), *Eating Disorders Review Part 1.* Oxford: Radcliff Publishing; 2005: 1–14.

21. Thompson RA. *Helping Athletes with Eating Disorders.* Champaign, IL: Human Kinetics; 1993.

22. Thompson RA. The last word: Wrestling with death. *Eating Disorders: The Journal of Treatment and Prevention*. 1998;6:207–210.

23. Thompson RA. *Athletes and Eating Disorders: Bridgingt Gap.* Keynote address presented at the Academy for Eating Disorders Athlete Special Interest Group Conference "Athletes and Eating Disorders: Bridging the Gap," Indianapolis, IN; October 2003.

24. Thompson RA, and Sherman RT. Reducing the risk of eating disorders in athletics. *Eating Disorders: The Journal of Treatment and Prevention*. 1993b;1:64–78.

25. Thompson RA, and Sherman RT. "Good athlete" traits and characteristics of anorexia nervosa: Are they similar? *Eating Disorders: The Journal of Treatment and Prevention*. 1999a;7:181–190.

26. Thompson RA, and Sherman RT. Athletes, athletic performance, and eating disorders: Healthier alternatives. *Journal of Social Issues*. 1999b;55:317–337.

27. Vaughn JL, King KA, and Csottrell RR. Collegiate athletic trainers' confidence in helping female athletes with eating disorders. *Journal of Athletic Training*. 1999b;39:71–76.

28. Zimmerman TS. Using family systems theory to counsel the injured athlete. In Ray R, and Wiese-Bjornstal DM (Eds.), *Counseling in Sports Medicine*. Champaign, IL: Human Kinetics; 1999b:111–126.

SECTION 4

Anatomical and Physiological Characteristics Unique to the Female Athlete

CHAPTER 13

Cardiac Complications Related to Eating Disorders

John MacKnight, MD

Introduction

Although athletes and nonathletes constitute two different populations, the effects of eating disorders on the heart and associated systems are the same to both groups. Therefore, this chapter will discuss the effects of eating disorders in general terms.

Cardiac Complications Associated with Eating Disorders

Eating disorders (ED) are common in the general population, with rates of incidence for anorexia nervosa and bulimia nervosa ranging from 1%–5% in adolescents and young adults,[14] and are much higher in athletes. As a result of the physiologic changes associated with starvation and dehydration, eating disorders are accompanied by a high incidence of medical complications. Of these, cardiac complications are common and include bradycardia, other electrocardiographic abnormalities including prolonged corrected QT interval (QTc) and cardiac dysrhythmias, congestive heart failure[7] and orthostasis.[56] Although many of these developments are benign, they may cause significant symptomatology and even death. In addition, the use of pathologic weight control behaviors, such as appetite suppressants, particularly stimulant diet pills, can lead to hypertension, palpitations, or stroke[17] while self-induced vomiting, laxative abuse, and diuretic abuse may create acid-base disturbances and electrolyte imbalances which can predispose to cardiac arrhythmias.

The mortality rate associated with eating disorders is the highest of any major psychiatric disorder. Patton[40] has reported in a cohort of eating disorder patients a mortality rate of 3.3% in patients with anorexia nervosa and 3.1% for bulimia nervosa; these values are consistent throughout the eating disorder literature. The mortality rate for anorexic women is 12 times greater than in age-matched normal women, often due to cardiac complications.[2] The most common cause of death in the anorexia group was suicide by substance overdose. Subsequent studies have revealed that approximately one-third of eating disorder deaths are due to cardiac complications.[22,36,49] Because of their prominent place in the secondary morbidity and mortality of eating disorders, cardiovascular complications are extremely important and are further explored in this chapter in order to aid practitioners and care providers in their recognition and management. Most cardiac complications are found in anorexic patients. The bulk of the following discussion is pertinent to anorexia nervosa except as specifically noted.

Assessment of Cardiovascular Function

An electrocardiogram, or ECG, is an electrical recording of the changes that occur in the heart during a cardiac cycle. The recording is acquired by placing multiple electrodes, usually 12 for best results, at specific locations on the chest and extremities. Once the ECG is obtained, it is analyzed for abnormalities including timing and rhythm dysfunction. For a review of the different components and interpretation of the ECG, please refer to Figure 13-1.

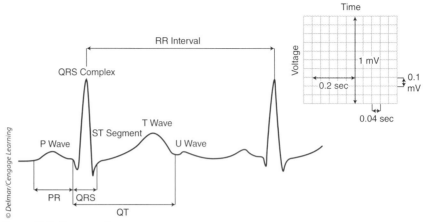

Figure 13-1 Electrocardiogram.
  - *P wave:* the *sequential* activation (depolarization) of the right and left atria
  - *QRS complex:* right and left ventricular depolarization (normally the ventricles are activated simultaneously)
  - *ST-T wave:* ventricular repolarization
  - *U wave:* origin for this wave is not clear – but probably represents "after-depolarizations" in the ventricles
  - *PR interval:* time interval from onset of atrial depolarization (P wave) to onset of ventricular depolarization (QRS complex)
  - *QT interval:* duration of ventricular depolarization and repolarization
  - *RR interval:* duration of ventricular cardiac cycle (an indicator of ventricular rate)
  - *QRS duration:* duration of ventricular muscle depolarization
  - *PP interval:* duration of atrial cycle (an indicator of atrial rate)

Cardiac Abnormalities Related to Disordered Eating

Table 13-1 lists the most common cardiac abnormalities seen in eating disordered patients. These include sinus bradycardia and a wide array of electrocardiographic abnormalities, hypotension and syncope, exercise dysfunction, chronic cardiovascular diseases, and sudden cardiac death. Any practitioner who works in an environment of eating disorder prevalence must have a full understanding of the deleterious physiology associated with starvation, and the potentially catastrophic cardiac conditions that may arise. Close involvement with medical personnel familiar with these issues is essential to ensuring the best care of every patient with an eating disorder.

Physiologic Alterations

While exercise can cause harmless conditions like bradycardia (a slowed heart rate) and hypotension (lower than normal blood pressure), individuals with eating disorders can experience the same cardiovascular effects, but these effects come from different mechanisms, which can prove to be pathological and/or lethal.

Bradycardia

Bradycardia is the most common electrical abnormality seen and documented in ED patients,[8,38] noticed many decades ago and found to be as low as 25 beats per minute[24] versus a normal heart rate of 70–0 beats per minute and it has been

TABLE 13-1 • **Cardiovascular Manifestations in Anorexia Nervosa**[31]

Physiologic alterations
Bradycardia
Hypotension and Syncope
Reduced cardiac output
Elevated total peripheral resistance
Exercise dysfunction
Electrocardiographic abnormalities
QT interval prolongation
Conduction delays
ST segment abnormalities
Arrhythmias
***Torsade de pointes* ventricular tachycardia**
Ventricular fibrillation
Structural cardiac alterations
Pericardial effusion
Mitral valve prolapse
Reduced left ventricular mass and volume
Atrial Failure
Sudden cardiac death
Chronic cardiovascular disease
Congestive heart failure (associated with re-feeding)

well described since. A bradycardic heart utilizes less energy and minimizes the workload of the heart to compensate for the negative energy balance and weight loss created by starvation. Abnormally high levels of cardiac vagal activity, perhaps added with altered arterial baroreceptor reflex sensitivity, have been demonstrated in anorexics and may play a contributing role in heart rate lowering.[26]

Mont et al.[34] demonstrated nocturnal bradycardia (<40 beats per minute) in the majority of anorexic patients studied. Four patients were even found to have minimum heart rates <30 beats per minute. Patients with heart rates in the 30–35 beat per minute range in the setting of moderate or severe anorexia should be considered for cardiac monitoring. If patients subsequently develop a high grade atrioventricular (AV) block (2nd or 3rd degree), then monitoring and consideration of pacemaker placement is appropriate. Fortunately, conduction delays of that magnitude are rare in this population.[37] The maximum, minimum, and mean heart rates all increase significantly with re-feeding and weight gain.

Hypotension and Syncope

Patients with severe anorexia nervosa may suffer syncope (loss of consciousness due to poor cerebral perfusion) secondary to postural hypotension, or a decrease in blood pressure due to change in position. Increased vagal tone (impulses from the vagus nerve producing an inhibition of the heartbeat), bradycardia, and low plasma volume from chronic dehydration favor the development of both low resting blood pressure and poor blood pressure maintenance with postural changes. Postural hypotension is best assessed by the presence or absence of postural dizziness as opposed to actual blood pressure readings, although patients who note postural dizziness should have postural blood pressures obtained to confirm the diagnosis.

Robinson[46] has suggested a scoring system for postural hypotension in anorexics: (0) no postural dizziness, (1) brief postural dizziness, (2) persistent postural dizziness, (3) unable to stand because of postural dizziness. This system may be useful in helping to quantify the severity of disease at a given point in time and determine an appropriate level of treatment intervention.

Studies, including tilt table testing (the "gold standard" testing modality for postural or vasodepressor syncope) provoked a vasovagal response in 35% of ED patients.[20] This vasovagal response usually is a transitory condition that is marked especially by fainting associated with hypotension, peripheral vasodilatation, and bradycardia resulting from an increased stimulation of the vagus nerve. Despite the increased vagal tone demonstrated uniformly in these patients, anorexia has not been shown to pose an additional risk for other common cardiac causes of syncope, namely neurocardiogenic or vasodepressor syncope.

Bulimics may also suffer syncopal attacks. Their causative factor classically, however, is hypokalemia-induced dysrhythmias that can deteriorate into lethal dysrhythmias. Other conditions may include a decreased cardiac output, which is a decreased amount of blood being ejected from the heart and increased peripheral resistance due to an increase in the contraction activity of the associated blood vessels in order to raise the individual's blood pressure. These both can be caused by extreme dieting and/or poor nutrition.

Electrocardiographic Abnormalities

Multiple electrocardiographic abnormalities can be demonstrated in anorexic patients. Over 50 years ago, some of the earliest studies in ED patients revealed sinus bradycardia, low QRS, P or T wave voltages, ventricular tachyarrythmias, and prolongation of the QT interval.[13] More recently, further study[6] confirmed the prior findings and identified a number of additional commonly encountered electrocardiographic findings in anorexic patients:

- Sinus bradycardia or tachycardia
- Low voltage of P waves and QRS complexes
- Rightward QRS axis
- Nonspecific ST-T wave changes
- Presence of U waves (follows the T wave, often associated with hypokalemia)
- Conduction disturbances

- QT interval prolongation
- Increased QT interval dispersion

These conditions are detailed later in this chapter.

QT Interval Prolongation

Panagiotopoulos et al.[39] studied the electrocardiographic characteristics of hospitalized women with eating disorders. In addition to sinus bradycardia, this group demonstrated longer QRS complex duration, shorter QTc (QT interval corrected for heart rate), lesser QTc dispersion, and lower amplitude of the QRS complex, particularly the R-wave (the electrically positive wave form in the QRS complex) in electrocardiogram lead V6. This decrease in R-wave amplitude may result from a reduction in left ventricular mass compared with the patient's actual body weight.[35] Animal studies have shown that such changes are the result of myocardial atrophy from extreme calorie restriction.

Increased clinical disease severity, as reflected by lower standardized BMI, was significantly related to: lower ventricular rate, shorter mean QTc, and lower amplitude of the R-wave in V6. QRS duration and QTc dispersion did not share this correlation. These findings suggest that selected electrocardiographic findings may be utilized to assess overall ED severity.

Of the potential deleterious cardiac manifestations of AN, corrected QT interval (QTc) prolongation is the most feared because of its association with malignant ventricular arrythmias and sudden cardiac death.[5] Studies have previously addressed this association,[7,25] but subsequent evidence linking the two has been conflicting. Cooke et al.[5] evaluated QT interval in a small number of adult anorexic patients. They found an incidence of 15% in the studied population with two patients suffering sudden death. They also found that weight gain and improvement in clinical status resulted in a shortening of the QT interval. Although improved, the QT interval did not return to normal.

There is also controversy regarding the contribution of electrolyte imbalance to electrocardiographic abnormalities and risk for serious arrhythmias. Some authors have found no QTc prolongation as long as electrolytes were normal,[39,59] while others documented QTc prolongation in patients with significant electrolyte abnormalities resulting from their weight loss behaviors.[5,11,55]

Depletion of potassium, chloride, and sodium is well known to create electrical instability in the cardiac system and generate abnormalities in heart rhythm. Simple cardiac ectopy is rarely problematic; however, electrolyte changes may predispose to serious rhythm disturbances that may degenerate into lethal arrhythmias. Frequent vomiting, laxative abuse, and diuretic abuse by ED patients can lead to depletion of these vital electrolytes. Hypokalemia (decreased potassium levels) resulting from vomiting, starvation, and abuse of potassium-depleting drugs is common in AN patients. This low potassium state may then result in an early after-depolarization phenomenon. The ECG may subsequently reveal a prolonged QT interval, which predisposes to arrhythmias, *torsade de pointes*, ventricular tachycardia, and ventricular fibrillation, especially superimposed on a baseline of bradycardia (Figure 13-2).

At present, the risk of malignant degeneration to *torsades de pointes* ventricular tachycardia appears to be quite low, if electrolyte balance is maintained and there are no drugs leading to QT prolongation (see below).[20] Vanderdonckt et al.[26] came to a similar conclusion after analyses of a series of AN patients. In this study population, QT and QTc interval prolongation were decidedly unusual, being demonstrated in only 1 of 47 studied cases. The sole variable which correlated with prolonged QTc duration was the potassium concentration. Their conclusion was that marked repolarization changes (either QT interval and/or T wave morphology) in anorexic patients should not be considered an intrinsic feature of the disease but rather an indicator of metabolic or electrolyte disturbances, drug effects, or genetic predisposition.

It is important to view each of the cardiac findings listed above as a physiologic manifestation of uncompensated anorexia nervosa. They often do not require cardiac-specific treatment for their correction unless there are negative physical manifestations associated with their presence. Addressing the primary changes associated with the eating disordered behavior itself (electrolyte imbalance and pathologic weight controlling behaviors) will result in resolution of these cardiac manifestations.

Conduction Delays

These delays appear on an ECG strip when the electrical conduction of the heart does not produce a normal conduction pattern and the timing is delayed. This can potentially lead to many different conduction pathologies, some of which can lead to death. Individuals who do not have an eating disorder and display these findings have been found to later have a heart attack.

ST Segment Abnormalities

These are specific abnormal findings (measurements) on an ECG strip that are associated with many different potentially fatal pathological conditions.

Arrhythmias

An arrhythmia is a general term given to a heart beat (pattern) that is not normal and can range from pathological to nonpathological conditions. The following conditions are pathological and are normally associated with more severe conditions:

- Torsade de Pointes. This in literal translation means "a twisting of the points" and is a lethal form of Ventricular Tachycardia.

- Ventricular Tachycardia. Ventricular Tachycardia (V-Tach) is a fast heart rhythm that originates in one of the ventricles of the heart instead of the atria and can prove to be fatal.

- Ventricular Fibrillation. This condition is an uncoordinated contraction of the cardiac muscle where the heart does not beat as one unit as it just quivers, which leads to decreased blood flow of the heart resulting in death.

(A) Prolonged QT Interval

Lead V₁

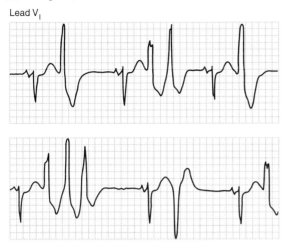

Multifocal PVC's, couplet, triplet in
patient with prolonged QT

(B) Torsade de pointes

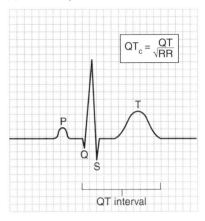

$$QT_c = \frac{QT}{\sqrt{RR}}$$

(C) Ventricular Tachydcardia

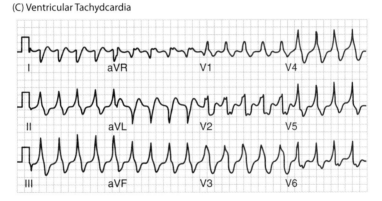

(D) Ventricular Fibrillation

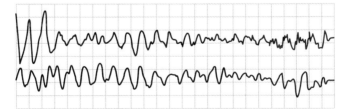

© Delmar/Cengage Learning

Heart Rate	Rhythm	P Wave	PR interval (in seconds)	QRS (in seconds)
300–600	Extremely irregular	Absent	N/A	Fibrillatory baseline

Figure 13-2 Various cardiac abnormalities as shown on an ECG (A) Prolonged QT Interval (B) Torsades de Pointes (C) Ventricular tachycardia (D) Ventricular fibrillation (E) normal sinus bradycardia.

(E) Normal Sinus Bradycardia

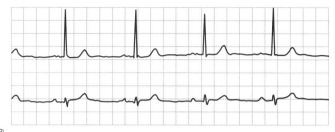

Heart Rate	Rhythm	P Wave	PR interval (in seconds)	QRS (in seconds)
< 60 bpm	Regular	Before each QRS, identical	0.12 to 0.20	< 0.12

© Delmar/Cengage Learning

Figure 13-2 (cont.)

Structural Cardiac Alterations

As a result of chronic starvation and low dietary protein status, ED patients are at risk to develop diffuse muscle loss; no such muscle loss is as vital as that related to the myocardium. Echocardiographic studies in this population have observed diminished wall thickness due to loss of cardiac muscle with a concomitant reduction in cardiac output.[42]

Pericardial Effusion

Further studies have revealed an incidence of silent pericardial effusion of 71% in studied anorexic patients vs. only 10% in controls.[45] Although the significance of this finding is still controversial, it is largely believed to be a cardiovascular marker of the physiologic disarray associated with AN, and not a primary cardiac complication. Inagaki et al. documented resolution of anorexia-associated pericardial effusion in response to weight gain.[21] Interestingly, these investigators also found that levels of brain natriuretic peptide (BNP) were elevated when the pericardial effusion was present and decreased with re-feeding and resolution of the effusion. They suggest that measurement of serum BNP may be a clinical parameter of use in cases of pericardial effusions.

Mitral Valve Prolapse

Structural changes in the mitral valve, with resultant prolapse and regurgitant (back flow) blood flow, are not uncommon in ED patients (Figure 13-3). With weight loss, a change in the anatomic relationship between the mitral valve leaflets and the ventricular chamber may arise as a result of loss of cardiac mass. The valve structures move closer together and become redundant, thus allowing for prolapse physiology.[9] de Simone demonstrated mitral valve motion

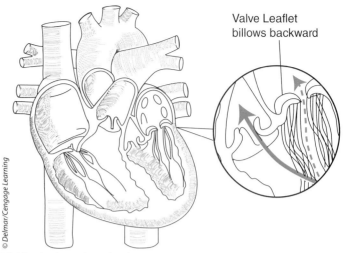

Valve Leaflet
billows backward

© Delmar/Cengage Learning

Figure 13-3 Mitral valve prolapse in a heart.

vvabnormalities in 62% of studied anorexic patients. Fortunately, clinically significant mitral regurgitation is very rare and no cases requiring mitral valve surgery have been described. With weight gain, the valvular changes in ED patients generally remit.[15,43]

Reduced Left Ventricular Mass and Volume

Mont et al.[20] found that 93% of studied anorexia nervosa patients had a decreased left ventricular mass relative to their age and body surface area. The thickness of the cardiac septum and free wall were diminished in 70% of patients; however, left ventricular diastolic and systolic diameters were within the normal ranges in 80% of them. Left atrial size was decreased in 50% of the individuals, and 80% showed a diminished cardiac index. After re-feeding and weight gain, there was a significant increase in systolic and diastolic diameters of the left ventricle, an enlargement of left atrial size, and an increase in left ventricular mass. Cardiac index improved significantly as well. These data suggest a high degree of reversibility for cardiac structural changes at early stages of anorexia. It is unknown whether this reversibility still exists in patients with long-standing anorexia.

de Simone et al.[9] performed echocardiographic evaluations on a small number of anorexic patients and again found a characteristic group of cardiac abnormalities. Left ventricular chamber dimension and mass were significantly decreased. They also found reduced cardiac index from both low stroke volume (the amount of blood ejected with each heart beat) and lower heart rate (relative bradycardia) with a decrease in overall exercise intolerance. Although not seen in all patients, decreases in left ventricular mass and systolic function have been demonstrated by other researchers as well.[41]

"Atrial Failure"

Extreme weight loss with AN has also been found to create atrial electrome-chanical dissociation (lack of atrial contraction despite normal electrical stimulation), or so-called "atrial failure."[33] Atrial failure should be appreciated as a potential clinical feature of anorexia nervosa that may contribute to decreased overall cardiac function. Weight gain during the treatment course resulted in complete resolution of such atrial dysfunction.

Congestive Heart Failure

Serious impairments in ventricular function resulting in frank congestive heart failure are uncommon in anorexic patients. Nevertheless, this complication can have lethal consequences and must be respected. It is most highly associated with rapid re-feeding (re-feeding is discussed separately below) of cachectic, or physically wasted patients.[37,19,16] Though the exact mechanism for the creation of heart failure is still unclear, it does appear that hypophosphatemia (decreased phosphorous levels) in association with rapid re-feeding plays an important role.[25] Some authors have suggested that hypomagnesemia (decreased magnesium levels) may play a role in the potential development of congestive heart failure in anorexic patients as well.[26]

Rapid sodium and volume repletion may be poorly tolerated in these patients because of small left ventricular chamber size and diminished baseline cardiac output. This may be further exacerbated by paradoxical elevations in peripheral vascular resistance, despite the relative hypotension that commonly accompanies severe fasting.[23] As a result, re-feeding must proceed in a slow, methodical fashion, allowing adequate time for fluid balance, sodium repletion, and electrolyte stability to be established, particularly with respect to phosphorous. This is critical, particularly in the early stages of inpatient weight restoration, in order to avoid serious cardiac complications.[3] High salt intake during this time must also be avoided.

Severely anorexic patients may develop a diffuse myopathy affecting skeletal muscle. Should the severity of their disease be great enough, they may also develop cardiac myocyte damage with resultant heart failure.[1]

Exercise Dysfunction

As would be expected from chronic and often severe calorie deprivation, exercise tolerance and exercise capacity are uniformly decreased in ED patients[52] and are more noticeable in athletes as their bodies do not have the calories to fuel their exercise. Some element of this dysfunction results from cardiac functional changes. Most of these patients demonstrate a blunted heart rate response, low baseline blood pressure, attenuated blood pressure response to exercise with a concomitant reduction in maximal work capacity[12] a significant incidence of ventricular ectopy, and decreased oxygen consumption. Diminished exercise capacity has also been attributed to a loss of cardiac muscle mass, dysfunction of the remaining cardiac muscle, and impaired cardiovascular responses to the initiation of exercise activities.

Evaluations of exercise capacity in anorexic patients have confirmed that this population demonstrates a blunted sympathetic response to maximal exercise. This is a frequent finding and is directly correlated to the degree of weight deficit or decrease in body mass index (BMI: weight[kg] / height[m²]). This "cardiac sympathetic withdrawal" is a manifestation of major autonomic nervous system derangement in anorexic individuals.[43]

In a study of exercise performance in a group of anorexia nervosa patients, abnormal work capacity and altered cardiovascular responses to exercise were observed.[3] The resultant low VO$_2$ max, both at rest and during exercise, allows these anorexic women to maintain a relatively high level of physical activity. This, unfortunately, allows these patients to foster additional pathologic weight loss by increasing their energy expenditure.

Sudden Death in Anorexia

"Sudden death" is defined as the sudden and unexpected occurrence of death for which no satisfactory explanation of the cause of death can be ascertained. It is now well established that cardiac involvement in anorexia nervosa may contribute to sudden death in some patients.[53]

Akin to the discussion of QT interval changes noted earlier, further insight into the risk of sudden cardiac death with ED can be derived from an understanding of the basic mechanisms contributing to "long QT syndrome." Two major pathogenic mechanisms have been postulated. The first suggests that arrhythmias are triggered by periods of increased adrenergic (sympathetic nervous system) activity driven by either physical or psychological stress. A second theory is based on a genetic change in potassium transport during the repolarization phase of the cardiac cycle.[48] Both of these mechanisms could be extrapolated to ED patients because of their severe physical stresses and potential for potassium deficiency from purging behaviors. As such, the substrate for abnormal electrical activity is prominent in this population and creates a high-risk physiologic milieu in which lethal arrhythmias may originate.[36]

Autopsy studies of anorexic patients with sudden death found interstitial hemorrhages of myocardial contraction bands with lipofuscin granule deposition in the myocardial cells of deceased anorexic patients.[44] This "aging" pigment is a marker of chronic myocyte damage induced by longstanding starvation and is an example of the fundamental cellular changes that eating disorders may generate within the heart. In addition, these patients had demonstrated severe hypokalemia, hypoglycemia, and ECG abnormalities including sinus bradycardia and downsloping ST segments, all of which are known to greatly heighten the risk for ventricular fibrillation. Similarly, Isner et al.[7] noted a connection with the degree of QT interval prolongation seen shortly before death in ED patients with severe calorie restriction.

Electrolyte Imbalance

As noted earlier, prolonged QT interval has been reported frequently, though not always, in anorexic patients and is considered a major risk factor for sudden death. Swenne et al.[28] found that nearly half of a sample of 58 patients demonstrated QT prolongation and also had a two-fold increase in QT dispersion (believed to be a better measure of arrhythmia risk) as compared to a control group. The propensity for an increased QT dispersion in this population predisposes them to a high risk of sudden death through generation of a *torsades de pointes* ventricular tachycardia. Clinical factors that correlated best with QT prolongation were low BMI, rapid rate of weight loss, and serum sodium level. Herzog et al.[18] previously had reported that a low level of serum albumin (<36 grams per liter) was the best predictor of a fatal disease course because of its association with severe starvation and disordered protein metabolism.

Further evidence linking the risk of anorexia and its associated electrolyte-dependent cardiac changes comes from data that suggests that there is a hormone-dependent decrease in potassium ion channel expression which may strongly control the tendency for women to have a higher incidence of QT prolongation and acquired *torsades de pointes*.[57] Torsades is often triggered during periods of bradycardia[27,35] which, unfortunately, is almost universally present in advanced cases of anorexia nervosa with associated starvation. Bradycardia, female gender, hypokalemia, and concurrent psychiatric medication use all contribute to creation of a favorable milieu for the generation of a lethal arrhythmia. The use of drugs with known arrhythmogenic potential, such as phenothiazine, clozapine, tricyclic antidepressants, and trazodone should be avoided,[60] and careful monitoring of fluid and electrolyte balance are essential to lessen the risk of sudden cardiac death in association with an eating disorder.

Autonomic Dysfunction

Autonomic nervous system imbalance has also been postulated as a potential causative factor for QT prolongation in anorexic patients.[7] An imbalance in sympathetic innervation of the heart may result in an enhanced susceptibility to sympathetic activity, which in turn may lead to malignant ventricular arrhythmias. As exercise induces activation of the sympathetic nervous system and naturally prolongs the QT interval, it is prudent to discourage anorexic patients from heavy exercise that could create electrical instability and significant, even lethal, cardiac rhythm disturbance.

With studied patients who have suffered sudden death in this population, ischemic heart disease does not appear to play a causative role.

Chronic Cardiovascular Concerns

Although the bulk of cardiovascular concerns in eating disorders are of an acute nature, there are long-term sequelae that may develop if the disordered physiology of starvation is manifest consistently over a prolonged period. Hypoestrogenemia (decreased estrogen levels) associated with the hormonal dysfunction of eating disorders, particularly anorexia, may result in a variety of metabolic derangements. When estrogen levels are low, changes in mineral, glucose, and fat metabolism accompany amenorrhea. No studies have addressed the risk of cardiovascular disease in young women with hypoestrogenic amenorrhea.

Nevertheless, estrogen decreases low-density lipoprotein, increases high-density lipoprotein, and likely directly affects vascular endothelial and smooth muscle function in favorable way. While some authors have subsequently suggested that chronic hypoestrogenemia in young women may increase their lifetime risk of cardiovascular disease,[28] others have presented contradictory data. Utilizing carotid intimal thickness as a surrogate marker for cardiovascular health and relative risk for coronary artery disease, Birmingham et al. found that anorexia nervosa patients demonstrated no significant differences in vascular status as compared to controls.[4] They conclude that the likelihood of atherosclerosis in anorexic patients is low. Further research is necessary to clarify this key question.

Myocardial infarction (heart attack) has been rarely reported in eating disorder patients during the re-feeding period as noted above. Acute cardiac events have also been described as a result of patient ingestion of weight loss products to aid in their eating disorder. Forman described the development of a subendocardial myocardial infarction in a 20-year-old bulimic as a result of a 20-gram-caffeine ingestion during a suicide attempt.

Re-feeding Syndrome

As noted earlier, the greatest period of risk for cardiac decompensation and congestive heart failure in an ED patient is with re-feeding during the first two weeks of recovery. The reductions in myocardial mass and function in association with starvation make it difficult for the myocardium to withstand the increased metabolic demands of the re-initiation of eating. In its most severe demonstration, rapid re-feeding, particularly with intake of highly caloric food sources and high glucose content, may result in cardiac collapse and death. This phenomenon was first described amongst World War II concentration camp survivors who died suddenly after receiving diets high in calorie-rich foods shortly after being released.

As cited earlier, the major mechanism of heart failure is re-feeding-associated hypophosphatemia. When glucose is ingested in significant quantities, it produces a shift of phosphate from the extracellular to the intracellular space. The transition toward an anabolic state, as a means of recovering from chronic starvation, results in prominent phosphate depletion as phosphate is prominently incorporated into newly synthesized tissues. This phosphate depletion then produces wide ranging abnormalities at the cellular level. The most important change is the subsequent depletion of the body's major energy source, adenosine triphosphate. This, in turn, results in depression of cardiac stroke volume and frank heart failure.[50]

Cardiac decompensation during the re-feeding phase may be heralded by a number of physical findings including:[32]

- sudden sustained increase in pulse rate
- pulse rate <40
- electrocardiogram showing something other than sinus rhythm
- systolic blood pressure <60 mm Hg
- evidence of congestive heart failure

Bulimia

Although eating disorders in general share a number of common features, bulimia nervosa, characterized by a repetitive pattern of binge eating followed by purging with vomiting and/or laxative abuse, is associated with several unique medical complications.

Hypokalemia occurs in approximately 5% of bulimic patients[15,58] and may predispose them to cardiac arrhythmias as discussed previously. Given its low sensitivity, however, screening for hypokalemia cannot be recommended as a means of detecting bulimia.[30] The finding of hypokalemia in an otherwise healthy young woman, however, is highly specific for bulimia and should raise concern about the possibility of occult BN. This is in contrast to *the purely restricting* anorexic patient who is not at risk for any metabolic abnormality, acid-base disturbance, or hypokalemia.[29]

Bulimic patients who abuse syrup of ipecac to induce vomiting may develop toxic reactions. Though reversible, these can be significant and have been associated with the development of a cardiomyopathy.[20]

Suri describes two cases in which patients with claimed remote histories of bulimia nervosa developed cardiac rhythm disturbances (short runs of torsade de pointes and prolonged QT interval) when given anesthesia for a surgical procedure.[54] One patient denied recent bulimic behavior but did have otherwise unexplained hypokalemia at the time of surgery. The other claimed no bulimic behavior for 16 years and had no electrolyte abnormalities. These cases raise questions about residual effects of prior eating disordered behavior on the cardiovascular system or the potential continuation of such behavior despite denial from the patient.

Bulimic patients are well known to demonstrate elevated cardiac vagal tone, giving rise to many of the common cardiovascular manifestations including bradycardia and risk for syncope. Rissanen et al. reported a beneficial effect on cardiac vagal tone in BN patients with the use of 60 mg of fluoxetine, a selective serotonin reuptake inhibitor commonly used in the psychiatric management of this condition. At the end of 8 weeks of treatment, fluoxetine-treated patients demonstrated vagal tone equivalent to control patients.[47] As many of the common symptomatic cardiac complications in eating disorders are derived from increased vagal tone, a trial of fluoxetine may be warranted in this patient population.

Summary

Eating disorders, particularly anorexia nervosa, carry with them a risk for a wide variety of physical complications. Arguably, the most serious and potentially life threatening are those involving the cardiovascular system. A thorough understanding of these potentially serious developments is essential for any care provider who is involved in the management of individuals with eating disorders. Only then can adequate measures be taken to ensure that the risk of ventricular tachyarrhythmias, congestive heart failure, and sudden death is minimized or eliminated and that recovery can be aggressively and safely pursued.

References

1. Alloway R, Shur E, Obrecht R, et al. Physical complications in anorexia nervosa. Haematological and neuromuscular changes in 12 patients. *British Journal of Psychiatry.* 1988;153:72–75.

2. American Psychiatric Association Work Group on Eating Disorders. Practice guidelines for the treatment of patients with eating disorders (revision). *American Journal of Psychiatry.* 2000;157:1–39.

3. Biadi O, Rossini R, Musumeci G, et al. Cardiopulmonary exercise test in young women affected by anorexia nervosa. *Italian Heart Journal.* 2001;2(6):462–467.

4. Birmingham CL, Lear SA, Kenyon J, et al. Coronary atherosclerosis in anorexia nervosa. *International Journal of Eat Disorders.* 2003;34(3):375–377.

5. Cooke RA, Chambers JB, Singh R, et al. QT interval in anorexia nervosa. *British Heart Journal.* 1994;72:69–73.

6. Cooke RA, and Chambers JB. Anorexia nervosa and the heart. *British Journal of Hospital Medicine.* 1995;54:313.

7. Crisp AH, Callender JS, C Halek, et al., Long-term mortality in anorexia nervosa. A 20-year follow-up of the St. George's and Aberdeen cohorts. *British Journal of Psychiatry.* 1992;161:104–107.

8. Dec GW, Biederman J, Hougen TJ., Cardiovascular findings in adolescent inpatients with anorexia nervosa. *Psychosomatic Medicine.* 1987;49:285–290.

9. de Simone G, Scalfi L, Galderisi M, et al. Cardiac abnormalities in young women with anorexia nervosa. *British Heart Journal.* 1994;71(3):287–292.

10. DiVasta AD, Alexander ME, Fainting freshmen and sinking sophomores: cardiovascular issues of the adolescent. *Current Opinion Pediatrics.* 2004;16(4):350–356.

11. Durakovic Z, Durakovic A, M Korsic. Changes of the corrected QT interval in the electrocardiogram of patients with anorexia nervosa. *International Journal of Cardiology.* 1994;45:115–120.

12. Einerson J, Ward A, Hanson P. Exercise response in females with anorexia nervosa. *International Journal of Eating Disorders.* 1988;7:253.

13. Ellis, L. Electrocardiographic abnormalities in severe malnutrition. *British Heart Journal.* 1946;8:53.

14. Fischer M, Golden N, Katzman DK, et al. Eating disorders in adolescents: a background paper. *Journal of Adolescent Health.* 1995;16:420–437.

15. Greenfeld D, Mickley D, Quinlan DM, et al. Hypokalemia in outpatients with eating disorders. *American Journal of Psychiatry.* 1995;152:60–63.

16. Hall RC, Hoffman RS, Beresford TP, et al. Physical illness encountered in patients with eating disorders. *Psychosomatics.* 1989;30:174.

17. Haller CA, Benowitz NL, Adverse cardiovasscular and central nervous system events associated with dietary supplements containing ephedra alkaloids. *New England Journal of Medicine.* 2000;343:1833–1838.

18. Herzog W, Deter HC, W Fiehn, et al. Somatische Pradiktoren im Langzeitverlauf der Anorexia nervosa. *Zeitschrift fur Kinder und Jugendpsychiatre.* 1993;27(Supplement 1):54.

19. Heymsfield SB, Bethel RA, Ansley JD, et al. Cardiac abnormalities in cachectic patients before and during nutritional repletion. *American Heart Journal.* 1978;95:584.

20. Ho PC, Dweik R, Cohen MC. Rapidly reversible cardiomyopathy associated with chronic ipecac ingestion. *Clinical Cardiology.* 1998;21:780-783.

21. Inagaki T, Yamamoto M, Tsubouchi K, et al. Echocardiographic investigation of pericardial effusion in a case of anorexia nervosa. *International Journal of Eating Disorders.* 2003;33(3):364–366.

22. Isner JM, Roberts WC, Heymsfield SB, et al. Anorexia nervosa and sudden death. *Annals of Internal Medicine.* 1985;102:49–52.

23. Johnson GL, Humphries LL, Shirley PB, et al. Mitral valve prolapse in patients with anorexia nervosa and bulimia. *Archives of Internal Medicine.* 1986;146:1525.

24. Keys A, Henschel A, Taylor HL. The size and function of the human heart at rest in semistarvation and in subsequent rehabilitation. *American Journal of Physics.* 1947;150:153.

25. Kohn MR, Golden NH, Shenker IR. Cardiac arrest and delirium: Presentations of the refeeding syndrome in severely malnourished adolescents with anorexia nervosa. *Journal of Adolescent Health.* 1998; 22:239.

26. Kollai M, Bonyhay I, Jokkel G, et al. Cardiac vagal hyperactivity in adolescent anorexia nervosa. *European Heart Journal.* 1994;15:1113.

27. Kurita T, Ohe T, Shimizu W, et al. Early after-depolarization-like activity in patients with class 1A induced long QT syndrome and torsades de pointes. *Pace.* 1997;20:695.

28. Mciver B, Romanski SA, Nippoldt TB, Evaluation and management of amenorrhea. *Mayo Clinic Proceedings.* 1997;72(12):1161–1169.

29. Mehler PS. Diagnosis and care of patients with anorexia nervosa in primary care settings. *Annals of Internal Medicine.* 2001;134:1048–1059.

30. Mehler PS. Bulimia Nervosa. *New England Journal of Medicine.* 2003; 349:875–881.

31. Mehler PS, and Krantz M. Anorexia nervosa medical issues. *Journal of Women's Health.* 2003;12(4):331–340.

32. Mehler PS, Chri Gray M, Schulte M. Medical Complications of Anorexia Nervosa. *Journal of Women's Health.* 1997;6(5):533–541.

33. Mizuno R, Fujii S, Kimura Y, et al. Anorexia nervosa with left atrial failure. *International Medicine.* 1998;37(10):857–860.

34. Mont L, Castro J, Herreros B, et al. Reversibility of cardiac abnormalities in adolescents with anorexia nervosa after weight recovery. *Journal of the American Academy of Child & Adolescent Psychiatry.* 2003;42(7):808–813.

35. Moodie DS, Salcedo E, Cardiac function in adolescents and young adults with anorexia nervosa. *Journal of Adolescent Health.* 1983;4:9–14.

36.   Neumarker, K. Mortality and sudden death in anorexia nervosa. *International Journal of Eating Disorders*. 1997;21:205–212.

37.   Nudel DB, Gootman N, Nussbaum MP, et al. Altered exercise performance and abnormal sympathetic responses to exercise in patients with anorexia nervosa. *Journal of Pediatrics*. 1984;105:34.

38.   Palla B, and Litt IF. Medical complications of eating disorders in adolescents. *Pediatrics*. 1988;81:613–623.

39.   Panagiotopoulos C, McCrindle BW, Hick K, et al. Electrocardiographic Findings in Adolescents with Eating Disorders. *Pediatrics*. 2000;105(5): 1100–1105.

40.   Patton, G. Mortality in eating disorders. *Psychological Medicine*. 1988;18:947–951.

41.   Powers PS. Heart failure during treatment of anorexia nervosa. *American Journal Psychiatry*. 1982;139:1167.

42.   Powers PS, Schocken DD, J Feld, et al. Cardiac function during weight restoration in anorexia nervosa. *Inernational Journal of Eating Disorders*. 1991;10:521–530.

43.   Roche F, Barthélémy JC, Garet M, et al. Chronotropic incompetence to exercise separates low body weight from established anorexia nervosa. *Clinical Physiology and Functional Imaging*. 2004;24(5):270–275.

44.   Rajs J, Rajs E, and T Lundman, Unexpected death in patients suffering from eating disorders. A medico-legal study. *Acta Psychiatrica Scandinavica*. 1986;74:587–596.

45.   Ramacciotti CE, Coli E, Biadi O, et al., *Silent pericardial effusion in a sample of anorexic patients*. EWD, 2003. 8(1): p. 68–71.

46.   Robinson, P., Review article: recognition and treatment of eating disorders in primary and secondary care. *Alimentary Pharmacology & Therapeutics*. 2000;4(4):367–377.

47.   Rissasnen A, Naukkarinen H, Virkkunen M, et al. Fluoxetine normalizes increased cardiac vagal tone in bulimia nervosa. *Journal of Clinical Psychopharmacology*. 1998;18(1):26-32.

48.   Schwartz PJ, Moss AJ, Vincent GM, et al. Diagnostic criteria for the long QT Syndrome- An update. *Circulation*. 1993;88:782–784.

49.   Sharp CW, and Freeman CP. The medical complications of anorexia nervosa. *British Journal of Psychiatry*. 1993;162:452–462.

50.   Solomon SM, and Kirby DF. The refeeding syndrome: a review. *Journal of Parenteral and Enteral Nutrition*. 1990;14:90.

51. Sours HE, Frattali VP, Brand CD, et al. Sudden death associated with very low calorie weight reduction regimens. *American Journal of Clinical Nutrition.* 1981;34:453–461.

52. St John Sutton MG, Plappert T, L Crosby, et al. Effects of reduced left ventricular mass on chamber architecture, load and function: a study of anorexia nervosa. *Circulation.* 1985;72:991–1000.

53. Sullivan PF. Mortality in anorexia nervosa. *American Journal of Psychiatry.* 1995;152:1073–1074.

54. Suri R, Poist ES, Hager WD, et al. Unrecognized bulimia nervosa: a potential cause of perioperative cardiac dysrhythmias. *Canadian Journal of Anaesthesia.* 1999;46(11):1048–1052.

55. Sweene I, and Larsson PT. Heart risk associated with weight loss in anorexia nervosa and eating disorders: risk factors for QTc interval prolongation and dispersion. *Acta Paediatrica*;88:304–309.

56. Wesley RC Jr, and Turnquest P. Torsades de pointe after intravenous adenosine in the presence of prolonged QT syndrome. *American Heart Journal.* 1992;123:794.

57. Wolbrette D, Nacarelli G, Curtis A, et al. Gender differences in arrhythmias. *Clinical Cardiology.* 2002;25:49.

58. Wolfe BE, Metzger ED, Levine JM, et al. Laboratory screening for electrolyte abnormalities and anemia in bulimia nervosa: a controlled study. *International Journal of Eat Disorders.* 2001;30:288–293.

59. Vanderdonckt O, Lambert M, MC Montero, et al. The 12-lead electrocardiogram in anorexia nervosa: a report of 2 cases followed by retrospective study. *Journal of Electrocardiology.* 2001;34(3):233–242.

60. Vannacci A, Baronti R, Masini E, et al. Anorexia nervosa and the risk of sudden death. *American Journal of Medicine.* 2002;112(4):327–328.

CHAPTER 14

Exercise and Fertility in the Female Athlete

John Storment, MD

Introduction

Physicians have known for centuries the adverse effects of stress and exercise on the reproductive system. Soranus, a Greek obstetrician and gynecologist, was the first to observe and describe the effect of over-activity on menstrual irregularity.[17] He also recognized the influence of undernourishment on menstruation. Late in the 20th century, a new awareness surfaced of the impact of strenuous recreational exercise and other forms of demanding activity on menstrual dysfunction. This interaction between physical activity and menses is primarily manifested through hypothalamic suppression.

The hypothalamus is a small organ located at the base of the brain which regulates certain metabolic processes and other autonomic activities. The hypothalamus links the nervous system to the endocrine system by synthesizing and secreting neurohormones, often called releasing hormones, that control the secretion of hormones from the pituitary gland. One such neurohormone, Gonadotropin-releasing hormone (GnRH) stimulates the pituitary gland to release Follicle Stimulating Hormone (FSH) and Luteinizing Hormone (LH). When secreted in appropriate amounts, FSH and LH stimulate the ovaries to produce estrogen and progesterone and stimulate ovulation. If this pathway is interrupted, menstrual irregularity ensues, and is often accompanied by other health consequences, such as osteoporosis.

Although the female athlete is most often confronted with the effects of overexertion on menstrual function, a greater number of women are affected by sedentary lifestyles and obesity. Given the rising prevalence of overweight and obese women in the United States,[5] menstrual dysfunction related to obesity and inactivity contributes much more to infertility than does being underweight and overactive. However, this chapter, will focus primarily on the female athlete and the effects of exercise on infertility. The main effect of exercise on the menstrual cycle is to either cause menses to become decreased in frequency (oligomenorrhea) or to stop completely (amenorrhea). The Female Athlete Triad of disordered eating, amenorrhea, and osteoporosis is well studied and becoming increasingly important to identify. This chapter will review the effect of the Female Athlete Triad (primarily amenorrhea) on normal menstrual function and fertility.

Amenorrhea

The pervasiveness of amenorrhea has perhaps been underestimated because of a lack of attention to anovulatory cycles or menstrual cycles in which ovulation is absent. Patients fulfilling any one of the following criteria should be evaluated for amenorrhea:

- no period by age 14 in the absence of growth or development of secondary sexual characteristics (breast growth, pubic hair growth, and the growth spurt)

- no period by age 16 regardless of the presence of normal growth and development with the appearance of secondary sexual characteristics
- the absence of periods for six months or more in a woman who has been menstruating

As many as two-thirds of recreational runners who have menstrual periods have either short luteal phases (fewer number of days between periods) or are completely anovulatory.[14] Even recreational runners with normal menstrual periods demonstrate great variability in cycle length from month to month, often with reduced hormonal function.[3] When physical training starts before menarche (a woman's first menstrual cycle), menarche can be delayed by as many as three years, and the subsequent incidence of lifetime menstrual irregularity is higher. When training begins after menarche, women can develop secondary amenorrhea (absence of periods for six months or more after the onset of menses). Therefore, anovulation is the primary means by which exercise influences fertility, a fact that is well supported in the medical literature.

A Penn State University study compared two groups of volunteers, 185 female varsity or club team athletes and 132 women who did not play team sports. About 30% of the athletes reported menstrual cycles shorter (less than 26 days) or longer (more than 32 days) than the normal range. Only 19% of the non-athletes reported abnormal cycle lengths.[6]

The interplay between physical activity and menstrual dysfunction is complex for several reasons. First, a number of factors, such as body weight and composition, energy balance, exercise behaviors, and physical and emotional stress levels contribute to the development of athletic menstrual dysfunction and infertility. Secondly, a high degree of variation exists in the extent to which these and other factors affect individual women.

Mechanisms of Athletic Menstrual Dysfunction and Fertility

While exercise and genetics can lead to conditions like amenorrhea, which can be both pathological and non-pathological in nature, there are other conditions that are more physiologically stressful. All of which are associated with menstrual disturbances. There are a range of variables that will affect the fertility of the female athlete. Some of them are genetic and some relate to environmental conditions and factors. These variables include body composition and weight, energy expenditure, climate and seasonal changes, and physical and emotional stress levels.

Body Weight and Composition

Young women who weigh less than 115 pounds and lose more than 10 pounds while exercising are the most likely to develop menstrual and ovulatory problems.[4] The critical weight hypothesis states that the onset and regularity

Health Risk Classification

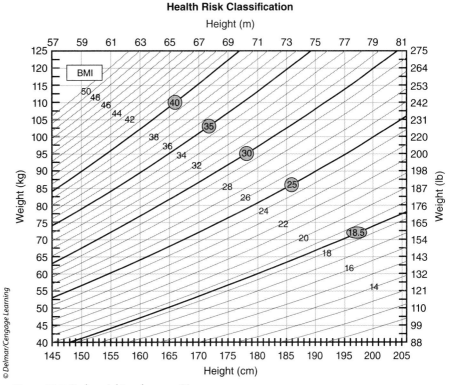

© Delmar/Cengage Learning

Figure 14-1 Body weight and composition.

of menstrual function necessitate maintaining weight above a critical level, and furthermore, above a critical amount of body fat. The 10th percentile at age 16 is approximately 22% body fat. Dropping below this level may result in abnormal menstrual function.[2] Although the chart in Figure 14-1 can help identify patients at risk of low body fat, the more reliable standard for calculating body composition is hydrostatic weighing of body density.

The competitive female athlete has about 50% less body fat than the non-competitor. Increasing the intensity of exercise significantly alters the body composition, but may not affect absolute weight. This is due to an overall increase in lean muscle mass. Therefore, the critical weight hypothesis is not reflective of a cause and effect relationship, (i.e., the decrease in fat does not cause menstrual dysfunction) but rather demonstrates that a correlation exists between body composition and normal menstrual function.

The hormone, leptin, which may also play a role in normal menstrual function, is a protein product of the obesity gene and is secreted by fat cells (adipocytes). Leptin levels fluctuate in response to fat stores and energy availability. For example, obese individuals have elevated leptin levels,[8] whereas athletes and patients with anorexia and delayed puberty have low levels.[12] Athletes with cyclic menses demonstrate a normal diurnal rhythm in leptin levels. However, athletes who do not menstruate do not have this same pattern. All female athletes (including women with normal menses and those with amenorrhea) have three times lower leptin levels, but only the athletes who have regular cycles show an increase in leptin after meals. (That is to say, those with no menses respond much differently than those with normal menses.) Therefore, the signal from the fat cells to the brain is likely through the leptin molecule. Additionally, this molecule is possibly responsible for a multitude of metabolic and developmental functions. Low levels of leptin may serve as a signal that fat stores are not sufficient for growth and reproduction.

Most likely, a critical body mass composition exists that helps to maintain normal reproductive function. Strenuous exercise interrupts normal signals through a variety of pathways (such as the leptin molecule) causing suppression of hypothalamic hormones. The end result is an alteration of normal menstrual cycles.

Energy Expenditure

One of the most important triggers for menstrual dysfunction, appears to be *energy drain* or *negative energy balance*; that is, failing to match energy expenditure with adequate food intake. A negative energy balance is the primary factor affecting hormones from the hypothalamus, specifically, the hormone GnRH. The mechanism is likely through both exercise and caloric restriction, as seen in athletes in aesthetic or lean build sports, gymnasts or figure skaters.[18] These young women report the highest incidences of menstrual dysfunction and frequently use long-term dieting to maintain a competitive weight.

In addition to their effects on body fat, stress and energy expenditure exert independent influences on the menstrual cycles. When available energy is excessively diverted, such as during exercise, or when insufficient, as with eating disorders, reproduction is temporarily suspended to support essential metabolism for survival. Dancers, for example, typically menstruate during intervals of rest, despite no changes in body weight or percentage body fat.[19] Leptin levels are lower in women with high energy output (even lower than expected due to low body fat alone).[1]

Education about energy balance may help healthy, active women avoid disordered eating and exercise patterns as well as prevents episodes of menstrual disturbance in their late teens and twenties when they appear to be more susceptible to such disturbances. Exercise should not be viewed as healthy if it results in a chronic energy debt (Figure 14-2).

Exercise Behaviors, Climate, and Seasonal Effects

Surprisingly, environmental factors and specific exercising behaviors can affect the menstrual cycle and subsequent fertility. Running in the dark as well as exercising during autumn and winter has been shown to affect menstrual function more

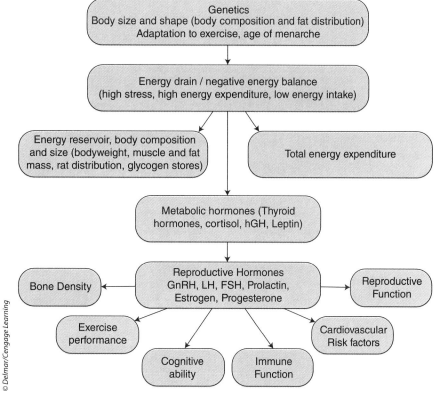

Figure 14-2 Energy balance. (Adapted from, C. M. et.al. The spectrum of eating disturbances. Int i eating disorders; 18: 29, 1995)

by increasing secretion of melatonin from the pineal gland. Melatonin can have a negative effect on the ovary and ovulation.[17] For example, the conception rate of women living in northern Scandinavia is higher during the summer (when there is more daylight) than in the winter.[9] Altering exercise behaviors when they influence normal menstruation is helpful, but sometimes difficult.

Physical and Emotional Stress Levels

Emotional and physical stress are also independent factors affecting menstruation. Many athletes report a "runner's high," or feeling of exhilaration and euphoria, during or after an extensive workout. Some sources have attributed these euphoric feelings to a psychological reaction or possibly an increase in endorphins (sometimes known as natural pain killers) produced by the body. The hypothalamus (where GnRH is produced) is very sensitive to opiates and endorphins. Endurance athletes demonstrate a continuous increase in endorphin output even after exercise,[16] which may partially explain the menstrual suppression associated with exercise. Emotional and physical stress also increases the body's opiod production. Not surprisingly, menstruation is restored in amenorrheic athletes who are given medicine to block opioids. Hence, endorphins and opioids play key roles in exercise-related amenorrhea and infertility.

Identifying the At-Risk Athlete

Early recognition, concentrated counseling, and confidential support are the central concepts in detecting and preventing a progressive problem. This is the ideal time to begin education about possibly future fertility problems and the long term effects of prolonged exercise. The high prevalence of eating disorders among female athletes indicates that the threat of progression should not be underrated. *Partia*, or sub-clinical eating disorders are estimated to occur 2-3 times more frequently than true anorexia nervosa. Without intervention, progression to the full syndrome may occur in as short as 1-2 years.[7] Coaches and teachers who have constant exposure to the teenage athlete must be aware of the importance of the short- and long-term effects of exercise and poor nutrition on the menstrual cycle. When physical activity has reached a level that alters the normal menstrual cycle, other organ systems have undoubtedly been affected as well.

Of the three abnormalities in the Female Athlete Triad, amenorrhea is the first to be evident. The woman with an eating disorder has a distorted body image and she does not consider herself underweight. She is often unaware of how severe her problem is until very late in the disease. The third part of the triad, osteoporosis, is diagnosed most often by special x-ray procedures (dual-energy x-ray absorptiometry or a DEXA scan) usually reserved for women above age 65. In the absence of any fractures, a young athlete is not likely to be tested by her physician. These factors present a challenge in identifying the at-risk athlete but a few simple strategies may aid in improved detection.

A logical method of identifying the "at risk" athlete is to have her document the intervals of her menstrual cycle in a menstrual diary. Any trend of 3-4 months of continuously irregular periods should be evaluated further. Another helpful tool is maintaining a training log to track physical activity and the days of menstruation. This allows an athlete to review her menstrual cycles in relation to a variety of influences over long time periods. The training log may also serve as excellent tool to also document caloric intake.

There are many samples on the internet, such as at *http://www.fitnessjournal. org,* but any formal system which tracks diet, menses, activity duration and intensity can be effective (Figure 14-3). Most coaches today should provide sample logs (which can be created using any simple computer worksheet) for every team member and reviewing them on a monthly basis. This provides an

DATE	MENSES (+/-; HEAVY/ LIGHT)	ACTIVITY (NUMBER OF MILES, MINUTES OF EXERCISE)	TOTAL CALORIES	SPECIFIC FOODS EATEN
3/15/2006	None	45 minutes run, 30 minutes weight	1300 cal	B: toast L; yogurt D: Pasta + sauce Snack: Fries
3/16/2006	Light sporting	90 minutes run	1500 cal	B: protein shake L: Turkey sandwhich D: Salad Snack: candy bars
3/17/2006	None	45 minutes walking	1200 cal	B: None L: Salad D: Sandwhich Snack: Yogurt

© Delmar/Cengage Learning

Figure 14-3 Sample training, diet, and menstruation log.

easy and objective method for helping determine if there is a problem with amenorrhea and opting for early intervention.

The diagnosis of exercise-associated amenorrhea remains a diagnosis of exclusion. Any young woman who demonstrates complete absence of menstruation or greater than 3-4 months between periods should be referred to a gynecologist or family physician. Serious problems with the uterus or pituitary gland must be ruled out first. On occasion, ovarian tumors (both benign and malignant) can lead to menstrual abnormalities. After a careful history and thorough physical examination, the physician will need to evaluate hormone levels in the blood to help determine the cause of the menstrual dysfunction. A pelvic ultrasound, and CAT (CT) scan or MRI of the head (to evaluate the pituitary gland) may also be warranted.

Once other more serious causes have been ruled out, the physician will likely want to review the athlete's menstrual calendar and training log as well as evaluate her daily dietary intake. Obtaining a bone mineral density test may also be prudent. This is a painless test that can be completed at most hospitals and many physicians' offices. The bone density will give the clinician a good idea of the chance of a fracture due to a lack of estrogen (if that is the problem) and help determine the best course of treatment.

In the patient who wishes to conceive completing the workup in her spouse to rule out male-factor infertility is also important. Further treatment will depend on whether ovulation dysfunction is the only cause of the couple's infertility.

Treatment of Amenorrhea in the Athlete

Treatment of any underlying nutritional deprivation may restore menses and stimulate an increase in bone density. Attention should also be focused on estrogen replacement to help increase bone density. As stated several times throughout this chapter, all other causes of amenorrhea must be ruled out before proceeding with treatment. Specific treatments may vary depending on several factors.

Peak Bone Mass or Maximal Height

Peak bone mineral density is achieved in late adolescence, usually by age 16. Girls with estrogen deficiency do not always achieve optimal peak bone density, and conflicting studies exist on how to treat the young patient who has not achieved maximal height. Some studies caution that giving these young women birth control pills (or any form of estrogen) may prematurely halt their overall growth by affecting the growth plates within the bones.[11] However, this theory has been challenged[13] and other researchers contend that maximal height is not affected by giving estrogen (or birth control pills) to girls who have not achieved their peak bone growth. Regardless of the disparity in these findings, these patients should be referred to a pediatric, medical or reproductive endocrinologist before starting any form of estrogen therapy or birth control pills. Current recommendations are that they also receive all of the appropriate nutritional counseling and supplements, such as calcium and vitamin D.

The Desire for Fertility

Infertility almost always accompanies menstrual irregularities. Therefore, if an athlete is trying to conceive but is not having spontaneous, regular menses, any ovulatory dysfunction must be corrected first. The main problem often lies with the pituitary gland not releasing the necessary hormones to stimulate ovulation. This may be caused by a central defect within the pituitary itself (e.g. a tumor) or by the effects of another medical problem (i.e. an eating disorder or thyroid disease). Unfortunately, amenorrhea may persist despite the correction of underlying disorders or excessive training regimens.

The next most appropriate step is to refer these athletes to a reproductive endocrinologist who has been trained to manage those patients with more complex dysfunction. This is especially important for the patient who is older than 35 because any significant delays in therapy may affect the chance of conception since egg quality begins declining at this age. The treatment of patients with infertility may vary tremendously depending on the specific cause of anovulation. The most commonly prescribed medicine to stimulate ovulation is clomiphene, but it is typically ineffective in women who are amenorrheic because of a hypothalamic problem (such as in the athletes described in this chapter). The most effective treatment for these patients are gonadotropins that contain both FSH and LH, the hormones normally required for ovulation to occur. Usually, only low doses are required for adequate response. Patients must be monitored carefully to prevent over stimulation of the ovaries that may result in multiple gestation or even life threatening illness.

For the athlete who does not desire fertility and has achieved maximal adult height, the standard treatment is a combination of estrogen and progesterone therapy. Several options are available:

- Birth control pills taken daily. This is a good option because they contain a sufficient amount of estrogen to initiate bone growth and prevent further bone loss and enough progesterone to prevent ovulation. The pill is convenient and may even be taken on a continuous basis if the athlete wants to avoid menstrual bleeding. (By skipping the seven placebo pills and only taking the active pills.) If the athlete has not achieved maximal growth, a lower dose pill (containing less estrogen) should be given, and bone density should be monitored more closely.

- Estrogen pills taken daily and progesterone pills taken for 2 weeks out of the month. In some individuals, the estrogen dosage may have to be increased in order to achieve menstrual bleeding.

- Estrogen and progesterone pills each taken daily. This therapy produces effects similar to the birth control pill.

Correcting the Negative Energy Balance

Improving an athlete's overall energy balance may reverse diet-induced menstrual problems.[5] An effective strategy is to increase energy intake (ideally by small increments of 200 Kcalories-300 Kcalories a day) while simultaneously reducing exercise energy expenditure, for example, by adding a rest day to the weekly routine.

Increasing energy intake in an athlete can be quite challenging. Ingesting adequate macro- and micro-nutrients to maintain good health and have the energy to fuel an intense training program on anything less than an 1800 calorie diet is almost impossible. Most female athletes require at least 2,300 Kcalories-2,500 Kcalories a day to maintain body weight, and those involved in endurance sports like marathon-running or triathlons may need as many as 4,000 Kcalories a day.

Female athletes are more likely to ingest low levels of protein (especially vegetarians), carbohydrates, essential fatty acids, pyridoxine, riboflavin, folate, calcium, magnesium, iron and zinc, and may need supplements to achieve an adequate intake. Dietary balance is especially concerning in those with menstrual irregularities because they are more susceptible to bone loss. These women need to be carefully monitored for appropriate intake of bone-building nutrients, and supplementation started if necessary, particularly if dairy products are not used on a regular basis.

Female athletes seeking to avoid the menstrual dysfunction that accompanies negative energy balance have a range of helpful strategies, which include the following:[16]

- Concentrate less on body weight and more on healthy nutritional habits such as making good food choices and eating regular meals and snacks.

- Don't constantly deprive yourself of favorite foods or set unrealistic dietary rules – remember that moderate amounts of foods can fit into a healthy lifestyle.

- Don't skip meals or let yourself get too hungry, which may lead to increased or overconsumption at subsequent meals.

- Consume fluids, especially water, throughout the day – dehydration is an unhealthy, transient means of reaching your goal weight.

- Always eat a nutritious breakfast – it will stop you overeating at lunch.

- Use a multivitamin and mineral supplement in preference to single nutrient supplements unless otherwise recommended by a health professional.

Adequate Counseling

Although addressing all of the psychological needs of the patient with a menstrual or eating disorder is beyond the scope of this chapter, it is a crucial component of the patient's management. Using a team of medical professionals including a physician, nutritionist, athletic trainer, and psychological counselor is essential to effective therapy. Athletes who experience irregular menstrual periods often have poor body images of themselves and more excessive training schedules than non-athletes. Psychological stress may exacerbate the effects of inadequate nutrition and excessive exercise. For some patients, antidepressant medications may be helpful adjuncts to counseling.

Counseling should also be initiated early in the recognition process with the amenorrheic athlete who desires fertility. The patient should be instructed to alter any excessive exercise regimens. If she is reluctant or unwilling to change her behavior, further treatment should be withheld until she has undergone appropriate psychotherapy to better prepare her for the stress associated with fertility treatment.

Infertility and Obesity

Although the athlete more commonly faces the problems of being underweight and overactive, the rising prevalence obesity among U.S. women may contribute more to infertility and being underweight.[10] Abnormal weight is often defined in terms of body mass index (BMI). A BMI greater than 25 kg/m² (appropriate for someone 5'4" and 150 pounds) is associated with ovulation problems. Some evidence suggests that being even moderately overweight increases the risk of ovulation problems that result in infertility.

Some medical conditions result in patients being overweight and amenorrheic. Patients with irregular or absent menses in combination with increased facial hair or obesity usually have polycystic ovary syndrome (PCOS). These patients have increased insulin resistance and increased testosterone. They release excess insulin when they consume any type of carbohydrate such as pasta or rice. The insulin then causes the ovary to produce more testosterone which can cause increased facial hair, acne, and irregular periods. (PCOS do not usually cause problems.) Although some of these patients have a normal BMI, weight loss can often cure the related infertility in a patient who is overweight. A weight loss of as little as 5% of the total body weight may improve ovulation almost as much as taking fertility medications.[20]

Infertility associated with being overweight and under active is far more common than that of overactivity. Treating the overweight infertile patient with increased activity and weight loss seems to be very effective in improving hormone levels, restoring regular menses, and sometimes correcting infertility.

Summary

Women are increasingly becoming active participants in competitive and recreational physical activity. Concern has arisen regarding the effect of physical training on the physiology of the menstrual cycle. As more women participate and training programs become more strenuous, physicians have seen more complaints of menstrual cycle disturbances.

Patient presenting with irregular or absent periods should be evaluated by their physician as they are at risk for osteoporosis and infertility. The nature and severity of the symptoms seen are dependent on a number of variables, such as the specific type of training, the intensity and duration of training, weekly mileage, and rate of progression of training program.

References

1. Aleandri V, Spina V, and Morini A. The pineal gland and reproduction. Human Reproduction Update. 1996 May-Jun;2(3):225–235.

2. Considine RV, Sinha MK, and Heiman ML. Serum immunoreactive-leptin concentrations in normal-weight and obese humans. *New England Journal of Medicine.* 1995;334: 292.

3. De Souza MJ, Miller BE, Loucks AB et al. High frequency of luteal phase deficiency and anovulation in recreational women runners: blunted elevation in follicle stimulating hormone observed during luteal follicular transition. *Journal of Clinical Endocrinology & Metabolism.* 1998;83:4220.

4.   Falsetti L, Pasinetti E, Mazzani. Weight loss and menstrual cycle: clinical and endocrinological evaluation. *Gynecological Endocrinology.* 1992;6:49.

5.   Flegal KM, Carroll RJ, and Johnson CL. Overweight and obesity in the United States: prevalence and trends, 1960-1994. *International Journal of Obesity and Related Metabolic Disorders.* 1998;22:39–47.

6.   Frisch RE. Body fat, menarche, and reproductive ability. *Seminars in Reproductive Endocrinology.* 1985;3:45.

7.   Hartard M, Kleinmond C, and Kirchbichler A. Age at first oral contraceptive use as a major determinant of vertebral bone mass in female endurance athletes. *Bone.* 2004 Oct;35(4):836–841.

8.   Holtkamp K, Herpertz-Dahlmann B, Mika C. et al. Elevated physical activity and low leptin levels co-occur in patients with anorexia nervosa. *Journal of Clinical Endocrinology & Metabolism.* 2003;88:5169.

9.   Howlett TA, Tomlin S, and Hgahfoong. Release of beta-endorphin and met enkephalin during exercise in normal eowmn: response to training, *British Medical Journal.* 1984;288:1950.

10.   Kiddy DS, Hamilton-Fairley D, Bush A, and Short F. Improvement in endocrine and ovarian function during dietary treatment of obese women with polycystic ovary syndrome. *Clinical Endocrinology.* 1992;36:105.

11.   Lloyd T, Taylor DR, and Lin HM. Oral contraceptive use by teenage women woes not affect peak bone mass: a longitudinal study. *Fertility and Sterility.* October 2000;74(4).

12.   Loucks AB. Exercise training in the normal female. In: Warren MP, and Constantini NW, Torowa (Eds.). *Sports Endocrinology.* NJ: Humana Press, Inc; 2000:165–180.

13.   Manore M. Dietary Recommendations and Atheletic Menstrual Dysfunction. *Sports Medicine.* 2002;32(14):887–890.

14.   Prior JC. Luteal phase defects and anovulation: adaptive alterations occurring with conditioning exercise. *Seminars in Reproductive Endocrinology.* 1985;3:27.

15.   Ronkainen H, Pakarinen A, and Kirkinen P. Physical exercise induced changes and season-associated differences in the pituitary-ovarian function of runners and joggers. *Journal of Clinical Endocrinology & Metabolism.* 1985;60:416.

16.   Shisslak CM, Crago M, and Estes LS. The spectrum of eating disturbances. *International Journal of Eating Disorders.* 1995;18:209.

17. Temkin O Soranus' Gynecology. Book III. I. *On the Retention of the Menstrual Flux and on Difficult and Painful Menstruation.* Baltimore: Johns Hopkins University Press; 1959:132–143.

18. Warren MP. Effect of exercise and physical training on menarche. *Seminars in Reproductive Endocrinology.* 1985;3:17.

19. Warren MP, Voussoughian F, Geer EB et al. Functional hypothalamic amenorrhea: hypoleptinemia and disordered eating. *Journal of Clinical Endocrinology & Metabolism.* 1999;84:873.

CHAPTER 15

Core Stabilization for the Female Athlete

Barb Hoogenboom, EdD, SCS, ATC and

Jolene Bennett, MA, PT, OCS, ATC

Introduction

Women and girls of all ages and abilities are participating in sports in record high numbers. In fact, 43% of high school athletes,[1] 43% of collegiate athletes[2] and approximately 40% of Olympic athletes[3] were female in 2004–2005.

The common prerequisite for participation and success in all types of sports is a strong and stable core of the human body, known as core stabilization. For the purpose of this chapter core stabilization will be defined as the muscular balance and control required about the pelvis, hips, and trunk (lumbar, thoracic and cervical spines) to maintain functional stability of the entire human body. Control of the segments of the spine during upright posture is required not only for activities of daily living, but also for balance, stability, and coordination during high level sports activity.[14] This stability enables athletes to transmit forces from the earth through the kinetic chain of the body and ultimately propel the body or an object using the limbs. The concept of core stabilization of the trunk and pelvis as a prerequisite for movements of the extremities was described biomechanically in 1991.[6] Subsequently, core training for stabilization has become a major trend both in treatment of injuries, as well as in training regimes used to enhance athletic performance and prevent injury.

This chapter will describe relevant anatomy, potential injuries to the core, mechanisms of injury, rehabilitation techniques, and application of concepts of prevention and wellness for the female athlete. The rehabilitation professional, as an important member of the sports medicine team, has valuable knowledge for rehabilitation and prevention of athletic injuries in the female athlete. Application of and sharing of knowledge related to core stabilization and "the butt and gut" will benefit female athletes in all sports at all levels by improving performance, increasing athleticism, and decreasing the potential for injury to the spine and extremities.

Overview of Core Stabilization

Many terms and rehabilitation programs are associated with the concept of core stability, including: lumbar stabilization, dynamic stabilization, motor control (neuromuscular) training, neutral spine control, muscular fusion, and trunk stabilization.[4] The authors use the term "butt and gut" to teach students, colleagues, and patients the concept of core stability in therapeutic exercise and prevention and wellness contexts. The core has been conceptually described as either a box or a cylinder,[43] because of its anatomical and structural composition. The abdominals create the anterior and lateral walls, the paraspinals and gluteals form the posterior wall, while the diaphragm and pelvic floor create the top and bottom of the cylinder, respectively (Figure 15-1).

Additionally, hip girdle musculature reinforces and supports the bottom of the cylinder. Envisioning this cylindrical system helps to understand its function as that of a dynamic muscular support system, described by some

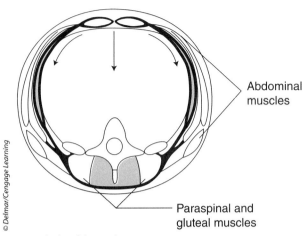

© Delmar/Cengage Learning

Figure 15-1 Anatomic cylinder of the trunk.

authors as the powerhouse, engine, or a "muscular corset that works as a unit to stabilize the body and spine, with and without limb movement."[4]

Static stabilization of the core is a prerequisite, but is not sufficient for athletic performance. Core stability must be further understood as the ability to stabilize the core musculature during *dynamic* movement tasks of the core and extremities.

Proximal stability for distal mobility is a commonly understood principle of human movement originally described by Knott and Voss and applied in the concepts associated with proprioceptive neuromuscular facilitation.[34] Nowhere is the concept of dynamic proximal stability more important than in sport. Without proximal control of the core, athletes could not use the lower extremities LEs to propel the body in running and jumping or use the upper extremities UEs to support or propel the body (in activities, such as gymnastics and swimming), manipulate, use and throw objects (such as throwing a shot put or using a tennis racquet). The core is in the middle of the human kinetic chain and serves a link between the UEs and LEs. This allows for transfer of energy from the LEs to the UEs and vice versa. According to Kibler:[33]

> "injuries or adaptations in some areas of the kinetic chain can cause problems not only locally but distally, as other distal links have to compensate for the lack of force or energy delivered through the more proximal links. This phenomenon, called *catch-up*, is both inefficient in the kinetic chain and dangerous to the distal link because it may create more load of stress than the link can safely handle."

Strength and coordination of the core musculature is vital to performance and generation of power in many sports. When the core is functioning optimally, muscles elsewhere in the kinetic chain also function optimally atllowing the athlete to produce strong, functional movements of the extremities.[33,5] (See Table 15-1).

TABLE 15-1   •   Core Demands, Kinetic chain relationships, and Outcomes of Example Sporting Activities

SPORTING ACTIVITY	CORE DEMANDS	KINETIC CHAIN RELATIONSHIPS	OUTCOME
Windmill softball pitch	Rotational and flexion/extension stability, acceleration and deceleration of trunk	Transmission of forces from ground to LEs through trunk to UEs to ball	Velocity, location, rotation of pitched ball (55-70 mph). Delivery of various types of pitches (drop, rise, breaking ball, etc.)
Gymnastics: vault event	Rotational and flexion/extension stability. Power with punch from horse	Transmission of forces from horse to UEs through trunk to propel body in airborne positions	Conversion of horizontal energy to vertical; speed, position, and trajectory of body through space
Tennis serve	Rotational and flexion/extension stability, acceleration and deceleration of trunk	Transmission of forces from ground to LEs through trunk to UEs through racquet to ball	Velocity, location, spin of served ball (80-120 mph). Delivery of various types of serves
Swimming: butterfly stroke	Flexion/extension stability	Transmission of forces from UEs to trunk to LEs to team with butterfly kick	Efficient propulsion of body through water, avoid excess trunk flexion and extension
Volleyball serve	Rotational and flexion/extension stability, acceleration and deceleration of trunk	Transmission of forces from ground to LEs through trunk to UEs to ball	Velocity, location, rotation of served ball. Various types of spins and serves (names)

Even small alterations in the kinetic chain have serious repercussions throughout other portions of the kinetic chain and thus on skills that are based upon efficient utilization of the entire chain.[33] Therefore, without proper stabilization and dynamic concentric and eccentric control of the trunk during athletic tasks the extremities or "transition zones" between the core and extremities can be overstressed (i.e., hip and rotator cuff).

A wide variety of movements are associated with sport performance, therefore, athletes must possess sufficient strength and dynamic motor control of the core in all three planes of movement (transverse, frontal, saggital).[35] Core stability, vital to athletic performance, is especially important for the female athlete. In a study of male and female runners, females were found to have greater hip adduction, hip internal rotation, and tibial external rotation movements during the stance phase of running. Ferber et al. believe that gender differences in lower extremity kinematics place greater demands on the core musculature of female athletes.[15]

Additionally, core stability may be more vital for the female athlete due to her overall decreased total extremity strength as compared to her age-matched male participant. (UEs 40%–75%, LEs 60%–80%).[5] Documented differences in proximal strength measures in female athletes suggest that females may have a less stable base upon which torque and force can be generated or resisted. This lack of core stability is a possible contributor to lower extremity injury.[20,29] Although important energy has been devoted to prevention of anterior cruciate ligament and other knee injuries in the female athlete, rehabilitation professionals must broaden their focus to the body as a whole and include core strengthening activities as a part of preparatory training for all female athletes.

Anatomy

Stability of the core requires both passive (offered by bony and ligamentous structures) and dynamic stiffness offered by coordinated muscular contractions. A spine without the contributions of the muscular system is unable to bear essential compressive loads associated with normal upright activities and remain stable.[36] Anatomists have known for decades that a compressive load of as little as 2 kg causes buckling of the lumbar spine in the absence of muscular contractions.[39] Likewise, significant microtrauma of the lumbar spine can occur with as little as 2° of rotation, demonstrating the vital stabilizing function of the muscles of the lumbar spine.[18,17] Core stabilization is important not only for protection of the lumbar spine, but also to resist the reactive forces, produced by moving limbs, that are transmitted to the spine and other muscles of the core.

Local and Global Muscles

Richardson, Jull, Hodges and Hides[7] have described classifications of local and global muscles, which together contribute to stability of the core (Table 15-2).

The local or intersegmental muscles are hypothesized to function primarily as stabilizers and the global or multisegmental muscles are hypothesized to function primarily as producers of movement.[31] Panjabi et al.[41] suggested that global muscles may play an important role in stabilization due to their ability to efficiently produce stiffness in the entire spinal column, as compared to local muscles acting on only a few levels. The global muscle system, although important for movement and total spinal stability, appears to be most limited in its' ability to control segmental shear forces.[43]

Consider the possibility that even if the global muscle system is performing adequately, the local system could be working insufficiently to control segmental motion. In fact, excessive use of global muscles in co-contraction during light functional tasks may indicate inappropriate trunk muscle control in patients with low back pain.[41] Global muscles that link the trunk to the extremities (e.g. the psoas in the lower extremity and the latissimus dorsi in the upper extremity) may actually challenge segmental core stabilization.[43] Spinal segment stability must be maintained in the presence of contractions of powerful global muscles during functional activities.[43] Certainly, local and global muscles both contribute

TABLE 15-2 · **Local and Global Muscles of the Core**

LOCAL MUSCLES (POSTURAL, TONIC, SEGMENTAL STABILIZERS)	GLOBAL MUSCLES (DYNAMIC, PHASIC, TORQUE PRODUCING)
Intertransversarii and interspinales (function primarily as proprioceptive organs) • **Multifidi** • **Transversus abdominis** • **Quadratus lumborum** • **Diaphragm** • **Internal oblique (posterior fibers)** • **Iliocostalis and longissimus (lumbar portions)** • **Psoas major (when working on the spine, not as a hip flexor)** • **Hip rotators** (disagreement exists about whether these are local or global)	• **Rectus abdominis** • **External oblique** • **Internal oblique (anterior fibers)** • **Longissimus (thoracic portion)** • **Iliocostalis (thoracic portion)** • **Latissimus dorsi** • **Hip rotators** (disagreement exists about whether these are local or global) • **Hip abductors** • **Hip adductors** • **Hip extensors** • **Quadriceps** • **Hamstrings**

Source: Bergmark A. Stability of the lumbar spine. A study in mechanical engineering. *Acta Orthopedica Scandinavica.* 1989;60:3-52 and Richardson C, Jull G, Hodges P, and Hides, J Therapeutic exercise for spinal segmental stabilization in low back pain: scientific basis and clinical approach. Edinburgh, NY: Churchill Livingstone; 1999.

to postural segmental control and general multisegmental stabilization during static and dynamic tasks.[4,43]

However, debate continues over which muscles are important stabilizers and how to best train the neuromuscular control system to provide sufficient stability to the core.[31] Cholewicki and McGill[7] and Cholewicki and VanVliet[9] reported on the basis of biomechanical analyses that no single local or global muscle owns a dominant responsibility for lumbar spine stability. Stability and movement likely depend on appropriate length and excursion, facilitated co-contractions, and coordinated muscular activity (both concentric and eccentric) in *all* muscles of the core. The emergent view by many prominent authors is that continual, low level, local muscle contractions, neuromuscular coordination, and control are requisite for all functional activities.[43]

The Abdominals

Although as a society we are fixated upon the rectus abdominis and its classic "6-pack" appearance, understanding of the importance of the local muscles diminishes its functional importance. The rectus abdominis, a global muscle, is a trunk flexor with a large movement capacity in the trunk that often substitutes for contractions of the important local muscles. Many fitness programs incorrectly overemphasize the training of the rectus abdominis[4] and inappropriately induce shear forces by the flexion moments produced by its contraction. The shear forces induced by the contraction of the rectus femoris are counterproductive to the goal of segmental and total core stabilization which is the real goal of core strengthening. Further discussion of Exercises and proper strategies for core strengthening are discussed further in section ""of this chapter.

Contemporary research has illuminated the roles of two important local muscle groups, the transversus abdominis (TA)[12,25] and the multifidus.[50,23] The TA, the deepest of the abdominal muscles, uses its horizontal fiber alignment and attachment to the thoracolumbar fascia to increase intraabdominal pressure (IAP) thereby making the core cylinder as a whole, more stable. Although increased IAP had been associated with the control of spinal flexion forces and a decrease in load on the extensor muscles,[49] it is probable that the TA is most important in its ability to assist in intersegmental control[7] by offering "hoop-like" cylindrical stresses to enhance stiffness and limit both translational and rotational movement of the spine.[4,37] Bilateral contraction of the TA performs the movement of "drawing in of the abdominal wall,"[43] and does not produce spinal movement. The TA is active throughout the movements of both trunk flexion and extension, suggesting a unique stabilizing role during dynamic movement, different from the other abdominal muscles.[10,11]

Also, electromyographic evidence suggests that the more internal muscles of the trunk (transversus abdominis and internal obliques) behave in an anticipatory or feed-forward manner to provide proactive control of spinal stability during movements of the upper extremities,[26,28] regardless of the direction of limb movements.[26]

Spinal Muscles

Among the posterior spinal muscles, the multifidus is important for its contribution to control of the neutral or stable position of the spine.[42,50] Due to its unique anatomical structure and segmental innervation, the multifidus is important for segmental stiffness and motion control. The tonically active multifidus is reported to offer two thirds of the increase in segmental stiffness at the L4-L5 segment when contracted.[50] Dysfunction of the multifidus that occurs after injury to the spine[23] makes this group an important focus for rehabilitation. Clinical and preliminary experimental evidence suggests a biomechanically beneficial co-contraction of the TA and multifidi that occurs during specific exercises (see Figure 15-2).[43]

This specific and specialized relationship provides increased stiffness within spinal structures, offering critical tonic cylindrical stabilization for the core, and is the basis for rehabilitation.

Internal Musculature

The importance of the top and bottom of the core of the human body, the diaphragm and the pelvic floor respectively, must not be underestimated. The diaphragm, like the TA, functions in anticipatory postural control by firing

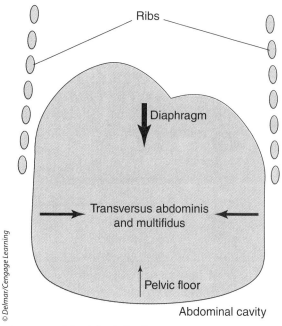

Figure 15-2 Muscular support of the abdominal cavity.

prior to extremity musculature during the movement of shoulder flexion.[27] Also, contraction of the diaphragm occurs concurrently with activation of the TA, independent of phase of respiration.[27] Although beyond the scope of this chapter discussion, diaphragmatic breathing techniques may be an important component of a core strengthening program.[4] The pelvic floor has been shown to be active during lifting tasks and to be instrumental in increased activation of the TA when voluntarily contracted.[43] Conversely, electromyography activity of the pubococcygeus increased during activation of the abdominal muscles.[43] Thus, the bottom of the cylinder, the pelvic floor, cannot be ignored during core strengthening.

Reviewing and considering the anatomy of the core allows the rehabilitation professional to best understand principles of injury and rehabilitation which will be presented next. It also sets the stage for attempting to persuade athletes, coaches, and other professionals to decrease the preoccupation with the training of the rectus abdominis and other "high profile" global muscles of the core which may in fact diminish effective sport performance and rehabilitation.

Mechanisms of Injury to the Core

Many potential mechanisms of injury exist for the athlete. Injury to the trunk, abdomen and low back is not gender specific, and male and female athletes are injured in similar mechanisms. Cholewicki et al.[8] suggested that a common factor for injury to athletes may be the inability to generate sufficient core stability to resist external forces imposed upon the body during high speed events. Other authors suggest a deficient endurance of the trunk stabilizing musculature that predisposes the athlete to traumatic forces over time,[43] motor control deficits and imbalances of the local muscles (TA and multifidus) and the global musculature (rectus abdominus and erector spinae) that occur during performance of functional activities. A weak core could result in inefficient movements, altered postures, and an increased potential for both macro- and micro-traumatic injury.[5]

Mechanisms of Injury to the Core

Like the extremities, the core may be injured in macrotramatic mechanisms such as contusions, muscle strains, muscle tears, and during other injuries such as fractures and dislocations. Subsequent to macrotramatic injuries development of laxity in spinal joints and ligaments could occur, which would contribute to segmental instability. The core can also be injured over time by repetitive microtrauma during activity due to poor posture, repetitive excessive movements (especially hyperextension, rotation), improper muscle activation patterns, and strength imbalances. Segmental instability of the lumbar spine has been implicated as a possible cause of functional limitations, strains and pain. Increased or excessive motion of segments results in the loss of sensory motor contributions to stability and the ability to maintain a neutral or supported position.

Olympic beach volleyball player Misty May suffered an abdominal muscle injury (macrotrauma) early in 2004 that decreased her ability to compete in the spring AVP volleyball season as well as to train for the 2005 Athens Olympics. She did however make an excellent recovery and was able to return to high level performance in her sport and together with her partner, earn a gold medal for the United States. Because the core musculature is so vital to sports performance, strains and contusions to the trunk, although not frequent, have the potential to produce muscular dysfunction, pain and imbalance over time in a wide variety of sports. Likewise muscular injuries have the potential to decrease the efficiency and accuracy of UE and LE movements during sport performance in activities such as the softball pitch or golf swing.

Microtraumatic Injuries

Spondylolysis and spondylolisthesis are two examples of microtraumatic injuries that occur in the female athlete are. The athletic population is more prone to these conditions and is more likely to be symptomatic from these injuries. Spondylolytic microfracture of the pars is believed to happen due to shear forces occurring during repetitive flexion and extension.[15] Athletes with high rates of this type of microtraumatic injury include: gymnasts,[21] divers, figure skaters, swimmers who perform the butterfly stroke,[15] and volleyball players,[21] due to the extreme extension/flexion reversals in trunk posture demanded by these sports. In fact, gymnasts younger than age 24 have a four times greater incidence of spondylolysis than the general female population.[15] Microtraumatic injuries may occur due to muscular imbalances, uncontrolled shear forces acting on the spine[15,21] or because of lack of muscular control and stabilization offered by the core stabilizers. Sports such as golf, diving, and softball provide potential for microtraumatic injury to the core induced similarly, but related to extremes of rotation, often in combination with extension. Careful assessment of motor strategies and subsequent corrective movement retraining by the rehabilitation professional may be a key to prevention of many microtraumatic injuries.

In a study by Leetun et al., the researchers found that male athletes had statistically greater core stability scores on tests of hip abduction, hip external rotation, and the side bridge when compared to female athletes.[35] Figure 15-3 illustrates how the side plank or side bridge exercise should be done, unless the athlete cannot hold herself sufficiently. If that is the case, the exercise can be modified by bending the knees and shortening the lever of resistance. It is imperative that the athlete maintain a straight body and not elevate or drop the hip.

Athletes who experienced injury to the core (spine/hip/thigh), knee or ankle and foot during an athletic season demonstrated lower core stability measures than those who did not.[35] Once again, this leads the sports physical therapist

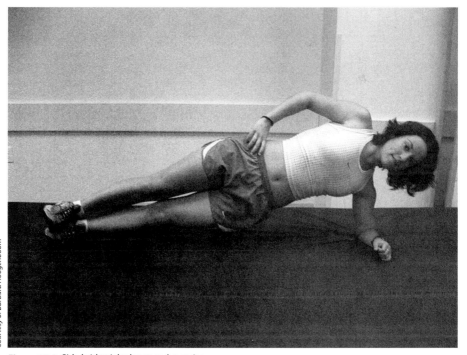

Courtesy of Barbara Hoogenboom

Figure 15-3 Side bridge/plank test and exercise.

to consider core strength, endurance and motor performance training as a possible intervention for prevention of injury, especially for the female athlete.

The Role of the Multifidus

Ultrasound findings from patients with acute LBP indicate that rapid multifidus atrophy, as measured by cross sectional area, occurred on the same side as the low back pain, even as quickly as within 24 hours post injury.[23] This effect is likely due to muscular inhibition. Also, it has been shown that after a first episode of acute low back pain, recovery of multifidus strength and cross sectional area does not occur without specific intervention.[24] In a study of male high performance rowing athletes, multifidus muscle dysfunction was present *despite* their rigorous training. In this same study, the fatigue rates of the multifidus were used to successfully discriminate between controls and subjects with low back pain.[44] Fortunately, regular training with specific, localized muscular contractions of the core, can facilitate recovery of the multifidus muscle.[44] Understanding the support function of the local muscles is relevant to treatment of a wide variety of conditions including generalized low back pain, disc dysfunction, facet irritation and dysfunctions, sacroiliac dysfunction, incontinence, and respiratory disorders.[43]

Further information about this concept will follow in the upcoming section on evaluation and rehabilitation.

Rehabilitation and Treating the Core

There are various tests that can be used to assess and evaluate core stability. After the evaluation of the core strength is assessed, training techniques can be implemented to improve and maintain stability of the core.

Evaluation

The functions of the deep, local muscles of the core are best objectively examined using fine wire electromyography[17,50,46] or real time ultrasound and MRI.[43] Recent evidence suggests that technologically advanced testing and training techniques using real time ultrasound may be useful for both examination and patient education.[22,48,16] Real time ultrasound has been used extensively in research settings and is a reliable tool for evaluating the activation patterns of various abdominal and spinal muscles.[22,48,16] Although real time ultrasound is not currently readily available in clinical settings, perhaps clinical practice of the future will allow for increased use of this tool for both examination and exercise training.

Objective Clinical Tests

Simple, reliable and objective clinical test procedures for dynamic motor control of the core are not readily available. Clinically, therapists utilize manual muscle tests that examine isometric holding of muscles (i.e., Kendall tests for upper and lower abdominals), some positional holding tests (the plank or side plank) for endurance in isometric positions, and pressure biofeedback to asses the ability of a patient to hold the core stable during some dynamic tasks. A clinical test for the multifidus was devised that involves the activation of the multifidus at various segments under the palpating fingers of a therapist.[43] This activation test is performed in the prone position using the command "gently swell out your muscles under my fingers without using your spine or pelvis. Hold the contraction while breathing normally."[43] This test includes both side-to-side and multiple level comparisons to assess for segmental activation or inhibition of the lumbar multifidi (Figure 15-4).

An inability to properly activate the segmental multifidus is indicated by palpating little or no muscle tension developing under the fingers after the verbal command. A rapid and superficial (non-sustained) development of tension is also unsatisfactory.

Richardson et al. adopted the *abdominal drawing in* motor skill as the test of function of the deep abdominal muscles, and subsequently developed the air filled pressure biofeedback unit to attempt to quantify this task. This clinical test of deep muscle co-contraction is performed in prone, by performing the drawing in task while concurrently using the pressure biofeedback device.[43] The authors are unaware of any reliability studies related to the use of the

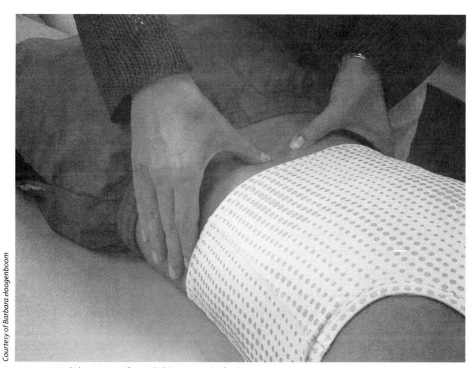

Courtesy of Barbara Hoogenboom

Figure 15-4 Palpation test for multifidus muscular facilitation.

pressure biofeedback device and future reliability studies would enhance of the use of this device. Figure 15-5 demonstrates the use of an air filled pressure biofeedback device. The device is centered with distal edge of the pad in line with the ASISs and inflated to 70 mmHg. The motor contraction test should attempt to draw the abdomen off the pad and be held for 10 seconds. Note the pressure change. A successful test reduces the pressure by 6-10 mmHg. A drop of less than 2 mmHg, no change in pressure, or an increase in pressure are considered poor results.

In addition to the basic performance of this task, the physical therapist must also monitor the task for the ability to hold a tonic, smooth contraction of the TA without resorting to use of the global muscles. The prone position is useful because it minimizes the ability of the patient to use the rectus abdominis for the contraction. In a single-blind study of non-back pain and back pain subjects, it was determined that only ten percent of patients with a history of LBP could perform the transversus abdominis test as compared to 82% of the non-low-back pain patients.[43]

The testing of control of lumbopelvic posture as a measure of core stability is accomplished clinically by performing various leg loading activities in supine, using the pressure biofeedback device (Figure 15-6 and Figure 15-7).

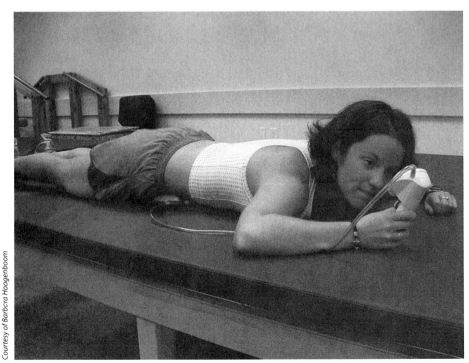

Courtesy of Barbara Hoogenboom

Figure 15-5 Prone use of air filled pressure biofeedback device. (The Stabilizer Pressure Biofeedback™, manufactured by Chattanooga Pacific, Queensland, Australia.)

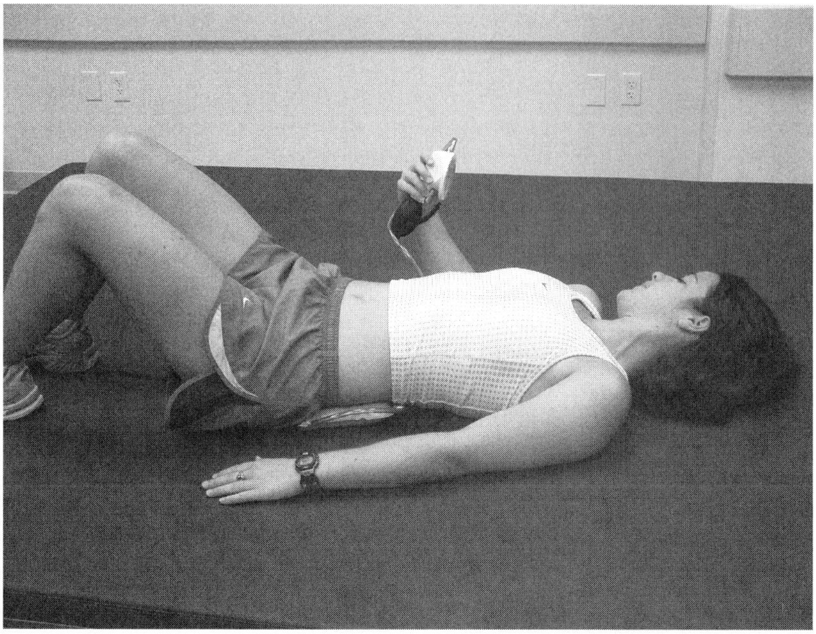

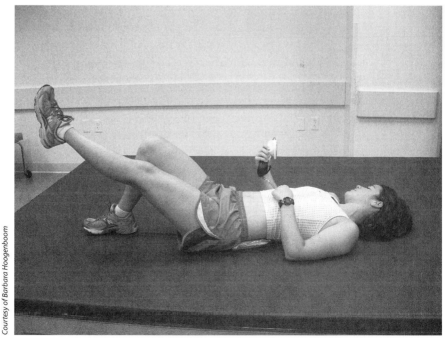

Courtesy of Barbara Hoogenboom

Figure 15-6 Supine biofeedback with varied levels of leg loading. Test is performed by inflating the cuff to approximately 40 mm Hg and positioning the patient in hooklying.

Courtesy of Barbara Hoogenboom

Figure 15-7 Begin with low load tests of short lever leg (bent knee) loading and progress difficulty, using larger load tests (unsupported and extended legs). The patient is asked to precontract the TA with the drawing in maneuver, then hold the pressure reading steady during various maneuvers including the single leg slide with contralateral support, single leg slide without contralateral support, and unsupported leg slide with contralateral support.

The test examines the ability of the core to hold the lumbopelvic region still or steady during various progressive leg loading activities as described by Sahrmann.[45] The pressure biofeedback device provides information to the patient about loss of support or neutral position during functional tasks. Posterior pelvic tilt motion of the pelvis results in an increase in baseline pressure while anterior pelvic tilt results in a decrease in pressure from baseline. Assessment of other tasks in prone and supine, such as movement of the extremities and loading activities, can be performed. Important to remember is that effective contraction of the TA solicits a co-contraction of the multifidus and vice-versa.[43]

Unfortunately, the use of the pressure biofeedback device is limited to activities that involve a surface to offer counterforce in order to read the pressure exerted onto the device. It is not yet clinically possible to evaluate dynamic core stability and measure activity of deep stabilizing musculature in the upright position and clinicians must rely on motor performance taught in other positions to carry over to more demanding positions. Richardson et al. advocate frequent repeat prone formal testing, using the biofeedback device to check efficiency of the local core stabilizers because "assessment in functional tasks by means of observation and palpation only does not give a reliable indication of the improvement in deep muscle capacity."[43]

As previously mentioned, real time ultrasound can be used for examination of the transversus abdominis. Henry and Westervelt[41] explored the use of real time ultrasound for teaching the abdominal "drawing in" or abdominal hollowing maneuver to healthy subjects. They found that this feedback tool decreased the number of trials needed to consistently perform this maneuver. The authors stated that real time ultrasound is a beneficial teaching tool for facilitating consistency of performance of the abdominal hollowing maneuver as compared to verbal and cutaneous feedback, which are the teaching methods used presently by most clinicians. Teyhen et al. demonstrated that real time ultrasound imaging can be used reliably to measure the thickness of the TA in both contracted and non-contracted states.[42] When such technology becomes readily available in clinical settings it should be considered for both the examination and education of patients.

Exercises and Training Techniques

Contemporary thinkers refer to the concept of *neuromuscular retraining* of the core (contributing to segmental stability and stiffness) rather than pure strengthening of muscles supporting the core.[14,4,43] To effectively provide core stabilization, the athlete must use the neuromuscular system to coordinate contractions of many muscles able to influence the position of the pelvis, hips, and spine. In vitro studies demonstrated that local muscles can effectively provide segmental stabilization of the lumbar spine.[50] Thus, recruitment and tonic activity of local musculature are the hallmark of contemporary rehabilitation and training activities, as compared to older programs that focused on contractions of global musculature. Motor control programs for functional performance of skills used by athletes (both healthy and injured) are widely varied, complex, and may involve alterations in both feedback and feed forward mechanisms.[43] Multifidus muscle dysfunction present in highly trained athletes despite their excellently trained condition supports the use of an alternate exercise approach rather than traditional exercise regimens often used for core strengthening with their focus on global musculature.[44] Jemmet[30] has described such an alternate approach as a shift away from treating multifidus dysfunction from a strengthening model to a model based on motor reeducation. This description is in harmony with the treatment philosophy advocated by Richardson et al.[43]

Gender Performance

Gender differences in performance of core stabilizers have been reported in the literature. Female athletes who have injured a lower extremity or the low back demonstrated greater side-to-side differences in hip extension strength symmetery.[40] Likewise, males demonstrated significantly greater endurance in the side bridge (see Figure 15-3: side plank) than females.[38] Thus, both healthy and injured female athletes should be educated in proper core stabilization techniques for prevention injury and decreased likelihood of reinjury.

Phases and Goals of the Program

According to Richardson, Jull, Hodges, and Hides[43] rehabilitation has three distinct phases: formal motor skill training; gradual incorporation into light functional tasks; and progression to heavy-load functional tasks. With the female athlete, the last phase must be modified to include high level sport specific demands in a wide variety of body positions, whether during a prevention or rehabilitation programs. Sport specific training of the butt and gut requires creativity and knowledge of sports demands. Therapeutic exercise in more advanced activities must have two different goals in mind:

- ensuring that the deep local muscles remain functional stabilizers of the lumbopelvic region when higher load exercises are added.

- assessing and treating any dysfunction that is identified in the global musculature during task performance.[7]

Current evidence supports the concept that training efforts should not focus on any single muscle, rather should have components of local and global muscle training.[7,9]

The Drawing in Exercise

The key to assessing and training the local stabilizers is teaching the abdominal drawing in or hollowing exercise, an action specific to the transversus abdominis. Drawing in of the abdominal wall was originally described by Kendall and McCreary[32] and later further described by DeTroyer et al.[13] as "drawing the belly in." The patient must be cued to "narrow your waist" or "pull your belly button away from your waistband" without using the other abdominal muscles or holding her breath. An important feature of teaching this skill is that the athlete understands the corset-like circular function of the TA so she can envision it working to draw in the waist or hollow the abdomen. The difficulty of core exercises must be tailored to the level of achievement of the abdominal drawing in exercise,[5] and progressed from there. She must also understand that this action occurs without producing any movement of the spine. Movement of the spine or pelvis indicates that she is using global muscles to attempt the task, rather than effectively recruiting and using the local TA. The authors often use the four point position to teach this task initially, and then add other positional instruction (i.e., prone, sitting, standing, and half kneeling). See Figure 15-8.

The difficulty of exercises should only be progressed by when the patient has the ability to maintain spinal stability and contraction of the TA while breathing normally.[5] The drawing in maneuver should then be taught in the plank exercise, which helps to develop endurance of the TA and multifudus in a semi functional position (Figure 15-9).

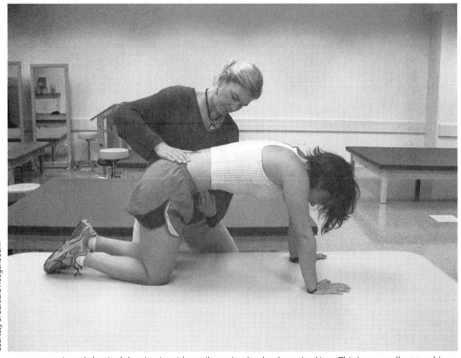

Courtesy of Barbara Hoogenboom

Figure 15-8 4-pt abdominal drawing in with tactile cueing by the therapist. Note: This is an excellent teaching position, but the athlete must progress to more functional positions such as standing and half kneeling (most difficult because it removes the LE contribution to stabilization).

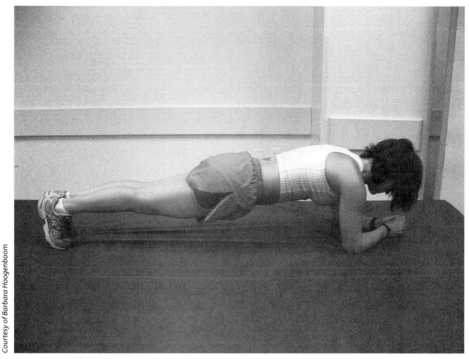

Courtesy of Barbara Hoogenboom

Figure 15-9 Full plank. Note: The position of the trunk. If the patient cannot maintain this position, can be done in a modified position, bearing weight on the knees, much like a modified push up).

Maintaining the drawing in maneuver during perfect lumbopelvic position is critical, as the athlete often has a tendency to be too flexed or too extended in the trunk. The authors use the cue "keep your back flat like a table top" while performing the plank exercise for a timed bout. Athletes with excellent core control and endurance have been known to hold this position for more than 3 minutes. The average athlete goes for bouts of 30-60 seconds and works up in time duration. For athletes who have trouble maintaining the position for 30 seconds, an alternate position with the knees flexed (modified position) may be utilized which decreases core demands by shortening the control lever arm.

Other Dynamic Exercises

Once the drawing in exercise has been mastered during static positions and the plank it must be transferred to dynamic functional tasks. Functional progression of core stabilization activities is the most important part of the program when used either for prevention or rehabilitation. Functional progressions require therapist knowledge of sport demands as well as creativity. Without progression through relevant functional tasks, appropriate motor learning cannot be achieved because carryover from lower functional level tasks cannot be assumed. The most basic functional task requiring tonic deep muscular support is walking. An early dynamic exercise is to teach the athlete to activate the TA and multifidus walking and breathing normally.[43] Difficulty can

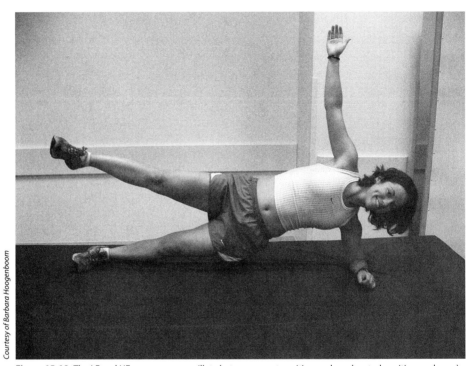

Courtesy of Barbara Hoogenboom

Figure 15-10 The LE and UE can move or oscillate between a rest position and an elevated position as shown).

be added to exercises by changing body positions, using less stable positions (i.e., therapeutic balls, foam rollers, dynadiscs or other unstable surfaces), adding equipment for perturbations, or increasing load during tasks. The plank can be made more difficult and somewhat dynamic in the side plank position by adding UE and LE challenges (Figure 15-10).

Examples of more dynamic exercises include the pike-up (Figure 15-11). The pike up exercise and the knee-up (same maneuver as pike up, but with knees flexed instead of extended) which are highly functional for gymnasts and divers. The authors also use many other types of equipment such as the Body Blade™ and the Sport Cord™ to add resistance to typical athletic maneuvers (Figure 15-12). The rehabilitation therapist may be limited only by their own creativity in designing advanced, functional core stabilization exercise. Table 15-3 shows exercise progression for core stabilization.

The practice of isolated training of a specific group of muscles to reduce compressive loads on the spine must be examined.[31] Strength training of the lumbar extensors has traditionally been a part of low back rehabilitation. The lumbar extensors are considered global muscles. They serve as prime movers into trunk extension and may need to be addressed in strengthening exercise programs for athletes following injury to the low back. Many exercises directed at strengthening the lumbar extensors as a group, however, fail to place the pelvis in a stable, neutral position and prevent substitution of the gluteals.

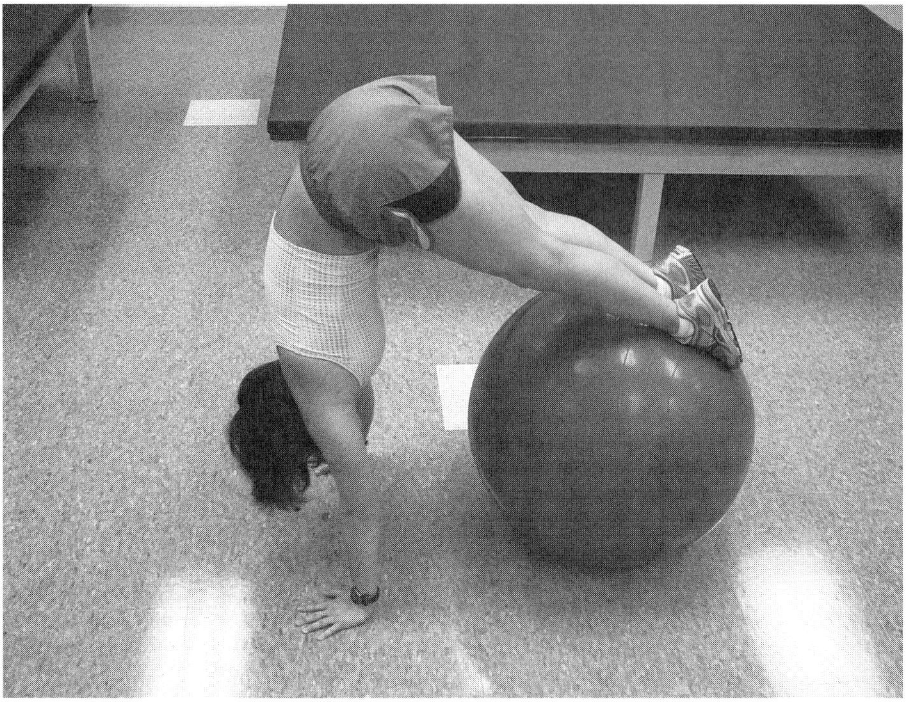

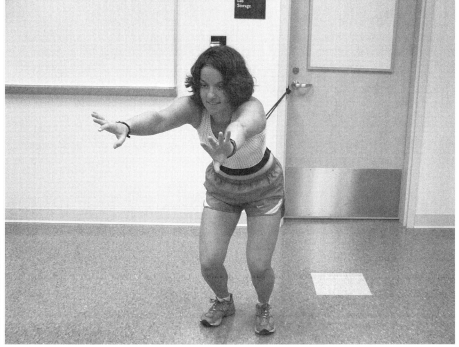

Courtesy of Barbara Hoogenboom

Figure 15-11 This dynamic exercise begins in a handstand with the LEs supported on the ball, flexion of the hips and trunk to a piked position completes the exercise.

Courtesy of Barbara Hoogenboom

Figure 15-12 Sport Cord activity of landing.

TABLE 15-3 · **Progression of Core Stabilization Exercises**

BEGINNING EXERCISES	INTERMEDIATE EXERCISES	ADVANCED EXERCISES
Isometric holding exercises: • **The abdominal hollowing exercise** • **Pelvic floor contractions, best started in supine, hook-lying** • **Lumbar multifidus contractions** • **Diaphragmatic breathing**	Dynamic positions with Stabilizer biofeedback: • **Movement of UEs** • **Movement of LEs into leg loading tasks, rotation** • **Resistance of LEs with tubing into rotation and extension**	Progress to advanced positions: Kneeling on ½ foam rollers with UE resistance demands Standing on dynadiscs or foam rollers. Add trunk or UE movements with or without resistance
Prone abdominal hollowing with the Stabilizer biofeedback static positions: • **Knees straight** • **Knees bent** • **Knees bent** • **(Slightly more difficult due to inability to counterbalance with LEs)**	Planks: • **Side planks, knees flexed** • **Side planks, LEs extended** • **Front planks, knees flexed (modified push-up position)** • **Full front planks**	Sport Specific Training postures: • **Use a tennis racquet with tubing attached for rotational stability** • **Sport postures with Body Blade in varied positions**
Abdominal hollowing alternate positions: • **Supine with Stabilizer biofeedback** • **Sitting** • **Four point**	Dynamic activities during side planks: • **LE movements** • **UE movements** • **UE/LE movements** • **Use of tubing and weights**	Dynamic sport positions: • **Ball activities in prone** • **UE weight bearing with ball, i.e. pike ups** • **Sport cord for landings**

Notes: It is important to provide the patient with clear explanations and use a variety of teaching "tools" such as verbal analogies/descriptors, visual aides, clinician demonstration, and tactile cues. The patient must be educated to the type of skill and motor retraining that needs to occur. This includes a discussion about precision and intensity of contractions (mild to moderate contractions of the involved musculature, rather than maximal contractions are indicated). The patient must understand from the outset the subtlety and precise natures of the contractions involved, and then apply to all activities.

Be certain to monitor for signs of unwanted global muscle activity during activities. These signs include: pelvic or spine movement, rib cage depression, no change in diameter of the abdominal wall (should draw in laterally and anteriorly), aberrant breathing patterns, inability to perform normal breathing during tasks, co-activation of thoracic portions of erector spinae. Methods of observation include visual observation, palpation and EMG assessment.

Be creative in designing and progressing activities of core stabilization, your only limitation is your own imagination!

In fact, many commercially available "low back strengthening" exercise machines do not attempt to stabilize the pelvis. Graves et al. studied the effect of pelvic stabilization on retraining of the lumbar extensors and found that strengthening should be performed with the pelvis stabilized.[19] It should be noted, however, that in their research they used a machine that provided passive external stabilization to the lumbar spine (due to machine design), while the authors of this chapter believe that a successfully maintained active pelvic stabilization may be more appropriate. Techniques of core stabilization using local musculature can be applied during various strengthening tasks involving global muscles of the trunk and extremities. Likewise, Kavcic et al. concluded that it is "justifiable to train motor patterns that involve the contribution of many of the potentially important lumbar spine stabilizers"[31] during rehabilitation, and that focus on a single muscle appears to be misdirected if the goal is the development of a stable spine.

Summary

Core stability training is increasing in popularity, as clinicians have become aware of the relationship that a weak core has to function and injury. The importance of the local muscular system for postural control, core stabilization and functional performance has been discussed. Indeed, many fitness and exercise regimens including Aquatic therapy, Swiss ball activities, Pilates, Yoga, Tai Chi, Feldenkrais, and Somatics all incorporate the concepts of core stabilization. Experts agree that retraining of the deep local muscles of the core must be incorporated into rehabilitation of patients with injury to the low back to effectively accomplish functional rehabilitation.[43]

It must be acknowledged that the concept of core stabilization is not intended to replace many other systems and philosophies of exercise, but may need to precede more general exercise and be incorporated in subsequent exercises in order to successfully educate or reeducate deep local muscles in their essential stabilizing function. Furthermore, local muscular exercises must be carefully taught and mastered prior to training the global muscles of the core. Successful utilization of local muscles during exercises and function will prevent or correct motor control problems that may contribute to recurrent injury and incorrect use of the muscles of the core.

No matter the exercise approach or applied theory, the clinical outcomes of core stability programs have not been well researched.[4] The specific exercises and theories described in this chapter need further investigation both for rehabilitation of injury to the low back, pelvis and associated core muscles and for utilization in strength training and performance enhancement programs. Incorporation of core stabilization techniques into both rehabilitative and fitness, prevention and wellness programs appears imperative for excellence in the ever evolving practice of rehabilitation. We owe our female athletes the application of cutting edge knowledge and principles of core stabilization for treatment of their injuries, development of athleticism and skilled performance, as well as injury prevention.

References

1. www.nhfs.org

2. www.ncaa.org

3. www.msnbc.org, retrieved 8/27/04.

4. Akuthota V, Nadler SF. Core Strengthening. *Archives of Physical Medicine and Rehabilitation.* 2004;85(Supplement 1):S86–S92.

5. Andrews JR, Harrelson GL, Wilk KE. Physical rehabilitation of the injured athlete, 3rd edition. Philadelphia, PA: Saunders; 2004.

6. Bouisset S. Relationship between postural support and intentional movement: biomechanical approach. *Arch Int Physiol Biochem Biophys.* 1991;99:77–92.

7. Cholewicki J, and McGill S. Mechanical stability of the in vivo lumbar spine: implications for injury and chronic low back pain. *Clinical Biomechanics.* 1996;11:1–15.

8. Cholewicki J, Simons APD, Radebold A. Effects of external trunk loads on lumbar spine stability. *Journal of Biomechanics.* 2000;33:1377–1385.

9. Cholewicki J, and Van Vliet J IV. Relative contribution of trunk muscles to the stability of the lumbar spine during isometric exertions. *Clinical Biomechanics.* 2002;17:99–105.

10. Cresswell AG. Responses of intra-abdominal pressure and abdominal muscle activity during dynamic trunk loading man. *European Journal of Applied Physics.* 1993;66:315–320.

11. Cresswell AG, and Thorstensson A. Change in intra-abdominal pressure pressure, trunk muscle activation and force during isokinetic lifting and lowering. *European Journal of Applied Physics.* 1994;68:315–321.

12. Cresswell AG, Oddson L, and Thorstensson A. The influence of sudden perturbations on trunk muscle activity and intra abdominal pressure while standing. *Experimental Brain Research.* 1994;98:336–341.

13. DeTroyer A, Estenne M, Ninane V, VanGansbeke D, and Gorini M. Transversus abdominis muscle function in humans. *Journal of Applied Physics.* 1990;68:1010–1016.

14. Ebenbichler GR, Oddsson LIE, Kollmitzer J, and Erim Z. Sensory-motor control of the lower back: implications for rehabilitation. *Medicine & Science in Sports & Exercise.* 2001;33(11):1889–1898.

15. Ferber RI, Davis M, Williams DS. Gender differences in lower extremity mechanics during running. *Clin Biomech.* 2003;18:350–357.

16. Frantz Pressler J, Givens Heiss D, Buford JA, and Chidley JV. Between-day Repeatability and Symmetry of Multifidus Cross-sectional Area Measured Using Ultrasound Imaging. *Journal of Orthopaedic and Sports Physical Therapy.* 2006;36:10–18.

17. Gardner-Morse M, and Stokes I. The effect of abdominal muscle coactivation on lumbar spine stability. *Spine.* 1998;23:86–92.

18. Gracovetsky S, Farfan H, and Helleur C. The effect of the abdominal mechanism. *Spine.* 1985;10:317–324.

19. Graves JE, Webb DC, Pollock ML, Matkozich J et al., Cirulli J. Pelvic stabilization during resistance training: its effect on the development of lumbar extension strength. *Archives of Physical Medicine and Rehabilitation.* 1994;75:210–215.

20. Griffin LY, Agel MJ, Albohm MJ, et al. Noncontact anterior cruciate ligament injuries: risk factors and prevention strategies. *Journal of American Academy of Orthopaedic Surgeons.* 2000;8:141–150.

21. Hall CM, and Thein Brody L. Therapeutic exercise: moving toward function. Philadelphia: Lippincott Williams & Wilkins; 1999.

22. Henry SM, and Wetervelt KC. Time Ultrasound FeedbackThe Use of Real-Time Ultrasound Feedback in Teaching Abdominal Hollowing Exercises to Healthy Subjects. *J Orthop and Sports Phys Ther.* 2005; 35:338–345.

23. Hides JA, Stokes MJ, Saide M, Jull GA, and Cooper DH. Evidence of lumbar multifidus muscle wasting ipsilateral to symptoms in patients with acute/subacute low back pain. *Spine.* 1994;19:165–172.

24. Hides JA, Richardson C, and Jull GA. Multifidus muscle recovery is not automatic after resolution of acute, first episode low back pain. *Spine.* 1996;21:2763–2769.

25. Hodges PW. Is there a role for transversus abdominis in lumbo-pelvic stability? *Manual Therapy.* 1999;4(2):74–86.

26. Hodges PW, and Richardson CA. Feedforward contraction of transverse abdominis is not influenced by the direction of arm movement. *Experimental Brain Research.* 1997;114:362–370.

27. Hodges PW, Butler JE, McKenzie D, and Gandevia SC. Contraction of the human diaphragm during postural adjustments. *Journal of Applied Physics.* 1997;505:239–248.

28. Hodges PW, and Richardson CA. Delayed postural contraction of transverse abdominis in low back pain associated with movement of the lower limb. *Journal of Spinal Disorders & Techniques.* 1998;1:46–56.

29. Ireland ML, Willson JD, Ballantyne BT, Davis IM. Hip strength in females with and without patellofemoral pain. *Journal of Orthopaedic and Sports Physical Therapy.* 2003;33:637–651.

30. Jemmet RS. Rehabilitation of lumbar multifidus dysfunction in low back pain: strengthening versus a motor re-education model. *Br J Sports Med.* 2003;37(1):91–92.

31. Kavcic N, Grenier S, and McGill S. Determining the stabilizing role of individual torso muscles during rehabilitation exercises. *Spine*. 2004;29(2):1254–1265.

32. Kendall FP, McCreary EK. Muscle: testing and function, 3rd Edition. Baltimore, MD. Williams & Wilkins, 1983.

33. Kibler WB, Herring SA, Press JM, and Lee PA. Functional rehabilitation of sports and musculoskeletal injuries. Gaithersburg, MD: Aspen Publishers; 1998.

34. Knott M, and Voss D. Proprioceptive neuromuscular facilitation: patterns and techniques. New York: Harper & Row; 1968.

35. Leetun DT, Ireland ML, Willson JD, Ballantyne BT, and Davis IM. Core stability measures as risk factors for lower extremity injury in athletes. *Medicine & Science in Sports & Exercise*. 2004;36(6):926–934.

36. McGill, S. Low back disorders: evidence-based prevention and rehabilitation. Champaign, IL: Human Kinetics; 2002.

37. McGill S, and Brown S. Reassessment of the role of intra-abdominal pressure in spinal compression. *Ergonomics*. 1987;30:1565–1588.

38. McGill SM, Childs A, Lieberman C. Endurance times for low back stabilization exercise: clinical targets for testing and training from a normal database. *Archives of Physical Medicine and Rehabilitation*. 1999;80:941–944.

39. Morris JM, Lucas DM, and Bressler B. Role of the trunk in stability of the spine. *Journal of Bone and Joint Surgery*. 1961;43:327–351.

40. Nadler SF, Malanga GA, DePrince M, Stitik TP, and Feinberg JH. The relationship between lower extremity injury, low back pain, and hip muscle strength in male and female collegiate athletes. *Clinical Journal of Sports Medicine*. 2000;10:89–97.

41. OSullivan PB, Twomey LT, and Allison GT. Evaluation of specific stabilizing exercise in the treatment of chronic low back pain with radiologic diagnosis of spondylolysis or spondylolisthesis. *Spine*. 1997;22:2959–2967.

42. Punjabi M, Abumi K, Duranceau J, et al. Spine stability and inter-segmental muscle forces: a biomechanical model. *Spine*. 1989;14:194–200.

43. Richardson C, Jull G, Hodges P, and Hides J. Therapeutic exercise for spinal segmental stabilization in low back pain: scientific basis and clinical approach. Edinburgh, NY: Churchill Livingstone; 1999.

44. Roy SH, DeLuca CJ, Snyder-Mackler L, Emley MS, Crenshaw RL, and Lyons JP. Fatigue, recovery and low back pain in varsity rowers. *Medicine & Science in Sports & Exercise*. 1990;22:463–469.

45. Sahrmann SA. Diagnosis and treatment of movement impairment syndromes. St. Louis: Mosby; 2002. muscle strength in male and female collegiate athletes. *Clinical Journal of Sports Medicine.* 2000;10:89–97.

46. Stokes IA, Henry SM, and Single RM. Surface EMG electrodes do not accurately record from lumbar multifidus muscles. *Clinical Biomechanics.* 2003;18(1):9–13.

47. Swedan N. Women's sports medicine and rehabilitation. Gaithersburg, MD: Aspen Publishers; 2001.

48. Teyhen DS, Miltenberger CE, Deiters HM, et al. TheUseofUltrasound The Use of Ultrasound Imaging of the Abdominal Drawing-in Maneuver in Subjects With Low Back Pain. *Journal of Orthopaedic and Sports Physical Therapy.* 2005;35:346–355.

49. Thomson KE. On the bending moment capability of the pressurized abdominal cavity during human lifting activity. *Ergonomics.* 1988;31: 817–828.

50. Wilke HJ, Wolf S, Claes LE, Arand M, and Wiesend A. Stability increase of the lumbar spine with different muscle groups. A biomechanical in vitro study. *Spine.* 1995;20:192–198.

CHAPTER 16

Anemia and the Female Athlete

James Cole, MD

Introduction

Normal levels of hemoglobin are essential for optimum physical performance. Anemia, or a level of hemoglobin less than the 5th percentile for a specific age, is commonly found in young female athletes and can result from a variety of issues. These range from spurious dilutional anemia, due to plasma expansion associated with training, to various pathologic conditions, such as blood loss, iron and other nutritional deficiencies, hemolysis, or hemoglobin disorders. Anemia can lead to impairment of optimum athletic performance. Athletes, coaches, and parents, therefore, should be aware of its potential existence, causes, and treatment options.

Causes of Anemia

The most common reason for low hemoglobin levels in young athletes (commonly referred to as "sports anemia") is due to the expansion of plasma volume that derives from prolonged participation in most athletic endeavors.[11] This is actually a dilutional psuedoanemia as it is not a true decrease in hemoglobin. The anemia results from the relative overexpansion of plasma volume in relation to the solid components of the blood.[14] The mass of red blood cells is usually normal to increased. Plasma volume, however, can increase more rapidly and to a greater extent, leading to an apparent drop in hemoglobin levels.[3] This finding is usually associated more with endurance athletes and generally results in a slightly below normal level of hemoglobin. Hemoglobin levels usually return to normal a few days after cessation of whatever activity led to the finding, and symptoms generally are not encountered.[4]

Iron Deficiency

The most prevalent cause of true anemia is iron deficiency. While iron deficiency is quite common, occurring in up to 20% of premenopausal females, actual iron deficiency anemia is only found in 1%-3% of female athletes, the same rate as the general population.[5] Iron is not only essential for hemoglobin formation, but is also found in myoglobin and electron transport molecules. Low levels of iron can subsequently lead to the impairment of VO_2 max, decreased exercise tolerance, and subsequent poor performance.[15]

Iron deficiency can result from nutritional deficiencies due to poor absorption or dietary habits, chronic blood loss, or increased destruction of red blood cells. While menstruation is the most common cause of iron deficiency due to blood loss in young women, other sources include the gastrointestinal tract, genitourinary system, childbirth, or severe hemolysis. Gastrointestinal losses may result from dehydration leading to intestinal ischemia and are seen more commonly with endurance sports, including long-distance running, swimming, cycling, and cross-country skiing.[13] Anti-inflammatory drugs used for musculoskeletal pain frequently lead to gastritis, or inflammation of the stomach lining, which can result in gastrointestinal blood loss.[3] Hematuria, due to either renal tubule ischemia or direct trauma to the bladder or kidneys, is also frequently encountered in endurance athletes.[12] The blood loss is minimal, however, and rarely results in significant anemia. While iron loss in sweat can measure 1 mg-2 mg per day, equal to the average dietary intake of iron, it is generally not felt to lead to iron deficiency.[2]

Hemolysis

Hemolysis, or the destruction of red blood cells, can sometimes be encountered with extreme athletic activity. If the hemolysis is severe or prolonged, it can sometimes lead to anemia. "Foot-strike anemia," or "march anemia" was first described in a European foot soldier that was found to have blood in his urine, or hemoglobinuria, after prolonged marches.[8] This phenomenon has been noted frequently in athletes, especially elite distance runners. The etiology of the destruction of red blood cells appears to be due to the actual trauma associated with the feet hitting the ground.[6] While this is a commonly described phenomenon in athletes, it rarely leads to actual anemia. Usually hemolyzed iron is scavenged by haptoglobin and recycled into new blood cell formation. It is only when hemolysis is severe enough to overwhelm the available haptoglobin that hemoglobinuria will occur, which eventually could lead to iron deficiency.[4] Exercise-induced hemolysis generally is mild however, and anemia due to hemolysis is usually indicative of a more significant disorder, such as the membrane disorders described below.

Impact of Diet

Dietary factors are a common factor in iron deficiency anemia. Endurance athletes may not have adequate caloric intake to obtain enough iron. Female athletes frequently restrict caloric intake for weight control or may be vegetarian, which may limit adequate iron ingestion.

Dietary habits may lead to deficiencies in other vitamins that are essential for red cell formation, notably folate and B12. Vitamin B12 is found in meat and certain vegetables and commonly can be a problem with strict vegetarians.

Impact of Genetics

Inherited hemoglobin disorders such as sickle cell disease or thalassemia can also be a cause for anemia. Sickle cell trait usually does not result in anemia, but can have implications for certain athletic activities. Endurance athletes with sickle cell trait have had problems with rhabdomyolysis, or the breakdown of muscle cells, with insufficient hydration. This could lead to kidney damage or failure, or even sudden death.[9] Less common causes of anemia include red blood cell membrane structural disorders such as hereditary spherocytosis or elliptocytosis, which lead to chronic red cell destruction. Even low levels of chronic hemolysis can lead to folate deficiency and subsequent anemia.

Evaluation of Anemia and Associated Clinical Tests

The Complete Blood Count (CBC)

The complete blood count (CBC) is the most useful screen for anemia. This reveals if an athlete is indeed anemic, as well as offer insight into various causes for the anemia. The hemoglobin level, measured in grams per deciliter, reveals the actual amount of hemoglobin within the blood, mostly within the red blood cells themselves. The hematocrit reveals the percentage of whole blood that is made up of solid red cells in relation to liquid plasma and other suspended proteins. The mean corpuscular volume (MCV), is a measurement of the size of red cells. Iron deficiency and hemoglobinopathies such as sickle cell disease and thalassemia are associated with a below normal MCV, while vitamin B12 and folate deficiencies and some hemolytic anemias usually produce an elevation in MCV. Finally, the red cell distribution width (RDW) indicates the variability in the size and shape of red cells. Situations where the bone marrow is producing blood inefficiently, such as in vitamin or mineral deficiency, or blood cells are breaking down quickly will cause an elevation in RDW.

Measuring Iron Levels

In suspected iron deficiency, measurement of ferritin, serum iron (Fe), total iron binding concentration (TIBC), and iron saturation percentage (Fe % sat) is helpful. Iron deficiency actually develops in three stages.[15] In the first stage, there is a decrease in ferritin, a storage form of iron. Stainable iron is also absent from the bone marrow, but hemoglobin levels remain normal. The second stage is associated with a decrease in serum iron levels, iron saturation percentage, and MCV with an increase in TIBC and RDW. The hemoglobin and hematocrit, however, still remain normal. Overt anemia, the third stage of iron deficiency, develops if there is further depletion of iron stores. One thing to keep in mind with iron deficiency is that while its cause is usually benign, it may be indicative of a more severe underlying problem such as gastrointestinal or genitourinary blood loss.

Counting New Red Cell Formation

The reticulocyte count is an indicator of new red cell formation. Elevated levels can suggest hemolysis where a stressed bone marrow is trying to compensate with increased red cell production. A low reticulocyte count in an anemic person, however, suggests inadequate production, possibly due to a substrate deficiency or a more significant bone marrow disorder.

Scavenger Proteins

Haptoglobin is a scavenger protein that binds free hemoglobin in the plasma and levels will be diminished in hemolytic anemias. The liver absorbs the haptoglobin-hemoglobin complex so iron can be recycled into new red blood cells. Iron deficiency anemia, subsequently, is rare in hemolytic states, unless there is so much free hemoglobin in the blood that haptoglobin is used up and substantial amounts of hemoglobin are lost in the urine. Another indicator of hemolysis is an elevation of lactate dehydrogenase (LDH) which is an enzyme found in intact red cells. When cells break down LDH is released into the bloodstream and can be detected in the serum.

Athletes with a macrocytic anemia, which results in an elevated MCV, should have measurement of vitamin B12 and folate levels. Of note, even with depleted vitamin B12 stores increased folate absorption can correct the anemia, sometimes leading to severe neurologic problems that can be encountered with vitamin B12 deficiency.

Suspected inherited hemoglobin disorders such as sickle cell disease and thalassemia are best evaluated with a hemoglobin electrophoresis. This test measures levels of normal Hemoglobin A and A_2, as well as detects hemoglobin variants such as Hemoglobin S.

Treatment of Anemia

Treatment of an athlete with anemia is dependent upon its cause and severity. As stated earlier in the chapter, dilutional psuedoanemia will resolve spontaneously within a few days of ceasing whatever activity led to its development. Foot-strike hemolysis can be combated by running on softer surfaces or by using shoes with more cushioning.

Athletes found to have iron deficiency should try to increase oral intake and maximize absorption of iron. Typically 10%-15% of dietary iron is absorbed.[16] Red meat has higher levels of "heme iron" which is more readily absorbed. Non-heme iron is found in leafy green vegetables, nuts, and cereals. Vitamin C may enhance absorption of iron as well. On the other hand, dietary products such as tea, coffee, antacids, and bran may inhibit absorption. Athletes with iron deficiency anemia should take oral iron supplementation, usually in the form of ferrous sulfate or ferrous gluconate.

An increased reticulocyte count 4–7 days after beginning iron supplement therapy is indicative of increased red cell production. Six–twelve months of therapy are generally adequate to replace iron stores. Iron supplementation can sometimes result in cramping or severe constipation, and some individuals do not absorb enough iron orally to overcome daily losses. Occasionally, iron must be replaced intravenously or intramuscularly under the direction of a hematologist.

While replenishing iron stores in a depleted individual is obviously important; too much iron can be just as detrimental. Approximately 10% of individuals of Northern European ancestry are heterozygous for the gene that causes hemochromotosis, and iron overload can be precipitated by too much dietary iron or supplementation.[16]

Strict vegetarians who do not eat any animal products do not have a reliable source of vitamin B12. Vitamin supplementation or fortified foods is therefore required.[1] Athletes with sickle trait should make sure they are well hydrated and should be closely monitored when exercising at altitude.[19]

Summary

In general, young athletes tend to have higher levels of hemoglobin compared to their less active counterparts.[10] As optimum performance is dependent upon adequate hemoglobin levels and the development of anemia can be insidious, active screening is warranted. Women are especially prone to iron deficiency because menstrual blood losses and more common dietary restrictions. Also, strict vegetarians are more likely to develop iron and B12 deficiencies and should be screened appropriately.

In elite female athletes, a CBC should be obtained every 6–12 months. As iron deficiency is relatively common and can precede anemia, regular ferritin monitoring is warranted as well.[7] Vegetarian and other diet-restricted athletes should have a baseline B12 and folate measurement, especially if there is any macrocytosis present. High activity and/or diet-restricted athletes should be educated in an iron-rich diet. Finally, young women with a family history of sickle cell disease or thalassemia should be evaluated for this as well.

While anemia in general, and iron deficiency anemia in particular, is no more common in female athletes than the general female population, its presence can have significant implications. Anemia can lead to decreased exercise tolerance and its correction can improve outcomes. Knowing the causes of anemia and how to correct them is an essential component of optimal athletic performance.

References

1. Barr SI, and Rideout CA. Nutritional considerations for vegetarian athletes. *Nutrition.* 2004;20:696-703.

2. Brune M, Magnusson B, Persson H, et al. Iron losses in sweat. *American Journal of Clinical Nutrition.* 1986;43:438-43.

3. Chatard JC, Mujika I, Guy C, and Lacour JR. Anemia and iron deficiency in athletes: Practical recommendations for treatment. *Sports Medicine.* 1999;1:229-240.

4. Clement DB, and Sawchuk LL. Iron status and sports performance. *Sports Medicine.* 1984;1:65-74.

5. Cook JD, Skikne BS, Lynch SR, et al. Estimates of iron sufficiency in the US population. *Blood.* 1986;68:726-731.

6.   Davidson RJ. Exertional Hemoglobinuria: A report on three cases with studies on the hemolytic mechanism. *Journal of Clinical Pathology.* 1964;17:536-40.

7.   Fallon KE. Utility of hematological and iron-related screening in elite athletes. *Clinics in Sports Medicine.* 2004;14:145-152.

8.   Fleischer R. Ueber Eine Neue Form von haemoglobinurie beim menschen. *Berl Klin Wochenschr.* 1881;18:691.

9.   Mercer KW, and Densmore JJ. Hematologic disorders in the athlete. *Clinics in Sports Medicine.* 2005;24:599-621.

10. Nikolaidis MG, Protosygellou MD, Petridou, A, et al. Hematologic and biochemical profile of juvenile and adult athletes of both sexes: Implications for clinical evaluation. *International Journal of Sports Medicine.* 2003;24:506-511.

11. Shaskey DJ, and Green GA. *Sports Hematology.* 2000;1:27-38.

12. Siegal AJ, Hennekens CH, Solomon HS, et al. Exercise-related hematuria. Findings in a group of marathon runners. *Journal of American Medical Association.* 1979;241:391-392.

13. Small E, and Bar-Or O. The young athlete with chronic disease. *Clinics in Sports Medicine.* 1995;14:709-726.

14. Weight LM, Darge BL, and Jacobs P. Athlete's psuedoanemia. *European Journal of Applied Physiology.* 1991;62:358-62.

15. Woodson RD, Wills RE, and Lenfent C. Journal of Applied Physiology. 1978;44:36-43.

16. Zoller H, and Vogel W. Iron supplementation in athletes-first do no harm. *Nutrition.* 2004;20:615-918.

CHAPTER 17

Anterior Cruciate Ligamentous Issues

Tab Blackburn, MPT, ATC

Introduction

Anterior cruciate ligament (ACL) injuries in athletes can be a devastating blow to, not only the athlete's career, but to the long term health of their knees. The non-reconstructed ACL deficient knee may suffer 'giving way' episodes, as well as meniscal tears,[10] and increased chances of degenerative joint disease (DJD).[26] The incidences of meniscal tears are estimated to be 40% in year one after injury, 60% at year 5 and 80% at year 10.[27] Injuries such as these may lead to radiographic changes in 10–15 years in 60%-90% of the patients.[1] This means that the athlete could be presented with DJD symptoms 15–20 years before their non-injured contemporaries.[42]

Epidemiology of ACL

The frequency of injury of the ACL in the general population is not as high as reported in the literature. It is estimated that 1 in 3,500 Americans suffer ACL injuries per year resulting in 95,000 new injuries per year,[11] although surgical reports indicate there are 100,000 ACL surgeries per year.[40] It is suggested that the ACL is the most frequently totally disrupted ligament in the knee;[33] this appears to be true for athletes, especially female athletes, according to literature that compares male and female injury rates.[4,5,25] The injury rates for females range from 2.4-9.7 times greater than that of males participating in similar sports.[7] Males have more ACL surgeries due to a larger number of males participating in high risk contact sports.[46]

In 1972, before the Title IX Educational Assistance Act, approximately 294,000 females and 2.6 million males participated in high school sports. The National Federation of State High School Associations reports there are now 3 million females and 4.3 million males participating in high school sports.[36] If injury estimates are accurate, some 38,000 females suffer ACL injuries in the upcoming years.[51] In economic terms, it costs approximately $17,000 for surgery and rehabilitation for the individual and as much as $646 million a year in the United States for the management of female ACL injuries.[20]

The National Collegiate Athletic Association (NCAA) injury data has been reviewed by Hootman et al.,[23] who examined the 1989–2004 academic school years. Basketball produced 665 ACL injuries (women 498 and men 167). Soccer produced 579 ACL injuries (women 411 and men 168). Three of the four sports with the highest rates were women's sports (gymnastics, basketball, and soccer), and, along with spring football, all had significantly higher ACL injury rates than any other sport. In basketball, women have an injury rate of 0.23 (per 1000 of Athlete-Exposures or A-E) with men at 0.07 A-E. In soccer, women have an injury rate of 3.7 with men at 1.3. Overall, ACL injury rates have significantly increased over the years, but still only account for 3% of all injuries. However, 88% of ACL injuries, resulted in 10+ days of time loss.

In a previous NCAA study,[3] it was found that 26% of the ACL injuries could not be categorized as to mechanism of injury. Contact ACL injury rates are significantly higher for women than men in both basketball (0.06 versus 0.02), and soccer (0.10 versus 0.04) with soccer being significantly worse than basketball for women and men. Non-contact injuries ranged from 29%-100% of total injuries over the 13-year review, with women averaging 67%, and men 58%. Non-contact ACL injury rates are significantly higher for women than men in basketball (0.16 versus 0.04) and soccer (0.13 versus 0.04), with basketball significantly worse than soccer for females. Still, it is puzzling that female rates have not changed since female athletes are much more experienced and effort has been exerted in the form of prevention programs.[3]

Researching Female ACL Injuries

Most studies have had a small number of subjects and larger studies are needed. Uhorchak et al. at the US Military Academy in West Point, New York, followed the graduating class of 1999 from first to last year. In that study, 739 males and 120 females were evaluated on admission to school for laxity, flexibility, strength, and notch ratios. Sixteen males and eight females suffered non-contact ACL injuries. This represented injury rates not different from Agel's report. Female cadets with hyper elasticity, body mass index's greater than 24.7, body weight greater than 68 Kg, and notch ratios shown to be consistent with ACL injury, were more likely to suffer an ACL injury. None of the men's characteristic related to their injuries.

Mechanism of Injury

Non-contact ACL injuries appear to be the biggest problem for women, which is where researchers have begun to develop programs to reduce these injuries. Soccer seems to be the sport most likely to produce an ACL injury in a woman. It appears that women ACL injury during deceleration, landing, or side step cutting with the knee slightly flexed, and in valgus. Many times the athlete has been pertubated, or the joint(s) stimulated before landing.[15]

Most of the literature points to three areas that may be the cause of non-contact injuries in females (and males):e anatomical and biomechanical, hormonal, and neuromuscular. None of these concepts are 100% proven and they all may play some role. Biomechanical changes to the body may be implemented by foot orthotics. There may be a case for hormonal intervention, but this could be prove to be complicated. It appears that neuromuscular components produce an adequate intervention.[52]

Anatomical and Biomechanical Influence

Some early anecdotal comments about women having more ACL injuries than men related back to Title IX legislation. Some felt that women just didn't have experience at sports, weren't in shape to play sports, and that they were the 'weaker' sex. Since the enactment of Title IX, women have progressed considerably in terms of conditioning, but their injury rate remains high compared to men in basketball and soccer.

Anatomical considerations were first discussed as 'scientific' reasons for female ACL injury rates. Many athletic training staffs looked at foot pronation as a major anatomical cause of ACL injury. Certified Athletic Trainers noted that their athletes with excessive pronation appeared to have more injury. Their thoughts are supported by descriptions of lower extremity biomechanics where increased pronation means increased valgus at the knee.

This supported other anatomical concepts that women have a different shaped pelvis with different anatomical and biomechanical alignment of the hip, femur, knee, foot, and ankle. There is usually (but not always) a more valgus knee, higher Q angles, more external tibial torsion, and more genu recurvatum than found in men. The fact that women were generally 'looser jointed' compared to men was also examined. Since on the average male athletes are stronger than female athletes, some thought this played a role.[16]

In a retrospective study, Souryal et al. discovered that male and females who had bilateral non-simultaneous ACL injuries had a much lower notch width index (NWI) (width of the femoral notch divided by the width of the femur) than those who had no injury or a unilateral injury (0.196-0.233).[49] In a prospective paper he presented in 1993, his group found that the average NWI was 0.233 and that those who suffered non-contact ACL injuries had a NWI of 0.189. So prediction of those predisposed to ACL injury may be possible;[48] however, other papers seem to disregard Souryal's theory.[50] It's possible that different age groups, types of athletes, levels of ability of athletes may all play a role in the importance of NWI.

If notch stenosis is an issue, is injury caused by the tight confines of the notch or does it mean that if there is a small notch, there is a small ligament? Shelbourne's et al. 1998 paper pointed out that the NWI was not reliable because notch width and bicondylar width did not correlate. He suggested that it is the absolute notch width that counts. Smaller widths appear to lead to more injuries in men and women. His results demonstrated that in his subjects, women overall had smaller notches than men. Women who have bilateral non-contact injuries have smaller notches than men in the same situation. Since ligament strength may be based on cross sectional width, smaller notches may mean smaller ligaments. His data was based on inter-operative measurements of the notch and suggests that the size or shape of the notch is not the causative factor to ACL injuries but reflects the size of the ligament.[47] Several researchers have noted that the shape of the notch may affect the injury of ACLs. MRI evaluation has also shown that larger notch mean larger ligaments in most subjects.[2,24,12] Anderson et al. found that when size and strength of the male and female athlete is taken into consideration, females have smaller ACL and this may make them predisposed to injury.[29] More work is required in this area.

Hormonal Influence

In 1991, Moller et al. found that the soccer players using oral contraceptives had fewer ACL injuries than those who were not taking this kind of drug.[32] Is it possible that ACL injuries in women could be altered by using oral contraceptives? What is the mechanism for this? Oral contraceptives in the early 1990s prevented follicular growth, ovulation, and corpus luteum by inhibiting pituitary producing follicle stimulating and luteinizing hormones and substituting synthetic estrogen and progesterone. New oral contraceptives do not have as much ovarian steroids and allow follicular growth but no ovulation. Some have suggested that the synthetic hormones found in these drugs affect the turnover of Type I and Type II collagen tissue because the anabolic/catabolic balance is altered.[56] Still, others postulate that there is a suppression of Type I and IV collagen fiber by estradiol leading to weaker connective tissue.[37]

Be aware of studies of female ACL injuries related to the menstrual cycle if urine or blood samples are not taken at the time of injury; these samples indicate where the athlete is in her menstrual cycle. In 2002, Wojtys et al. reported that with proper analysis of the menstrual cycle, women are more likely to injure their ACL during ovulation than in the follicular or luteal phases. His group also found that those subjects taking oral contraceptive had a 2.5 times less chance of ACL injury.[54]

Liu et al. described the estrogen and progesterone sites on the ACL itself. That could mean that hormones in the woman's body directly affect the collagen of the ACL.[28,29] There is information that indicates that estrogen affects the formation, metabolism, and function of collagen tissue.[18] But no one has been able to show a clear mechanism of how the ACL is affected by hormones.

Neuromuscular Influences

Research indicates that, besides the direct affect that hormones may have on the ACL, there are secondary effects on the neuromuscular system of the female.[44] The ability to contract the quadriceps and the strength of the quadriceps have been shown to be affected. This may translate into a limited protective stiffening around a joint which is accomplished through muscle contractions.[55]

Other Involved Mechanisms

While there are many factors which contribute to ACL injury, the following information can shed some light on other research that may explain the "how" and the "why" of this injury. Several older studies indicate that decision-making and full body coordination may also be involved.[57,6] The average male athlete has more lean body mass than the average female. Quad hamstring ratios are different. Some have suggested that women and men use their quads and hamstrings differently with different firing patterns. Others point to differences in balance and proprioception. Women may not be able to co-contract their muscles about their knee as quickly as men. This could be due to the elasticity of their tendons which causes a lag time with associated reflexes.[45] It appears though, that the real issue is the valgus position of the knee and the lack of knee flexion in women when they land. Certainly, the other ideas play some role, but any female or male that lands with their knee in valgus is at risk.

Markoff et al. pointed to valgus loading at the knee as a cause of increased stress on the ACL.[31] Fukuda et al. quantified these forces across the knee. These studies were done using cadavers.[14] It was Hewett's et al.[22] prospective research on the landing behaviors of males and females that has given us real world measurements of the forces and then followed the athletes to see who was injured. He found knee abduction angles or valgus position of the athlete's knees on landing to be 8.4° more at initial contact and 7.6° more at maximum knee flexion in the injured group than the uninjured group. There were also significant correlations between knee abduction angles and ground reaction forces in the injured group. The other interesting finding from Hewett was that of knee flexion angle upon landing. The initial knee flexion angle was similar in both the injured and non-injured groups. But the maximum knee angle was 10.5° less in the injured group. There was a significant correlation between maximum knee flexion angle and peak forces in the non-injured group. Ground reaction forces were 20% higher in the injured group. Female athletes who went on to ACL injury had a 16% shorter stance phase, or the process by which the body catches itself so it does not fall to the ground when landing. In other words, they are landing more stiff legged.

Predisposition

Is it possible to predict those who may have predisposition for non-contact ACL injury and can anything be done about it? In Hewett's reported research in 1996,[44] he looked at quadriceps and hamstring strengths and rations, balance and landing forces to determine who needs to go in his prevention program. In later studies, it appears landing forces are most likely to predict who might be predisposed for injury. Of course this requires expensive biomechanical equipment to analyze the landing forces. Visually, those with the highest valgus forces will demonstrate valgus knees upon jumping and landing. This could be a guide for clinicians.

Prevention

Certainly looking at the examination of quadriceps and hamstring strengths could be a part of the equation of injury prevention. Wilkinson et al. found that normal strength ratios at 60° and 300° per second were 0.6 and 0.8, respectively for hamstring quadriceps ratios. Quadriceps to body weight ratios were 1.0 and 0.5 at 60° and 300° per second, respectively. Hamstrings to body weight ratios were 0.6 and 0.4 at those same speeds, respectively.[53]

Balance and proprioception has also been considered as a part of several ACL prevention programs. Rozzi et al.[43] found that collegiate female basketball and soccer players had excessive laxity and that this may possibly lead to diminished proprioception, predisposing the athlete to ACL injury because the athlete would not be able to recognize potentially damaging forces on their knees. A number of the prevention programs include balance training as one of their activities.

There have been many discussions over the past 10 years about prevention strategies for ACL injuries. Initial thoughts concerned bracing and its role in injury prevention. No definitive study has been done to show that ACL braces prevent non-contact ACL injuries. Nor is there is any definitive study to show reduction in ACL injuries using orthotics or special shoes.

Newer Prevention Strategies

Other suggestions have surfaced. These include such ideas as enhancing neuromuscular control, enhancing strength and endurance, developing better co-contraction about the knee and faster reaction times, developing better hip and trunk control as well as controlling knee extension and valgus. Does this mean that there been any activities that change the biomechanics of landing? Hewett [44] found after an eight-week jump training program, females had a 22% decrease in peak landing forces, a 50% decrease in abduction and adduction movements at the knee, a 13%-26% increase in the hamstring quad ratio and a 21%-44% increase in hamstring strength.

Noyes et al.[38] looked at 325 untrained females and 130 untrained males with a specified protocol between the ages of 11–19. The majority of these untrained athletes had valgus knees, knocked knees upon landing from a jump. They were trained for six weeks in a plyometric, balance, and strength training programmed. They were educated on how to land with there knees in a neutral position. The females improved their lower extremity landing techniques while the males showed no changes. Onate et al.[39] studied training educational techniques involving ACL prevention programs. He found that almost all types of instructional forms worked better than no instruction at all. Instructional forms included an expert teacher, self taught with script and a combination of the two.

Myer et al.[34] attempted to find the difference between plyometric training and balance training on ACL prevention programs. He found that both techniques appear to change lower extremity biomechanics. Plyometrics affected sagittal plane kinematics when the subject jumped down off of a box. Balance training affected sagittal plane kinematics when the subject jumped down medial from a box. He concludes both activities must be included in an ACL prevention program.

Biomechanical landing characteristics can be changed by training. In 1990, Henning and Griffis produced a video of a prevention program they utilized over eight years designed to change basketball player's techniques of running, jumping and landing. While working with two, Division I basketball teams, they trained the players to flex their knees more upon landing, attempt to make rounded cuts, and to decelerate with multiple steps (similar to 'pumping' your brakes when stopping your car). They noted an 89% reduction in the rate of occurrence of ACL injuries in their intervention group.[19]

In 1996, an Italian researcher named Caraffa implemented a training program consisting of proprioception balance training on over 600 semiprofessional and amateur soccer players (Caraffa et al.).[8] The program consisted of 20 minute training activities that progressed through five phases of difficulty. After three years of training, the result was an 87% decrease in ACL injuries with the injury rate of the trained group at 0.15 and the control group at 1.15. Ettlinger and associates suggested a knee ligament injury prevention program for skiing. After over 20 years of collecting data via videotaping and biomechanical analysis of more than 1,400 ACL injuries, they developed an instructional program and video tape program for the prevention of the two most common ACL injury situations in skiing. With an experimental and control group, they trained 'on-slope' personnel with the program. While monitoring ACL injuries over the next three years, they found a 62% reduction in ACL and severe knee ligament injury.[13]

In Norway, ACL injuries devastated the Olympic Handball Team. Mykelbust et al.[35] implemented a proprioception training program over a two year span. There were 855 athletes in the first year and 850 during the second year of the program. There were 29 ACL injuries in the control group and 23 in the training group. At the end of the second year, the trained group dropped to 17 ACL injuries. Hewett et al.[21] based their prevention program on stretching, plyometrics and resistance training programs. 1263 males and females participated in the program. Each received instructions and a video tape on the program. Each participated in six weeks of trainings before the season started. The results showed that only five ACLs occurred in the untrained female group and none in the trained female group. The injury rate for untrained females was 3.6 times higher than in trained females and 4.8 times higher than males.

Heidt et al.[17] followed 300 soccer players aged 14–18 over a one year period after 42 of them trained with the Frappier Acceleration Program. The program included strength, flexibility, cardiovascular training, and plyometrics over a seven-week period. The untrained athletes had a 3.1% ACL injury rate versus the trained group at 2.4%.

Soccer is very popular in Southern California. Mandelbaum et al.[30] managed many ACL injuries in young female soccer players. They instituted the Prevent injury, Enhance Performance (PEP) program to 1041 athletes and utilized another 1905 athletes as controls. The program consisted of educational information, stretching, plyometrics and sports specific activities. At the end of the first year the untrained group had 32 ACL tears and the trained group had two. By the second year, the untrained group suffered 35 ACLs and the trained suffered 4. It was a resounding success for the program.

Although these studies do not have many subjects and there does not seem to be a specific program that is better than another, there is no doubt that training makes a difference. Those who wish to integrate a program into their athletic teams may find several logistical problems. Many times coaches don't want extra activities for their athletes. They are already short on time.

Summary

It appears that most of the successful programs include resistance training for generalized strengthening, especially for the hips and thighs. Flexibility and balance training are also very important. Plyometric training is usually at the foundation of many of the programs. It is important that the athletes are trained to maintain an athletic position or bent knee position. Standing with the knees in hyperextension can be dangerous to the health of the ACL.

Athletes should be taught to land softly, and flex their knees as far as possible. They should be mid-foot rockers and roll over their feet for less impact and coaches need to teach "drop like a shock absorber, and jump like a spring." Above all, don't let the knees fall into valgus. Keep the knees apart when jumping and landing. Remember that these programs aren't conditioning programs, but training programs that teach how to jump and land, dissipate forces evenly, and to anticipate injury situations. Researchers are slowly proving what activities can be done to prevent ACL injuries in males and females and will eventually be fine-tuned to fit most athletes and the sports in which they participate.

References

1. Anderson AF, Dome DC, Gautam S, Awh MH, and Rennirt GW. Correlation of anthropometric measurements, strength, anterior cruciate ligament size, and intercondylar notch characteristics to sex differences in anterior cruciate ligament tear rates. *American Journal of Sports Medicine.* 2001;29:58-66.

2. Anderson AF, Lipscomb AB, Liudahl KJ, et al. Analysis of the intercondylar notch by computed tomography. *American Journal of Sports Medicine.* 1987:15:547-552.

3. Agel J, Arendt E, and Bershadsky B. Anterior cruciate injury in National Collegiate Athletic Association basketball and soccer: A 13 year study. *American Journal of Sports Medicine.* 2005;33:524-532.

4. Arendt E, and Dick R. Knee injury patterns among men and women in collegiate basketball and soccer: NCAA data and review of literature. *American Journal of Sports Medicine.* 1995;23:694-701.

5. Arendt EA, Agel J, and Dick R. Anterior cruciate ligament injury patterns among collegiate men and women. *Journal of Athletic Training.* 1999;34:86-92.

6. Backstrom T, Landgren S, Zetterlund B, et al. Effects of ovarian steroid hormones on brain excitability and their relation to epilepsy seizure variation during the menstrual cycle, in Porter RJ et al. (eds): *Advances in Epileptology: The XVth Epilepsy International Symposium.* New York, Raven Press, 1984, pp. 269-277.

7. Beynnon B, Johnson R, Abate J, Braden C, Fleming B, and Nichols C. Treatment of Anterior Cruciate Ligament Injuries, Part I, *American Journal of Sports Medicine.* 2005;33:1579-1602.

8. Caraffa A, Cerulli G, Projetti M, Aisa G, and Rizzo A. Prevention of anterior cruciate ligament injuries in soccer: a prospective controlled study of proprioceptive training. *Knee Surgery, Sports Traumatology, Arthroscopy.* 1996;4:19-21.

9. Chimera N, Swanik K, Swanik B, and Straub S. Effects of Plyometric Training on Muscle-Activation Strategies and Performance in Female Athletes. *Journal of Athletic Training.* 2004;39(1):24-31.

10. Conteduca F, Ferretti A, Mariani PP, Puddu G, and Perugia L. Chondromalacia and chronic anterior instabilities of the knee. *American Journal of Sports Medicine.* 1991;19:119-123.

11. Daniel DM, Stone ML, Dobson BE, Fithian DC, Rossman DJ, and Kaufman KR. Fate of the ACL-injured patient: a prospective outcome study. *American Journal of Sports Medicine.* 1994;22:632-644.

12. Davis TJ, Shelbourne KD, and Klootwyk TE: Correlation of the intercondylar notch width of the femur to the width of the anterior and posterior cruciate ligaments. *Knee Surg Sports Traumatol Arthrosc.* 1999;7:209-214.

13. Ettlinger C, Johnson R, and Shealy J. A method to help reduce the risk of serious knee sprains incurred in alpine skiing. *American Journal of Sports Medicine.* 1995;23:531-537.

14. Fukuda Y, Woo SL, Loh JC, et al. A quantitative analysis of valgus torque on the ACL: a human cadaveric study. *Journal of Orthopaedic Research.* 2003;21:1107-1112.

15. Griffin LY, American Academy of Orthopaedic Surgeons. *Prevention of Noncontact ACL Injuries.* Rosemont, Ill: American Academy of Orthopaedic Surgeons; 2001.

16. Griffin LY, Agel J, Albohm MJ, et al. Noncontact anterior cruciate ligament injuries: risk factors and prevention strategies. *Journal of American Academy of Orthopaedic Surgeon.* 2000;8:141-150.

17. Heidt RS, Sweeterman LM, Carlonas RL, Traub JA, and Tekulve FX. Avoidance of soccer injuries with preseason conditioning. *American Journal of Sports Medicine.* 2000;28:659-662.

18. Heitz NA, Eisenman PA, Beck CL, et al. Hormonal changes throughout the menstrual cycle and increased anterior cruciate ligament laxity in females. *Journal of Athletic Training.* 1999:34:144-149.

19. Henning CE, and Griffis ND. *Injury Prevention of the Anterior Cruciate Ligament* [videotape]. Wichita, Kan: Mid-America Center for Sports Medicine; 1990.

20. Hewett TE, Stroupe AL, Nance TA, and Noyes FR. Plyometric training in female athletes: decreased impact forces and increased hamstring torques. *American Journal of Sports Medicine.* 1996;24:765-773.

21. Hewett TE, Lindenfeld TN, Riccobene JV, and Noyes FR. The effect of neuromuscular training on the incidence of knee injury in female athletes. *American Journal of Sports Medicine.* 1999;27:699-706.

22. Hewett TE, Myer GD, Ford KR, et al. Biomechanical measures of neuromuscular control and valgus loading of the knee predict anterior cruciate ligament injury risk in female athletes: a prospective study. *American Journal of Sports Medicine* 2005;33:492-501.

23. Hootman JM, Dick R, and Agel J. Epidemiology of Collegiate injuries for 15 sports: summary and recommendations for injury prevention initiatives. *Journal of Athletic Training.* 2007;42(2):311-319.

24. Houseworth SW, Mauro VJ, Mellon BA, et al. The intercondylar notch in acute tears of the anterior cruciate ligament: A computer graphics study. *American Journal of Sports Medicine.* 1987: 15: 221-224.

25. Ireland ML. Anterior cruciate ligament injury in female athletes: epidemiology. *Journal of Athletic Training* 1999;34:150-154.

26. Kannus P, and Järvinen M. Conservatively treated tears of the anterior cruciate ligament: long-term results. *Journal of Bone and Joint Surgery (Am).* 1987;69:1007-1012.

27. Levy AS, and Meier SW. Approach to cartilage injury in the anterior cruciate ligament-deficient knee. *Orthopedic Clinics of North America.* 2003;34:149-167.

28. Liu SH, Al-Shaikh RA, Panossian V, et al. Estrogen affects the cellular metabolism of the anterior cruciate ligament: A potential explanation for female athletic injury. *American Journal of Sports Medicine.* 1997:25: 704-709.

29. Liu SH, Al-Shaikh RA, Panossian V, et al. Primary immunolocalization of estrogen and progesterone target cells in the human anterior cruciate ligament. *Journal of Orthopaedic Research.* 1996:14:526-533.

30. Mandelbaum BR, Silvers HJ, Watanabe DS, et al. Effectiveness of a neuromuscular and proprioceptive training program in preventing the incidence of anterior cruciate ligament injuries in female athletes: 2-year follow-up. *American Journal of Sports Medicine.* 2005;33:1003-1010.

31. Markolf KL, Burchfield DM, Shapiro MM, Shepard MF, Finerman GA, Slauterbeck JL. Combined knee loading states that generate high anterior cruciate ligament forces. *Journal of Orthopaedic Research.* 1995;13: 930-935.

32. Moller Nielson J, and Hammar M: Sports injuries and oral contraceptive use: Is there a relationship? *Sports Meicine*.1991;12:152-160.

33. Muneta T, Sekiya I, Yagishita K, Ogiuchi T, Yamanoto H, and Shinomiya K. Two-bundle reconstruction of the anterior cruciate ligament using semitendinosus tendon with endobuttons: operative technique and preliminary results. *Arthroscopy*. 1999;15:618-624.

34. Myer G, Ford K, McLean S, and Hewett T. The effects of plyometric versus dynamic stabilization and balance training on lower extremity biomechanics. *American Journal of Sports Medicine*. 2005:33(3):1-11.

35. Myklebust G, Maehlum S, Holm I, and Bahr R. A prospective cohort study of anterior cruciate ligament injuries in elite Norwegian team handball. *Scand J Med Sci Sports*. 1998;8:149-53.

36. National Federation of State High School Associations. *High School Sports Participation Increases Again; Girls Exceeds Three Million for First Time*. National Federation of State High School Associations; 2007.

37. Neugarten J, Acharya A, Lei J, et al. Selective estrogen receptor modulators suppress mesangial cell collagen synthesis. *American Journal of Physiology-Renal Physiology*. 2000:279 F309-F318.

38. Noyes F, Barber-Westin S, Fleckenstein C, Walsh M, and West J. The drop-jump screening test: Difference in lower limb control by gender and effect of neuromuscular training in female athletes. *American Journal of Sports Medicine*. 2005:33 (2):197-207.

39. Onate JA, Guskiewicz KM, Marshall SW, et al. Instruction of jump landing technique using videotape feedback: altering lower extremity motion patterns. *American Journal of Sports Medicine*. 2005;33: 831-842.

40. Owings MF, and Kozak LJ. Ambulatory and inpatient procedures in the United States 1996. *Health Statistics. Vital Health. Stat 13* 1998;139: 1-119.

41. Paterno MV, Myer GD, Ford KR, and Hewett TE. Neuromuscular training improves single-limb stability in young female athletes. *Journal of Orthopaedic & Sports Physical Therapy*. 2004;34:305-317.

42. Roos H, Adalberth T, Dahlberg L, and Lohmander LS. Osteoarthritis of the knee after injury to the anterior cruciate ligament or meniscus: the influence of time and age. *Osteoarthritis Cartilage*. 1995;3:261-267.

43. Rozzi S, Lephart S Gear W, and Fu F. Knee joint laxity and neuromuscular characteristics of male and female soccer and basketball players. *American Journal of Sports Medicine*. 1999;27:312-319.

44. Sarwar R, Niclos BB, and Rutherford OM. Changes in muscle strength, relaxation rate and fatigability during the human menstrual cycle. *The Journal of Physiology*. 1996;493:267-272.

45. Scoville CR, Williams GN, Uhorchak JM, et al. Risk factors associated with anterior cruciate ligament injury. In: *Proceedings of the 68th Annual Meeting of the American Academy of Orthopaedic Surgeons*. Rosemont, Ill: American Academy of Orthopaedic Surgeons; 2001:564.

46. See reference 40.

47. Shelbourne KD, Davis TJ, Klootwyk TE, et al. The relationship between intercondylar notch width of the femur and the incidence of anterior cruciate ligament tears. A prospective study. *American Journal of Sports Medicine*. 1998:26: 402–408.

48. Souryal T, and Freeman T. Intercondylar notch size and anterior cruciate ligament injuries in athletes: A prospective study. *American Journal of Sports Medicine*. 1993;21:535-539.

49. Souryal T, Moore H, and Evans J. Bilaterality in anterior cruciate ligament injuries: associated intercondylar notch stenosis. *American Journal of Sports Medicine*. 1988;16:449-454.

50. Teitz C, Lind B, and Sacks B. Symmetry of the femoral notch index. *American Journal of Sports Medicine*. 1997:25:687-690.

51. Toth AP, and Cordasco FA. Anterior cruciate ligament injuries in the female athlete. *Journal of Gender-specific medicine* 2001;4:25-34.

52. Uhorchak J, McDevitt D, Taylor M, Williams G, Arcerio R, St. Pierre P, and Taylor D. Risk factors associated with non-contact injury of the ACL: A prospective four-year evaluation of 859 West Point cadets. *American Journal of Sports Medicine*. 2003:Vol 31:831-842.

53. Wilkerson G, Colston M, Short N, Neal K, Hoewischer P, and Pixley J. Neuromuscular Changes in Female Collegiate Athletes Resulting From a Plyometric Jump-Training Program. *Journal of Athletic Training*. 2004:39(1):17-21.

54. Wojtys E, Houston L, Boynton M, Spindler K, and Lindenfeld T. The effect of the menstrual cycle on anterior cruciate ligament injuries in

women as determined by hormone level. *American Journal of Sports Medicine.* 2002;30:182-188.

55. Wojtys EM, Huston LJ, Schock HJ, Boylan JP, and Ashton-Miller JA. Gender differences in muscular protection of the knee in torsion in size-matched athletes. *Journal of Bone and Joint Surgery (Am).* 2003;85: 782-789.

56. Wreje U, Brynhildsen J, Aberg H, et al. Collagen metabolism markers as a reflection of bone and soft tissue turnover during the menstrual cycle and oral contraceptive use. *Contraception.* 2000;61:265-270.

57. Zimmerman E, Parlee MB: Behavioral changes associated with the menstrual cycle: An experimental investigation. *Journal of Applied Social Psychology.* 1973;3:335-344.

Index